D0217852

Infection Control in Home Care

Emily Rhinehart, RN, MPH, CIC, CPHQ
Vice President
AIG Healthcare Management Services
Atlanta, Georgia

Mary M. Friedman, MS, RN, CRNI
Principal and Home Care Consultant
Home Health Systems, Inc.
Marietta, Georgia
Nurse Surveyor
Joint Commission on Accreditation of Healthcare Organizations
Oakbrook Terrace, Illinois

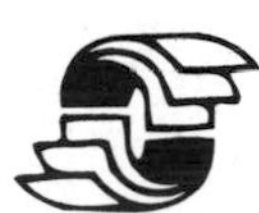

AN ASPEN PUBLICATION®
Aspen Publishers, Inc.
Gaithersburg, Maryland
1999

The authors have made every effort to ensure the accuracy of the information herein. However, appropriate information sources should be consulted, especially for new or unfamiliar procedures. It is the responsibility of every practitioner to evaluate the appropriateness of a particular opinion in the context of actual clinical situations and with due considerations to new developments. The authors, editors, and the publisher cannot be held responsible for any typographical or other errors found in this book.

Library of Congress Cataloging-in-Publication Data
Rhinehart, Emily,
Infection control in home care / Emily Rhinehart, Mary Friedman.
p. cm.
Includes index.
ISBN 0-8342-1143-2
1. Home care services. 2. Nosocomial infections—Prevention.
3. Communicable diseases—Prevention. I. Friedman, Mary.
II. Title.
[DNLM: 1. Home Care Services. 2. Infection Control—methods. WY
115 R473i 1999]
RA645.3.R46 1999
362.1′4—dc21
DNLM/DLC
for Library of Congress 98-32394
CIP

Orders: (800) 638-8437
Customer Service: (800) 234-1660

About Aspen Publishers • For more than 35 years, Aspen has been a leading professional publisher in a variety of disciplines. Aspen's vast information resources are available in both print and electronic formats. We are committed to providing the highest quality information available in the most appropriate format for our customers. Visit Aspen's Internet site for more information resources, directories, articles, and a searchable version of Aspen's full catalog, including the most recent publications: **http://www.aspenpublishers.com**

Aspen Publishers, Inc. • The hallmark of quality in publishing
Member of the worldwide Wolters Kluwer group.

Editorial Services: Ruth Bloom
Library of Congress Catalog Card Number: 98-32394
ISBN: 0-8342-1143-2

Printed in the United States of America

1 2 3 4 5

To Randy,
my wonderfully supportive
husband and partner.

Emily Rhinehart

To my husband Dan
and our sons,
Evan and Mark,
for their love and support.

Mary Friedman

Table of Contents

Foreword

As health care professionals, we are all concerned with the quality of the care and services we provide. We strive to deliver the most appropriate care in the most effective and efficient manner, optimizing intended outcomes of care and minimizing adverse outcomes. We also strive to provide a safe environment for the patient, his or her family and for the home care providers. Infection control is critical to these goals for home care. Prevention and control of home care-acquired infections in patients, as well as exposures and occupational illnesses in staff, is critical to this effort and key to performance measurement and improvement. The Joint Commission's accreditation process for home care and hospice organizations has, since its inception in 1988, included very specific standards related to infection control. In fact, an entire chapter is dedicated to the function.

But, there has been a particular struggle within home care and hospice to develop and implement infection control programs. This challenge is due to the lack of surveillance data on home care-acquired infections as well as the lack of guidelines specifically addressing the prevention and control of infection in home care patients. Nonetheless, home care professionals have made an outstanding effort to address these issues. Now they will have Infection Control in Home Care to assist them in this important endeavor.

This book will assist home care and hospice organizations in their infection control programs with information for applying and adapting strategies for infection, prevention, control and surveillance. I applaud the author's for their practical and effective approach as a guide for practice in the home setting. It has been sorely needed and will positively contribute to our mutual goal of improving the quality of health care provided to individuals in the home!

Maryanne L. Popovich, RN, BSN, MPH
Executive Director
Home Care Accreditation Services
Joint Commission on
Accreditation of Healthcare Organizations
Oakbrook Terrace, Illinois

Preface

The application of infection control principles and practices to home care has been challenging. As home care has grown and expanded its scope of services to include more high-technology practices in the care of more acutely ill patients, the need for a more formal approach to infection control has become increasingly evident. The Joint Commission on Accreditation of Healthcare Organizations acknowledged the need for a systematic infection control program with the advent of the home care standards in 1988. These standards require an organized approach to infection control planning as well as performance measurement, including surveillance of home care–acquired infections. In light of this mandate, as well as the home care industry's recognition that infection control efforts must be improved, everyone seems to be struggling with the development and implementation of specific infection control practices and, even more so, performing surveillance. This book is intended to provide some assistance in this struggle as well as to serve as a reference source.

The home care experience seems to parallel the history of infection control in acute care to some degree. Although efforts to prevent infections (e.g., handwashing and aseptic technique) have always been a part of patient care, formal infection control programs did not come into existence in modern American hospitals until the early 1970s, when more intensive care units were being opened and patients were surviving critical illnesses and shock. In addition, there were more medical devices being employed in their care. This combination of prolonged survival and the use of invasive devices resulted in the development and recognition of an increase in hospital-acquired infections. The benefits of improved survival were threatened by increased mortality due to nosocomial infection. Thus the discipline of hospital infection control was born.

Similar circumstances have been observed in home care: longer survival of more acutely and chronically ill patients being cared for in their homes with more invasive devices. At this point, however, we do not know the incidence of infections resulting from home care (home care-acquired infections). We assume that they are occurring based on what is known about the risk of nosocomial infection. Home care providers have a professional, moral, and ethical responsibility to reduce the incidence of home care-acquired infections through infection control strategies.

Unfortunately, the same strategies used in a hospital to prevent and control infection cannot be incorporated into home care practice without adaptation and consideration of the limitations of the setting. The home is not a clinical setting and does not ordinarily have the benefits of an institutional setting, such as sufficient handwashing facilities, air handling, and a central supply department. Space may be limited, maintenance of aseptic technique may be difficult, and there are generally no support staff available for on-site consultation and assistance. In contrast to the rather controlled hospital environment, the home is an uncontrolled, unpredictable environment in which to provide care.

Thus, although home care nurses are knowledgeable in the basics of infection control, they face a significant challenge when having to adapt acute care practices to the home. In our experience, this adaptation has resulted in a wide variation of practice (e.g., isolation precautions and cleaning and disinfection of equipment) as well as many ritualistic, arbitrary practices that have been codified and standardized in policies and procedures. Although these practices were developed with the best of intentions, they frequently lack a scientific basis. For example, nursing bag technique (i.e., placing a barrier, such as newspaper, between the nursing bag and the surface on which is it placed in the home) is found in the policy and procedures manual of most home care organizations but is unknown in the infection control literature. Although this technique was developed to address a perceived risk ("contamination" of the nursing bag), it is ritualistic, unscientific, and unnecessary. Other arbitrary practices that have become standard were also developed to decrease risk but are contrary to published data and recommendations. Many home care organizations arbitrarily require the indwelling urethral catheter and drainage system to be changed every 30 days. This issue is specifically addressed in the Centers for Disease Control and Prevention (CDC) *Guideline for Prevention of Catheter-Associated Urinary Tract Infections* (Wong, 1983). Written and published more than 15 years ago, the guideline states that there are no scientific data to show that routine change is advantageous; routine catheter changes are not recommended. Nonetheless, the practice continues and is reinforced by the Health Care Financing Administration, which provides reimbursement to Medicare-certified home health agencies to change a Foley catheter every 30 days (HCFA, 1996). With a lack of experience, lack of scientific data specific to home care experience, and little or no data on the incidence of home care acquired infection, however, home care nurses have done the best they can to address these issues and protect their patients.

We hope that this book will play some role in advancing the application and adaptation of strategies for infection prevention, control, and surveillance in home care. We have attempted to incorporate scientific knowledge and data from hospital infection control into our experience and knowledge of home care to formulate effective, practical, and scientifically sound recommendations. We have relied on the information in the infection control literature as well as our own experience in home care. In many cases we have had to adapt the recommended acute care practices for application in the home care setting while incorporating additional, common-sense strategies. For example, rather than routinely discard irrigation solution after 24 or 48 hours or 1 week, we recommend that an attempt be made to select solution in a quantity that will be used within a reasonable period of time (150 mL versus 500 mL). In addition, the bottle should be stored in a manner that will minimize potential for contamination. We have had to recognize that some patient care practices requiring aseptic technique in the hospital can be provided safely in the home using clean technique, although there may be no references or data for this practice. We have also recognized that, without other patients in the care setting, isolation precautions focus more on protection of the home care staff member, not other patients.

Surveillance of home care-acquired infections continues to present significant challenges. Although definitions and methods for nosocomial infection surveillance are well advanced and appear valid and reliable, for many reasons they are not well suited to the home care setting and require significant revision. We have not attempted to provide specific definitions for home care-acquired infections. That formidable task should be undertaken by a national effort for consensus development and field testing. Rather, we have provided some key considerations for the development of definitions as well as recommended methods for surveillance and analysis of data. We are conscious of the limited resources for surveillance in home care and especially the lack of laboratory data for confirming and defining infections.

We are hopeful that this book will accomplish several goals. First, we hope that it will serve as a reference for home care nurses as they care for patients, develop policies and procedures, and undertake surveillance efforts. We also hope that it will encourage infection control professionals to become more familiar with home care practice and enable them to understand that the "way we do it in the hospital" may not be practical or possible in the home. Although the scientific principles must be preserved as much as possible, there must be adaptation of practice suitable to the setting and degree of risk.

Second, we hope that home care staff can improve their knowledge of the principles underpinning infection control practice so that they can adapt their practice to the situation at hand. We could not address each and every situation that may arise, but by understanding the principles, actual infection risks, and rationale for recommended practices, the home care nurse can determine the best course of action in a given situation. The basic elements for acquisition of infection (discussed in Chapter 2) are critical to this concept. If home care nurses can think in terms of the chain of infection, their problem-solving abilities related to infection control should be significantly enhanced.

Third, we hope that this book can serve as a starting point for discussion, debate, and study of infection control in home care. Although we can all contribute what we think is the "best way" to approach home care infection control, none of us really knows without data. At this point in time, we do not have reliable data on the incidence of home care-acquired infection. Acquiring these data will be costly and will probably require a government agency, such as the CDC, to fund and guide the cause, just as the CDC did for nosocomial infection surveillance. It will also require a national commitment from the home care industry and the infection control discipline. Until then, surveillance efforts by individual home care organizations will be difficult. Only the large, corporate agencies will be able to mount a sufficiently organized and funded program. Nonetheless, we encourage efforts such as those of the Missouri Home Care Alliance and others. More experience and data from home care surveillance efforts must be published for discussion and debate. Until we have a better idea of the frequency of home care-acquired infection, we cannot estimate its cost, nor can we determine the effects of risk reduction strategies.

Finally, we hope that those of you who use this book will find it helpful and practical. We appreciate the encouragement we have received from friends and colleagues to write this book. We did so with few directly applicable references; therefore we have adapted recommendations and science to suit the needs of home care. We hope that this effort will provide information and knowledge to home care providers as well as result in improved services and care for home care patients.

REFERENCES

Health Care Financing Administration (1996, April). *Medicare Home Health Agency Manual.* Revised. Material transmittal No. 277, 14-14–14-15, Washington, DC: U.S. Government Printing Office.

Wong, E.S. (1983). Guideline for prevention of catheter-associated urinary tract infections. *American Journal of Infection Control, 11,* 28–31.

CHAPTER 1

Infection Control as a Health Care Discipline

HISTORICAL PERSPECTIVE

Although the modern era of infection control began in the early 1950s, the recognition and awareness that the provision of medical and nursing care in an institutional setting (e.g., a hospital) could result in an increased risk for the acquisition of infection occurred more than 100 years ago. In the 1840s, Dr. Ignaz Philip Semmelweiss was caring for postpartum women in a lying-in hospital in Vienna. He was concerned about the incidence of puerperal fever and its related mortality. Eighteen percent of the women who acquired the infection died. As the first "hospital epidemiologist," Semmelweiss observed, studied, and proved that the postpartum infection was related to care provided by the medical students. His theory was that the medical students carried an infectious agent from their work in the autopsy suite to the maternity wards, where they infected patients through direct transmission via their unwashed hands. Because the science of microbiology was in its infancy, Semmelweiss could not perform cultures to identify the source of the infection (cadavers), the mode of transmission (hands of the medical students), or the causative agent of infection (*Streptococcus* organisms) in the postpartum women. Through a simple case-control study, however, he did demonstrate the relationship (time, place, and person) of the medical students working in the necropsy suite and then going directly to the postpartum ward and transmitting infection. Semmelweiss showed that the uninfected private patients (controls) had significantly less risk for puerperal fever than ward patients (cases) who were cared for by the medical students. When medical students began washing their hands before going from their anatomic studies to the patient ward, the incidence of puerperal fever declined measurably (Rotter, 1996). This classic epidemiological study is the earliest evidence we have of the identification and analysis of nosocomial infection. *Nosocomial* is the term that specifically refers to hospital-acquired infection.

Some time after Semmelweiss reported his observations and findings, other physicians and scientists furthered his work; among these were Louis Pasteur's development of germ theory and Robert Koch's contributions to the science of microbiology. In England, Joseph Lister added to the work of Semmelweiss with his study and development of surgical asepsis. These scientific pioneers provided the initial scientific theories and foundations for modern infectious disease epidemiology.

INFECTION CONTROL PROGRAMS IN THE UNITED STATES

Infection control as an organized discipline in American health care dates back to the 1950s. In the post-World War II years, hospital-based outbreaks of infection caused by *Staphylococcus aureus* were being frequently recognized and reported. Many of these outbreaks were occurring in newborn nurseries. This increased incidence of nosocomial infection in outbreak situations demanded an organized response for investigation and control. Thus the discipline of hospital infection control was born. Teams of nurses, physicians, and microbiologists worked together to investigate the occurrence of the outbreaks and develop and implement measures to control them. Strategies to prevent further outbreaks were also developed and implemented, as were methods to reduce the risk of endemic infection.

In 1958, the American Hospital Association (AHA) recommended that surveillance of nosocomial infections be undertaken in all hospitals. Many large hospitals undertook this task. It was not until 1970, however, when the Center for Disease Control (CDC), as it was then called, recommended that hospitals establish and support specific job descriptions and roles for an infection control nurse (ICN) and a hospital epidemiologist that formal programs and training for infection control began to emerge. The CDC held its first course for ICNs (course 1200G) in 1972. Support for the role of the ICN and the discipline of infection control was enhanced in 1976, when the Joint Commission on Accreditation of Hospitals (now the Joint Commission on Accreditation of Healthcare Organizations) included in its accreditation standards a requirement for a formal, organized infection control program.

Because there was little in the scientific literature to guide prevention and control strategies, early hospital infection control programs concentrated time and efforts on surveillance of nosocomial infections. The CDC, through the National Nosocomial Infection Surveillance (NNIS) study, supported this effort. Using standardized definitions and methods for nosocomial infection surveillance, ICNs performed continuous, hospitalwide surveillance (Garner, Jarvis, Emori, Horan, & Hughes, 1988; Horan, Gaynes, Martone, Jarvis, & Emori, 1992). Some hospitals reported their results to the CDC NNIS program for aggregation and analysis, establishing a national database. This provided the opportunity to establish benchmarks for the incidence of nosocomial infection, allowing individual hospitals to compare their data with those of other institutions (Gaynes, Edwards, Jarvis, Culver, Tolson, & Martone, 1996; Martone et al., 1995; Jarvis et al., 1998).

In addition to surveillance, infection control programs developed policies and procedures for the prevention and control of nosocomial infections. Initially these policies and procedures focused on patient care practices such as handwashing, care of surgical wounds, insertion and care of urinary catheters, care of tracheotomies and endotracheal tubes, and other invasive procedures. Surveillance data provided early recognition of risk related to the use of indwelling medical devices.

Isolation precautions were also developed and implemented by the infection control program. Again, the CDC provided guidance and standardization through its publication *Isolation Techniques for Use in Hospitals* (CDC, 1970). Isolation precautions were used to prevent the transmission of infection from a patient known to have a potentially communicable disease to other patients and health care providers. As infection control programs grew and developed, increased attention to prevention of occupationally acquired infections among hospital staff was expanded and is currently a major part of any infection control program (see Chapter 12).

In 1972, the Association for Practitioners in Infection Control (APIC), a national professional organization, was chartered to support communication among infection control professionals through conferences, meetings, and newsletters. In 1983, APIC published its first major document to support infection control and assist individuals in their preparation for certification in infection control. Through the development of the *APIC Curriculum for Infection Control Practice* (Soule, 1983), APIC established eight essential domains for infection control practice:

1. Patient care practices
2. Microbiology
3. Infectious diseases
4. Occupational health
5. Sterilization, disinfection, and cleaning
6. Epidemiology and statistics
7. Communication and management
8. Education

These eight distinct areas continue to provide the foundation for the professional practice of infection control in all segments of health care delivery.

EPIDEMIOLOGY OF NOSOCOMIAL INFECTION

The current epidemiology of nosocomial infection is based on more than 20 years of NNIS data and many studies in the published literature, and is therefore well known. Descriptive information about the endemic (usual) rate of nosocomial infection as well as epidemics (a greater than expected number of infections or unusual occurrences) is easily obtained.

Nosocomial infection is defined by the site of infection. Although both intrinsic (host) factors and extrinsic (environmental) factors must be considered, endemic rates of nosocomial infection are well established. The reliability of these data depends on the application of standard definitions and methods as developed and published by the CDC NNIS study (Garner et al., 1988; Horan et al., 1992). Therefore, if a hospital infection control program applies the same definitions and methods (Emori, Culver, & Horan, 1991), it can compare its endemic rate at specific body sites with national data to determine whether its rate is significantly higher or lower than that of others. Epidemiological methods to control for additional factors that are known to affect the rate of infection can be applied to ensure a more reliable comparison. Such extrinsic factors include the type and size of the hospital, level of care, length of surgery, duration of exposure to medical devices, and others. Intrinsic factors may include such considerations as underlying severity of illness, age, immunologic status, other infections, and current antibiotic therapy. Some of these risk factors are well studied (e.g., duration of indwelling urinary catheter), whereas many others require further investigation and analysis.

STATUS OF INFECTION CONTROL IN HOME CARE

It is evident that the discipline of hospital infection control is well developed and has a significant body of knowledge and epidemiologic data. The practice has been an acute care-based discipline and has evolved with the support of the CDC, NNIS, APIC, and other professional organizations, such as the Society for Healthcare Epidemiologists of America (SHEA) and the American Society for Microbiology. Physicians, nurses, microbiologists, and others have worked diligently to perform original research on risks related to the acquisition of nosocomial infection and to report outbreak investigations. Both these approaches have resulted in a body of knowledge on which the discipline is based and that has provided support to the CDC in its guidelines development. Since the publication of the first guideline, *Guideline for the Prevention of Catheter-Associated Urinary Tract Infections* (Wong, 1983), the CDC and APIC have supported development of additional guidelines and updates (Table 1–1).

The work has contributed significantly to the improvement of care and reduction of risk of infection in hospitalized patients. There are no similar bodies of work or epidemiologic data pertaining to home care-acquired infection, however. As the health care delivery system continues to shift more severely ill patients

Table 1–1 CDC and APIC Guidelines for Prevention of Nosocomial Infection

Guideline	*Year of Last Revision*
CDC	
Guideline for the Prevention of Catheter-Associated Urinary Tract Infections	1983
Guideline for Handwashing and Hospital Environmental Control	1985
Guide for Preventing Transmission of *Mycobacterium tuberculosis* in Health Care Facilities	1994
Recommendations for Preventing the Spread of Vancomycin Resistance	1995
Guideline for Prevention of Intravascular Device–Related Infections	1996
Guideline for Isolation Precautions in Hospitals	1996
Guideline for the Prevention of Surgical Site Infection	1985 1997 (draft)
Guideline for the Prevention of Nosocomial Pneumonia	1997
Guideline for Infection Control in Health Care Personnel	1998
APIC Guidelines	
APIC Guideline for the Selection and Use of Disinfectants	1990
APIC Guideline for Infection Prevention and Control in the Long-Term Care Facility	1991
APIC Guideline for Handwashing and Hand Antisepsis in Health Care Settings	1995

with greater high-tech care needs into home care, home care providers and infection control professionals will need to develop a body of knowledge and data more specific to the risks of infection in home care. Risk analysis for infections and outbreak investigations will be reported. Surveillance systems and databases will eventually be developed and improved. Organizations such as APIC and SHEA will focus more attention on home care; agencies such as the CDC and the Department of Health and Human Services (HHS) will support efforts to write guidelines and develop surveillance systems. The National Association for Home Care (NAHC) will provide information, education, and services as its members demand them. The Joint Commission will continue its requirements for an organized infection control and surveillance program in home care.

Until this evolution occurs, home care providers and infection control professionals must rely on previously established principles found within the eight core areas of infection control practice. Principles and knowledge of infectious diseases and their transmission can be directly applied. Practices related to the prevention and control of infection in patient care, however, require modification and adaptation. Although principles of microbiology remain the same, application and use of microbiologic methods for identification and diagnosis of home care-acquired infection must be modified or developed. New sterilization methods are needed for easy and safe application in home care as well as other ambulatory settings. Occupational health practices for prevention and control of exposures and infections in staff members can generally be applied to home care. Some modifications in regulatory requirements have already occurred, however, such as the reduced requirement of enforcement of the Occupational Safety and Health Administration standard for use of personal protective equipment (OSHA, 1991). The basic principles of adult education as well as management and communication for infection control can be directly applied to home care practice.

Perhaps the greatest challenge is in the area of epidemiology and statistics. First, increased effort to describe and analyze the epidemiology of home care-acquired infections is critically needed. Before this body of data-based evidence can be produced, however, definitions and methods for the surveillance of home care-acquired infections must be developed and standardized. Although definitions of nosocomial infection are standardized (Garner et al., 1988; Horan et al., 1992), these definitions are not feasible for unmodified application in home care. Surveillance methods that were developed for hospitals also require significant modification for use in home care. Fortunately, investment in information systems and databases for home care is increasing. These efforts will help support the implementation of home care surveillance systems.

Surveillance data, once they are standardized and become widespread, can be used to begin to measure the incidence of home care-acquired infection. Additional efforts for the analysis of risk can be instituted to determine what practices in what patients increase the risk for home care-acquired infections and what practices in what patients decrease risk. These data and the information they provide will be used to reduce risk. Specific patient care practices, especially those involving an indwelling device, will be modified and improved.

It has been demonstrated that nosocomial infection increases the overall cost of health care. As more skilled care and a higher intensity of services shift to the home setting, home care-acquired infection will correspondingly increase the cost of home care and may increase the utilization of acute care and other resources. Without sufficient data on the incidence of home care-acquired infections, the actual cost of this adverse outcome will remain unknown. As more information about the incidence and cost of home care-acquired infection becomes available, more informed decisions can be made to provide the lowest-risk care in the most appropriate setting.

REFERENCES

Centers for Disease Control and Prevention. (1970). *Isolation techniques for use in hospitals*. Atlanta, GA: Department of Health, Education, and Welfare.

Emori, G., Culver, D., & Horan, T. (1991). National Nosocomial Infections Surveillance system (NNIS): Description of surveillance methods. *American Journal of Infection Control, 19*, 259–267.

Garner, J., Jarvis, W., Emori, T., Horan, T., & Hughes, J. (1988). CDC definitions for nosocomial infection, 1988. *American Journal of Infection Control, 23*, 128–140.

Gaynes, R., Edwards, J., Jarvis, W., Culver, D., Tolson, J., & Martone, W. (1996). Nosocomial infections among neonates in high-risk nurseries in the United States. National Nosocomial Infections Surveillance system. *Pediatrics, 98*, 357–361.

Horan, T., Gaynes, R., Martone, W., Jarvis, W., & Emori, T. (1992). CDC definitions of nosocomial surgical site infections, 1992: A modification of CDC definitions of surgical wound infections. *Infection Control and Hospital Epidemiology, 13,* 606–608.

Jarvis, W., Gaynes, R., Horan, T., Alonso-Echanove, J., Emori, T., Fridkin, S., Lawton, R., Richards, M., Wright, G., Culver, D., Abshire, J., Edwards, J., Henderson, T., Peavy, G., Toslon, J., & Wages, J. (1998). National Nosocomial Infections Surveillance (NNIS) system report: Data summary from October 1986–April 1998, issued June 1998. *American Journal of Infection Control, 26,* 522–533.

Martone, W., Gaynes, R., Horan, T., Danzig, L., Emori, G., Monnet, D., Stroud, L., Wright, G., Culver, D., Banerjee, S., Edwards, J., Henderson, T., Tolson, J., & Peavy, G. (1995). National Nosocomial Infections Surveillance (NNIS) semiannual report, May 1995. *American Journal of Infection Control, 23*, 377–385.

Occupational Safety and Health Administration. (1991). Occupational exposure to bloodborne pathogens: Final rule. 29 CFR 1910.1030. *Federal Register 56,* 64003–64282.

Rotter, M. (1996). Hand washing and hand disinfection. In G. Mahall (Ed.), *Hospital epidemiology and infection control* (pp. 1052–1068). Baltimore: Williams & Wilkins.

Soule, B. (Ed.). (1983). *The APIC curriculum for infection control practice.* Dubuque, IA: Kendall/Hunt.

Wong, E. (1983). Guideline for the prevention of catheter-associated urinary tract infections. *American Journal of Infection Control,* 11, 28–31.

CHAPTER 2

The Infectious Disease Process

AGENT, HOST, AND ENVIRONMENT

Humans live in their environment with many other species. Many members of the animal and plant kingdoms are microscopic and can cause human illness; this is called an infection. The presence of microscopic organisms does not always cause infection, however. The physical environment is abundant with microscopic organisms, such as bacteria, fungi, molds, and viruses. Under certain circumstances, some microorganisms cause disease; under the same circumstances, others do not. There are many microorganisms regularly found on and within human beings; these are referred to as normal or resident flora.

The infectious disease process provides a scientific explanation for the factors that determine the relationships among humans, the many microorganisms that are in the environment, and normal flora. There are many variables that determine the relationship between microorganisms and the human host. This interaction has been illustrated in various ways, including the epidemiologic triangle (Figure 2–1). The triangle portrays the three key elements in infection—agent, host, and environment—and their dynamic interaction. This model can be used to demonstrate this interaction for other types of disease as well. Specific characteristics or changes in any one of the three elements that can lead to the development of an infectious disease are discussed in this chapter.

TYPES OF INFECTION

The term *infection* refers to the presence and multiplication of microorganisms in the tissue of the host. The host response to this invasion and replication varies. When there are signs and symptoms caused by this invasion, such as fever, swelling, pain, and inflammation, we recognize these as characteristics of infection. Some infectious diseases are evident and produce acute signs and symptoms. For example, an acute urinary tract infection in a normal host results in pain, frequency, urgency, and burning on urination. An acute skin infection produces pain, swelling, warmth, and redness of the tissue. Other infections may occur without observable signs; these are referred to as subclinical infections. For example, a mild case of chicken pox may be unrecognized in a child if no rash occurs or if there are only a few concealed lesions that go unnoticed.

Some viruses can cause an asymptomatic, chronic infection. For example, approximately 10% of individuals who are infected with hepatitis B virus become chronically infected, and the majority remain asymptomatic. Hepatitis C virus is thought to result invariably in a chronic infection. Either of these viral infections may remain asymptomatic for a long period of time. This is called the *carrier state*. The infection can be diagnosed or documented by serological blood testing, which detects the viral antigen or antibody to show evidence of the infection. Although no signs and symptoms of an illness are evident, the host can potentially transmit hepatitis to another susceptible individual. Carriers of hepatitis B and hepatitis C viruses can transmit infection to others through sexual contact or contact with their blood.

NORMAL FLORA

The term *normal flora* describes the bacteria that are frequently found in everyone in specific parts of the

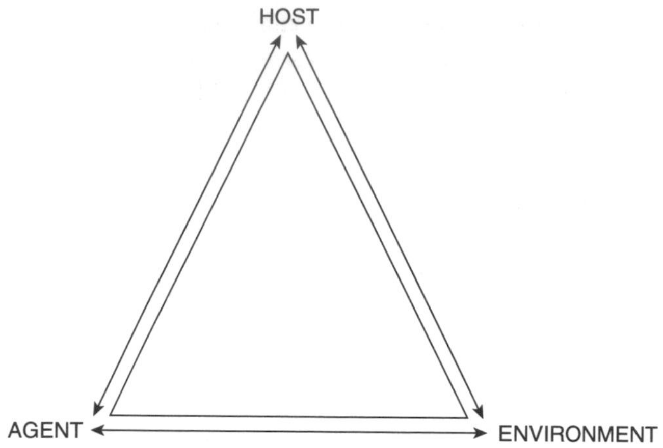

Figure 2–1 The Epidemiologic Triangle

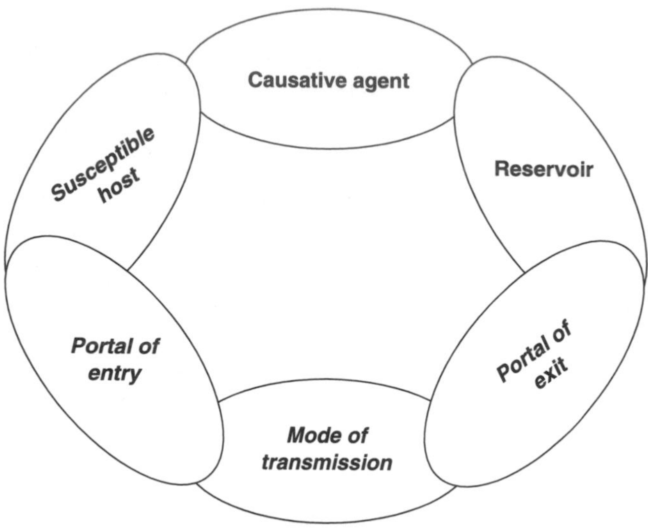

Figure 2–2 The Chain of Infection

body. For example, millions of *Escherichia coli* are normally found in the bowel. *Streptococcus viridans* is also normal flora present in the upper respiratory tract and mouth. *Colonization* is the term that describes the presence of bacteria without multiplication and damage to the host tissue. Sometimes bacteria that are not normal flora can be isolated from patients who are colonized. An example is when patients become colonized with multidrug-resistant microorganisms, such as methicillin-resistant *Staphylococcus aureus* (MRSA) or vancomycin-resistant enterococci (VRE). Patients with these organisms may have infections or may be colonized; as asymptomatic carriers, like asymptomatic hepatitis carriers, they can serve as the source of infection or colonization of others.

CHAIN OF INFECTION

The interaction among the agent, the host, and the environment leading to infection has been described in a model called the chain of infection (Figure 2–2). Specific conditions and characteristics affecting each element in the chain and each element's interaction with the other elements determine whether an infection will result.

CAUSATIVE AGENT

The causative agent of infection may be one of several classes of microorganisms causing human infectious disease. These include bacteria, viruses, fungi, protozoa, rickettsia, chlamydia, mycoplasma, and helminths. Each has various characteristics that influence its ability to cause an infection (Table 2–1). First, a sufficient number of organisms (infective dose) must be present to cause an infection. It takes only a few *Shigella* bacteria to cause an infection in the gastrointestinal (GI) tract, leading to severe diarrhea. In contrast, it takes many *Salmonella* organisms to cause a GI tract infection. Pathogenicity is the ability of the agent to cause disease (*Staphylococcus epidermidis* has low pathogenicity); the term *virulence* refers to the severity of the disease. *Shigella* species are considered more

Table 2–1 Characteristics of Causative Agents

Characteristic	*Definition*
Infective dose	Number of organisms required to cause infection
Pathogenicity	Likelihood that exposure to an organism will lead to infection
Virulence	Capacity to produce disease
Invasiveness	Ability of organism to breech natural barriers
Viability	Ability of organism to survive in environment
Host specificity	Ability of organism to infect specific animal hosts
Antigenic variation	Changes in organism make-up
Resistance	Ability of organism to develop resistance to antimicrobials through molecular changes

virulent than *Salmonella* species because they cause a more severe form of diarrhea. Invasiveness is the ability of the organism to enter the host tissues. Viability is the organism's ability to survive in the environment. Viruses, for example, are like parasites because they cannot survive independently, and thus require a living host (such as blood cells) to replicate. Other organisms, such as spore-forming bacteria, can survive in hostile environments and endure a wide range of conditions, such as high and low temperatures as well as exposure to low-level disinfectants. *Mycobacteria tuberculosis* (MTB) is a spore-forming bacterium that can survive for many years in dust particles.

Infectious agents cause disease in specific animal hosts. This is referred to as host specificity. There are various viruses, such as canine parvovirus, that cause disease in certain animals but do not affect humans. Others, such as varicella virus, cause human infectious disease (chicken pox) but are harmless to animals. In addition, viruses such as influenza A virus and bacteria such as streptococci can change their virulence through natural alterations in their antigen make-up. Thus in some years the flu season is worse than others as a result of antigenic variation in the influenza virus in those years.

Finally, the organism's ability to develop resistance to specific antimicrobial agents may also affect its ability to cause an infection. There are many biological mechanisms by which organisms such as bacteria can develop or acquire resistance. Once this resistance develops, the frequency of colonization and infection by the organism may increase, as has been observed with MRSA over the past two decades.

A list of common microorganisms that cause human infections is provided in Table 2–2. Bacteria are divided into categories of Gram negative and Gram positive based on their appearance when a particular stain—Gram's stain—is applied to them and they are examined under a microscope. Their shape can also be determined with a Gram's stain test. Round organisms are called *cocci*. Bacteria that are longer and in the shape of a rod are called *bacilli*. There are Gram-positive cocci, such as streptococci, and Gram-negative rods or bacilli, such as *Pseudomonas* species. Many other variations and shapes also exist. The results of Gram's stain are used as a preliminary test to determine what type of bacteria are present. For some sites of infection, the stain is used to determine whether white blood cells are also present, providing further evidence of infection. Other microorganisms can be initially identified by different microscopic examinations and staining techniques. For example, MTB in the sputum is identified by an acid-fast stain. These various stains may be used for a preliminary identification of an infectious organism. In most cases, however, the identification of the specific organism causing an infection is made by performing a culture.

RESERVOIR OF INFECTION

The source of a causative agent (e.g., bacterium, fungus, or virus) is referred to as the reservoir. This is a place where the organism can survive but may or may not multiply. Organisms causing infectious disease may be found in other humans, animals, or the physical environment. Human reservoirs may have a symptomatic or asymptomatic infection, or they may be colonized with a potentially infective agent. In health care settings, the human reservoir includes other patients as well as health care providers. In home care, because there are usually no other patients in the setting, this reservoir is less important. Home care staff, however, can transmit organisms from one patient who is infected or colonized to other patients on their hands. Animals can also carry or be infected with agents of human infection. This reservoir is more important in home care than in care provided in other settings (see Chapter 5). Animals infected with rabies can transmit the disease to humans; turtles and other reptiles are frequently colonized with *Salmonella* organisms, which can be transmitted to humans and cause disease.

The environment, including patient care equipment and devices, can also serve as a reservoir for infectious agents. Although this has not been studied or confirmed as an important source of infecting organisms in home care, there are many examples from other settings. In intensive care units, outbreaks have been traced to antibiotic-resistant Gram-negative bacteria contaminating sinks (Dandalides, Rutala, & Sarubbi, 1984). When health care workers used these sinks, their hands became contaminated, and they transmitted the organisms to patients. Ventilator tubing frequently becomes contaminated with bacteria from the patient's respiratory tract that may be transmitted to other patients via the hands of health care workers. Reusable devices may also serve as a reservoir of potentially infectious agents. If a bronchoscope used to examine a patient with tuberculosis is not sufficiently cleaned and disin-

Table 2–2 Common Pathogenic Agents

Agent	Type	Disease or Infection
Bacteria		
Acinetobacter spp.	Gram-negative rod	Upper respiratory tract infection, urinary tract infection (UTI), wound infection
Campylobacter jejuni	Gram-negative rod	Diarrhea, abdominal pain, fever
Clostridium difficile	Gram-positive rod (forms spores)	Diarrhea, pseudomembranous colitis
Clostridium tetani	Gram-positive rod (forms spores)	Tetanus
Cornybacterium diptheriae	Gram-positive rod	Cause of diptheria; skin, eye, ear infections
Enterobacter aerogenes	Gram-negative rod	UTI; respiratory tract, wound, blood, central nervous system (CNS) infections
Enterococcus faecalis (formerly *Streptococcus faecalis*)	Gram-positive coccus	UTI, subacute endocarditis
Escherichia coli	Gram-negative rod	Diarrhea, UTI, septicemia
Klebsiella pneumoniae	Gram-negative rod	Bacterial pneumonia, UTI, respiratory tract infections
Listeria monocytogenes	Gram-positive rod	Meningitis, encephalitis, septicemia
Mycobacterium tuberculosis	Acid-fast mycobacterium	Tuberculosis
Proteus vulgaris	Gram-negative rod	UTI, burn wound infection, respiratory tract infection
Proteus mirabilis	Gram-negative rod	UTI, bacteremia
Pseudomonas aeruginosa	Gram-negative rod	Eye, wound, burn wound infections; diarrhea
Salmonella choleraesuis, S. paratyphi, S. schottmuelleri	Gram-negative rod	Gastroenteritis, enteric fever, bacteremia, pneumonia
Serratia marcescens	Gram-negative rod	Wound, blood, CNS, respiratory tract infections; UTI
Shigella dysenteriae	Gram-negative rod	Bacterial dysentery
Staphylococcus aureus	Gram-positive coccus	Wound infection, boils, carbuncles, impetigo, pneumonia, bacteremia, food poisoning, toxic shock syndrome
Staphylococcus epidermidis	Gram-positive coccus	Skin abscesses, ventriculitis, meningitis, bacteremia
Streptococcus pneumoniae	Gram-positive coccus	Pneumonia, scarlet fever, meningitis
Streptococcus pyogenes	Gram-positive coccus	Tonsillitis, impetigo, rheumatic fever, skin infection
Streptococcus salivarius	Gram-positive coccus	Endocarditis
Viruses		
Adenovirus	Intermediate	Upper and lower respiratory tract infection, conjunctivitis
Coxsackievirus	Hydrophilic	Herpangina, aseptic meningitis, pleurodynia, myalgia
Cytomegalovirus	Lipophilic	Usually asymptomatic in immunocompetent adults (may infect unborn fetus)
Echovirus	Hydrophilic	Aseptic meningitis, encephalitis, exanthema, respiratory disease
Hepatitis A (formerly infectious hepatitis)	Hydrophilic	Low-grade fever, fatigability, myalgia, anorexia, vomiting
Hepatitis B (formerly serum hepatitis)	Lipophilic	Acute and chronic hepatitis
Hepatitis C (formerly non-A, non-B hepatitis)	Lipophilic	Acute and chronic hepatitis
Herpes simplex type 1	Lipophilic	Skin lesions; eye, ear, face infections
Herpes simplex type 2	Lipophilic	Skin lesions on and around genitalia
Human immunodeficiency virus	Lipophilic	Acquired Immunodeficiency Syndrome

continues

Table 2–2 continued

Agent	*Type*	*Disease or Infection*
Influenza A2 and B	Lipophilic	Headache, chills, fever, muscular pain, lower respiratory tract infection, pneumonia
Parainfluenza	Lipophilic	Upper respiratory tract infection
Poliovirus	Hydrophilic	Poliomyelitis, aseptic meningitis
Respiratory syncytial virus	Lipophilic	Lower respiratory tract infection
Rhinovirus 39	Hydrophilic	Common cold, upper respiratory tract infection
Rotavirus	Hydrophilic	Diarrhea, vomiting, fever
Rubella	Lipophilic	German measles
Vaccinia	Lipophilic	Used as model for smallpox virus
Fungi		
Aspergillus niger	Mold	Lower respiratory tract infection in immunosuppressed patients
Candida albicans	Yeast	Mouth, skin, hand, lung infections; thrush
Tricophyton mentagrophytes	Fungus	Athlete's foot

Courtesy of Reckitt & Colman, Inc., Wayne, New Jersey.

fected, it may serve as the reservoir of infection for a patient who is subsequently examined with the same instrument.

PORTAL OF EXIT

If a human is serving as the reservoir of an infectious agent, the means by which the agent leaves the original host is the portal of exit. Orifices that are part of each body system may serve as portals of exit. For example, the portal of exit for influenza is the mouth and nose (upper respiratory tract), from which secretions carrying the virus are excreted through coughing and sneezing. The upper respiratory tract (coughing through the mouth) is the portal of exit for pulmonary tuberculosis. Viruses and bacteria that cause diarrhea leave the host via the GI tract through feces and, occasionally, vomitus. Sexually transmitted diseases exit via the genitourinary tract. Blood and other body secretions that are contaminated with blood are also reservoirs of infectious disease. In this case, the portal of exit may vary. Blood may exit a wound or a break in the skin, or it may exit via bloody respiratory secretions.

PORTAL OF ENTRY

The portal of entry is the means by which the infectious agent enters the susceptible host. The portal of entry may be the respiratory tract, GI tract, genitourinary tract, or skin or mucous membranes. Breaks in the skin or mucous membranes may create a portal of entry, such as may occur with needlesticks or sharps injuries.

MODE OF TRANSMISSION

The mechanism by which an organism moves from the portal of exit (from an infected or colonized person) or an environmental reservoir to the susceptible host and through the portal of entry is referred to as the mode of transmission. Recognizing the mode of transmission is a critical component of infection control. There are four modes of transmission: contact, airborne, vehicle, and vector. Contact spread and airborne transmission are the most common modes of transmission in home care.

Contact Transmission

Infections can be transmitted through direct or indirect contact with the infected or colonized source. Direct contact occurs when there is actual physical contact and person-to-person transmission occurs. Sexually transmitted diseases are spread through direct contact. Infectious droplets from the upper respiratory tract that go from one person to another is another form of direct contact transmission. This is called droplet spread or droplet transmission, and it is the mode of transmission for common upper respiratory infections such as colds and flu. These respiratory droplets can travel about 3 feet before gravity causes them to fall. This makes it different from airborne transmission (discussed in the next section). Indirect contact transmission occurs when the infectious agent is carried from one person to another on an object. As mentioned above, a contaminated bronchoscope may be the inanimate object involved in indirect contact transmission. The hands of a home care staff member may also be involved in the indirect contact transmission of multidrug-resistant microorganisms such as MRSA or VRE.

Airborne Transmission

Airborne transmission can occur with a few infectious agents that can travel on tiny respiratory particles called droplet nuclei, which can be carried through the air. Other organisms, such as MTB, may be carried on dust particles and through ventilation systems. Some fungi and molds, such as *Aspergillus* species, may also be airborne. Tuberculosis may be droplet spread or airborne spread, as can measles and varicella. More infections are droplet spread than airborne spread because they are spread by respiratory droplets rather than droplet nuclei.

Vehicle Transmission

Vehicle transmission refers to infections that are spread through a common reservoir, such as food. Foodborne illnesses are frequently caused by vehicle transmission and occur when a number of people ingest the same contaminated food (e.g., staphylococcal food poisoning related to potato salad) or contaminated water. Infection from contaminated blood is also considered vehicle transmission. In home care, vehicle transmission may occur in contaminated intravenous fluid.

Vector Transmission

Vectorborne spread refers to infectious diseases that are transmitted through insects or rodents. For example, deer ticks transmit Lyme disease, and malaria is transmitted by mosquitoes. Vectorborne spread is not a common concern in home care in the United States.

REDUCING THE RISK OF INFECTION

Many of the home care policies and procedures for infection control are adopted to prevent infection by breaking the chain of transmission. That is why it is so important for home care staff to understand this model. Once the chain of infection model is understood, there can be a better comprehension of many of the infection control strategies, such as transmission-based precautions. As different situations arise, a home care professional can determine the best course of action to prevent infection based on this understanding. Not all circumstances can be addressed in written policies and procedures, but if the basic principles of infection control and the chain of infection are understood, all home care staff will be better prepared to make decisions and to apply interventions to protect themselves and patients. In addition, this understanding may reduce practices that are unnecessary and costly. In applying these principles, however, home care staff must also understand that each patient is different, and that his or her particular risk for infection also may be different.

SUSCEPTIBLE HOST

The host is the final and most important link in the chain of transmission. There are many variables that can determine whether a host will be susceptible to an infectious agent. Home care staff routinely assess patients for host factors to determine their specific risk for acquiring an infection. Some factors are specific to the patient (host) and are referred to as intrinsic risk factors. The risk for infection is also dependent on extrinsic factors. These are the external factors in the delivery of care, including the devices and procedures, the care provider, and the environment, that may increase or decrease risk.

The home care nurse can also recognize increased risk based on the physical assessment. Any break in the natural barriers to infection, including the skin and mucus membranes, may increase risk. Any indwelling catheters, tubes, or drains increase risk by breaching normal barriers and providing a portal of entry for infecting organisms. This includes catheters anywhere in the urinary system, wound drains and catheters, tracheotomies, and gastrostomy tubes for enteral feeding.

INTRINSIC RISK FACTORS

There are many recognized factors that can increase a patient's risk for developing or acquiring an infection. A basic consideration is age. It is well recognized that there is greater risk for infection at the extremes of age, that is, in the very young and the very old. In newborns and infants, increased risk is related to the immaturity of the immune system as well as lack of experience with and exposure to infectious agents. Newborns and infants have not yet developed antibodies to commonly seen agents. Even a full-term infant does not have a fully functioning immune system. This does not occur until around the age of 6 months. Infants, toddlers, and children frequently get community-acquired infections, especially as they enter day care and preschool, because they have not been exposed to these agents before and do not have immunity. The most common of these are called childhood diseases because most individuals used to get them sometime during their childhood, before vaccines were widely available.

In older people, increased susceptibility is related to the aging of the immune system. White blood cell function is not as efficient or effective in older individuals. Changes in anatomic structures, including the integumentary system, also increase risk because the natural physical barriers to infection are not as effective. Older patients are also more likely to have poor cough reflexes and therefore are more prone to aspiration; this increases risk for pneumonia. Poor circulation delays healing, which also increases the risk for infection.

Gender may also increase a patient's risk for infection. Females have a greater risk for urinary tract infections than males as a result of an anatomically shorter urethra. In addition to gender, a person's ethnic background may increase risk for certain diseases, including sickle-cell anemia and Tay-Sachs disease, which may increase risk for infection.

There are many studies that demonstrate the effect of socioeconomic status on the risk for infection. Cytomegalovirus infection occurs more frequently at a younger age in people of lower socioeconomic status than in those of higher status; this is attributed to crowded living conditions. There are many other infections that are acquired as a result of crowded living conditions. In addition, poor nutrition in lower socioeconomic status groups increases risk for infection. Similarly, lifestyle and marital status may affect risk for infection. Increased stress (e.g., as a result of homelessness) appears to affect the immune system. Other lifestyle issues, such as sexual behaviors, may also increase risk through increased exposure to infectious agents.

Occupation may also increase risk. Individuals involved in occupations that expose them to hazardous or carcinogenic agents that may affect their immune function may have increased risk. Chronic pulmonary diseases (e.g., brown lung) increase risk for pulmonary infection. Health care workers experience occupational exposures to infectious diseases.

The overall immune status of an individual is extremely important in determining risk for infection. Immune status can be affected by nutrition as well as by inherited and acquired immune diseases. Other chronic diseases, such as diabetes mellitus, affect immune system function. Some treatments, such as chemotherapy and radiation therapy, cause immunosuppression, as can drugs. Pregnancy also affects the immune system and increases risk for infection; anatomic changes may also be related to increased risk.

In assessing home care patients for risk of infection, the home care nurse considers the patient's history (congenital, underlying, acute, or chronic illness) and immune status as well as any current treatments or medications that may reduce immune response or increase susceptibility. It is well recognized that a patient who has an infection at one site is at significantly greater risk for another infection. There may be some interventions that home care staff can undertake to reduce this intrinsic risk (e.g., provide education to improve nutritional status, provide influenza vaccine, etc.), but for the most part there is little that home care staff can do to improve host immunity.

EXTRINSIC RISK FACTORS

There are various extrinsic risk factors that may affect a home care patient, including devices involved in home care, invasive procedures, exposure to home care staff, and the environment. Home care minimizes the extrinsic risk of exposure to other patients that exists in inpatient care. It is assumed that this is one reason the incidence of home care-acquired infection is lower than that of nosocomial infection. Home care staff, however, may transfer organisms from an infected or colonized patient to another patient on their hands, clothing, or inanimate objects that are used from one patient to another. Again, this occurs less frequently in home care than in hospitals or long-term care facilities because most of the inanimate objects that are used from one patient to another are noncritical items (see Chapter 8).

Devices are the most important extrinsic risk for home care-acquired infections. Devices that are left in place present the greatest risk because they breech a natural barrier and serve as a portal of entry for microorganisms. Indwelling urinary drainage catheters (i.e., urethral and suprapubic), intravenous devices, drainage tubes in surgical sites (e.g., Jackson-Pratt closed wound drainage systems), feeding tubes (e.g., gastrostomy tubes), and breathing tubes (e.g., tracheotomy tubes) are devices that are related to an increased risk for infection. Various interventions are necessary to reduce this extrinsic risk. First, the placement of a device into a sterile space (e.g., urinary bladder or venous system) must include the use of aseptic technique and antiseptic solutions in preparation of the site to reduce the number of bacteria that could be introduced with the device. For this purpose, antiseptics are used to prepare the skin or to cleanse the area around the urinary meatus before the device is introduced. If a device is left in place and involves a sterile space, the drainage or infusion system must be maintained in a sterile fashion. Other tubes and drains that are not introduced into a sterile space (e.g., gastrostomy tubes) must be maintained in a clean fashion to decrease extrinsic risk (see Chapter 3). Appropriate care of the insertion site, such as an intravenous exit site, a gastrostomy tube site, or a surgical wound drain site, is also important.

A single invasive event or procedure may also increase extrinsic risk. This may occur when a blood sample is obtained or when a urine sample is obtained from a urinary catheter. These procedures also include skin preparation or cleansing of the local area with an antiseptic to reduce the number of bacteria. When some devices, such as electronic thermometers, are used, protective covers (e.g., probe covers) are applied as a barrier to reduce the risk of contaminating the object and also to reduce the risk of transmitting infectious organisms to the patient.

The experience and skill of the home care staff member can also increase or decrease extrinsic risk for infection. Skill may affect risk in the performance of sterile, invasive procedures in the home. A more experienced, skillful nurse may accomplish the task in an efficient manner that reduces the risk of introduction of bacteria. Skill may also reduce the risk of trauma to the surrounding area or tissue.

Many times, home care staff must provide care in a home environment that is not well maintained or clean; often, the home may be infested with rodents and insects. Although this is frequently perceived to create an increased extrinsic risk for infection, there is no evidence that it does increase risk. If the lack of sanitary facilities, including sinks with running water and toilets, affects the patient's and family's ability to maintain an appropriate level of personal hygiene, this may affect risk for infection. For example, if there is no running water, handwashing may not be accomplished by caregivers in the home in an effective manner.

IMPACT OF HOME CARE STAFF

Home care staff can identify both intrinsic and extrinsic risks, but their ability to control and reduce risk is limited. As discussed above, there are limited interventions that can be undertaken to improve the patient's ability to resist infection. Many of these strategies are related to patient and family education; provision of vaccines for prevention of infection may also contribute to reducing risk. Home care staff also have limited ability to control or reduce risks related to the patient's environment. Therefore, the focus of risk reduction is related to the delivery of care. Handwashing (see Chapter 3) is the most important factor for minimizing the risk of transmission of organisms from one patient to another and from the home care staff member to the patient. Use of gowns and gloves for standard precautions and transmission-based precautions is also important. When home care involves skilled nursing procedures, risk is reduced by using the level of technique (e.g., clean or aseptic) that is appropriate to the specific procedure and level of risk. When inanimate objects are used, cleaning is the minimal risk reduction strategy. If the item is semicritical or critical, then disinfection or sterilization may be necessary (see Chapter 8).

REFERENCE

Dandalides, P., Rutala, W., & Sarubbi, F. Jr., (1984). Postoperative infection following cardiac surgery: Association with an environmental reservoir in a cardiothoracic intensive care unit. *Infection Control, 5,* 378–384.

CHAPTER 3

Patient Care Practices

Any home care that involves direct, hands-on care of the patient has some infection control ramification. It may be as simple as handwashing, or it may involve strict adherence to sterile technique. As a home care organization develops policies and procedures for care, it must determine what will be the standard of practice. This is guided by the experience of the nursing staff as well as written resources and references. Much of the written material on infection control is based on care provided in hospitals and other settings that home care professional staff must adapt for home care. Although many of the structural advantages of an institutional setting are not present in the home, neither are many of the potential risks for infection. In most home care settings, there are no other patients being cared for in the same room or area. This decreases the risk of transmission of microorganisms from one patient to another, but it does not eliminate the source of infection risk. Transmission can still occur from one patient to another on the hands of the home care staff member. Potential environmental reservoirs are eliminated, such as contaminated sinks, shared urine measurement devices, contaminated ventilator tubing from other patients, and other inanimate objects that have been implicated in infections within hospitals and other settings. Although practices should be performed in a manner to decrease infection risk, patient care practices in the home must also be feasible, sensible, practical, and cost effective. Infection control principles should be employed in a manner appropriate to the level of risk. The following discussion and recommendations for patient care practices have been developed with these guiding principles in mind.

HANDWASHING

Handwashing is the single most important patient care activity that a home care staff member can do to prevent cross-contamination and a home care acquired in fection. Handwashing is simply a vigorous, brief, rubbing together of all surfaces of soap-lathered hands followed by rinsing of the hands under running water. In home care, the staff member's hands are the greatest potential source for transmission of potentially infectious organisms to other patients.

Resident and Transient Microorganisms

The skin on the hands carries both resident and transient microorganisms. The resident (colonizing) microorganisms are normally located on the skin, whereas transient (noncolonizing) microorganisms are recent contaminants that can only survive for a limited amount of time on the skin and are readily removed by handwashing. Resident microorganisms (e.g., *Staphylococcus epidermidis*) rarely cause infections unless they enter the body through an invasive procedure, such as during the placement of a peripherally inserted central catheter. Most resident microorganisms are located in the superficial skin layers, but 10% to 20% can invade the deep epidermal layers. Handwashing with plain soaps or detergents and water will not remove resident microorganisms in the deep epidermal layers, but will remove many transient microorganisms. Only handwashing with antimicrobial agents can kill or inhibit resident microorganisms in the deep epidermal layers. For patients at high risk for infection, resident microorganisms can cause infections. *Staphylococcus aureus* is an example of a resident organism. Home care staff members may carry *S. aureus* on their hands and can spread the infection to the home care patient if the microorganism comes in contact with a portal of entry (e.g., nonintact skin, urinary drainage system, etc.).

Transient microorganisms survive less than 24 hours on the skin and can be removed easily by handwashing. Examples of transient microorganisms are *Escherichia coli* and *Pseudomona*, *Salmonella*, and *Shigella*. These transient organisms can be found on home care staff members' hands and may cause a home care-acquired infection. The reservoir of transient microorganisms is usually colonized or infected patients or contaminated patient-care equipment.

Indications for Handwashing

The home care staff member can serve as a role model for the patient and family to promote handwashing while performing the patient's care. The indications for handwashing depend on the type, intensity, duration, and sequence of home care activities. The indications for handwashing are listed in Exhibit 3–1.

Handwashing is not required for the following activities (Garner & Favero, 1986):

- superficial contact with a source not suspected of being contaminated (e.g., touching an object that is not visibly soiled, such as the doorknob of a patient's front door to enter the home)
- routine, brief patient care activities involving direct patient contact other than those listed in Exhibit 3–1 (e.g., taking the patient's blood pressure)
- routine home visit activities involving indirect patient contact (e.g., picking up medication bottles to review medications that the patient is currently taking to update the medication profile, completing paperwork, or talking with the patient and family)

Exhibit 3–1 Indications for Handwashing

Handwashing is indicated:

- before performing any invasive procedure, such as inserting an intravenous catheter or indwelling Foley catheter
- before taking care of patients at high risk for infection (e.g., premature infants)
- when there is prolonged or intense contact with any patient (e.g., after bathing a patient)
- between tasks and procedures on the same patient
- before and after touching a wound, whether surgical or associated with an invasive device
- after gloves are removed
- after situations in which microbial contamination of hands occurred or is likely to occur (e.g., after contact with contaminated items, secretions, excretions, or blood and body fluids whether or not gloves are worn)
- after touching inanimate sources that are potentially contaminated (e.g., after emptying a suction canister)
- after taking care of a patient who is infected or colonized with a multidrug-resistant microorganism
- when hands are visibly soiled
- after using the toilet, blowing the nose, or covering a sneeze
- after assisting a patient in using the toilet or changing diapers
- before eating, drinking, handling food, or serving food

When in doubt, wash your hands.

Source: Adapted with permission from J. Garner and M. Favero, CDC Guideline for Handwashing and Hospital Environmental Control. *American Journal of Infection Control,* Vol. 14, No. 3, pp. 110–129, © 1985, Mosby-Year Book, Inc.

Handwashing Facilities

In home care, staff members do not have the luxury of caring for the patient in a health care facility. Staff members may find themselves caring for a patient who has no access to clean or running water or having to bring water to the patient's home to give the patient a bath. When running water is not available, staff members should use a waterless handwashing product. The waterless handwashing product should be used when it would be appropriate to wash the hands, such as after performing patient care. Once the staff member has access to running water, either at the next patient's home (before providing any patient care) or at the office, his or her hands should be washed thoroughly with soap and running water.

When To Use Plain Soaps versus Antimicrobial-Containing Handwashing Products

A dilemma for home care staff members is when to use an antimicrobial agent and which agent to use. The choice of using plain soap, an antimicrobial agent, or a waterless handwashing product should be based on the degree of hand contamination, whether it is important

Table 3–1 Handwashing and Skin Cleaning Guidelines

Home Care Procedure	*Type of Soap*	*Gloves*	*Patient Skin Preparation*
Insertion of Foley catheter	Antimicrobial soap	Sterile	Antimicrobial
Insertion of peripheral short-line or midline IV device	Antimicrobial soap	Clean—short-line Sterile—midline	If skin is visibly dirty, wash with soap and water. Clip excess hair. Apply 70% alcohol and 10% povidone-iodine (must be applied thoroughly for 30 seconds and allowed to dry completely). Do not wipe off excess povidone-iodine with alcohol (Intravenous Nurses Society, 1998).
Insertion of PICC	Antimicrobial soap	Sterile	If skin is visibly dirty, wash with soap and water. Clip excess hair. Apply 70% alcohol and 10% povidone-iodine (must be applied thoroughly for 30 seconds and allowed to dry completely). Do not wipe off excess povidone-iodine with alcohol (Intravenous Nurses Society, 1998).
Insertion of needle for purpose of obtaining laboratory specimen	Plain soap	Clean	70% alcohol
Insertion of nasogastric tube	Plain soap	Clean	None
Suctioning oral cavity	Plain soap	Clean	None
Suctioning trachea	Plain soap	Sterile	None
Performing wound care	Antimicrobial soap	Sterile	Per physician's orders
Performing personal care services	Plain soap	Clean	None

to maintain a minimal number of resident microorganisms or to decrease the number, and whether it is important to remove the transient microorganisms mechanically. Table 3–1 contains guidelines as to when plain soap and antimicrobial soap should be used in the home. For routine patient care, washing the hands with plain soap and water for 10 to 15 seconds is sufficient to remove most transient contaminants from the skin. Plain soap removes microorganisms from the skin by suspending them and allowing them to be rinsed off the skin.

Antimicrobial handwashing products should be used only on intact skin and when the staff member is caring for patients on contact precautions or severely immunosuppressed patients and before performing any invasive procedures. The Food and Drug Administration considers antimicrobial soaps to be drugs because they kill or inhibit both transient and resident microorganisms. Even when an antimicrobial agent is used, there is a maximum level of reduction in bacterial counts that can be reached regardless of handwashing frequency or intensity (Larson, 1995). Antibacterial soap not only kills microorganisms but also can bind to the skin and continue to suppress microbial growth. Characteristics of antimicrobial agents are listed in Table 3–2.

Waterless Handwashing Products

Antimicrobial agents that do not require water for use, such as foams, gels, or rinses, should be used when there is no running water available (Larson, 1995). Antimicrobial products that are used as waterless handwashing products kill transient microorganisms, but do not remove soil or organic material. If the home care staff member's hands are visibly soiled and there is no running water available, single-use towelettes can be used first to remove the physical dirt, and then the hands can be cleaned with a waterless handwashing product. The hands should be washed with soap and water as soon after as possible. When alcohol-based waterless handwashing products are used, an alcohol

Table 3–2 Characteristics of Antimicrobial Agents

Disinfectant	*Features*
Alcohol	Concentrations between 60% and 90% by weight are optimal Active against most Gram-positive and Gram-negative bacteria, respiratory syncytial virus, hepatitis B virus, human immunodeficiency virus, fungi, *Mycobacterium tuberculosis* Not recommended in the presence of physical dirt Major disadvantage is its drying effect
Chlorhexidine gluconate	Active against Gram-positive and Gram-negative bacteria, viruses Activity against *Mycobacterium tuberculosis* is minimal Antimicrobial activity lasts longest after application
Hexachlorophene	Active against Gram-positive bacteria Activity against *Mycobacterium tuberculosis,* Gram-negative bacteria, fungi, viruses is minimal Antimicrobial activity lasts for several days after application Excessive absorption in infants can create neurotoxicity
Iodophors	Active against Gram-positive and Gram-negative bacteria, *Mycobacterium tuberculosis,* fungi, viruses Not commonly used for handwashing
***p*-Chloro-*m*-xylenol**	Active against Gram-positive bacteria Activity against *Mycobacterium tuberculosis,* Gram-negative bacteria, fungi, viruses is minimal
Triclosan	Active against Gram-positive and Gram-negative bacteria, viruses Activity against fungi and *Mycobacterium tuberculosis* is minimal

Source: Adapted with permission from E.L. Larson, APIC Guideline for Handwashing and Hand Antisepsis in Health Care Settings. *American Journal of Infection Control*, Vol. 23, © 1995, Mosby-Year Book, Inc.

concentration between 60% and 90% by weight is the most effective. An alcohol concentration greater than 70% by weight should not be used, however, because it can cause the skin to dry out and result in a chemical dermatitis (Larson, 1995).

The literature generally states that hands should be washed with soap and running water after gloves are removed. In some circumstances, it may not always be feasible to leave the patient and wash the hands with soap and water after removing gloves. When gloves are removed, "soap and water handwash or an antiseptic handrub should be used" (Larson, 1995, p. 258). In home care under certain circumstances, hand cleaning may be done with an alcohol-based antimicrobial hand rinse in lieu of handwashing with soap and water. For example, if the patient is left unattended in the home during wound care while the home care staff member goes into the bathroom or kitchen to wash the hands, the patient may be at greater risk for infection because the wound is left exposed, or a family pet may walk through a sterile field. Examples of when an antimicrobial agent may be used in lieu of handwashing with soap and water include the following:

- during a dressing change for a patient with multiple wounds when the staff member's gloves are removed several times
- after changing gloves to begin wound care at another site
- after removing a dirty dressing with nonsterile gloves and applying a sterile dressing with sterile gloves

An antimicrobial hand rinse also may be used, along with handwashing with soap and water, when it is important to reduce the number of resident and transient microorganisms, such as when caring for a patient at increased risk for infection.

Bar Soap versus Liquid Soap

Contrary to popular belief, bacteria can grow on soap. When plain soap is selected for handwashing, bar soap is not recommended for use if it is stored in the staff member's supply bag. Bar soap should not be carried by staff members making home visits because it may not have sufficient time to dry. Pooled moisture in a staff member's home care supply bag may support the growth of Gram-negative bacteria. Plain soap is acceptable, but it should be used in liquid form from a small container.

Liquid soap pump dispensers also can become contaminated. For that reason, a small soap container is recommended because liquid soap containers can become contaminated and serve as a reservoir of microorganisms. A small container can be cleaned when empty and brought back to the office to be refilled. A container that is almost empty should be completely emptied, cleaned, and dried before it is refilled. Liquid soap should not be added to a partially full soap dispenser. Refilling a pump dispenser is a more cost-effective approach and can be an indicator of the frequency with which the home care staff members are washing their hands in the home.

Side Effects of Handwashing

Frequent handwashing with plain soap or antimicrobial agents can cause skin dryness, cracking, irritation, or dermatitis, especially in geographical locations where the weather is cold and dry. This is caused by the soap stripping away the skin's natural oils. Home care staff members with cracked skin or dermatitis are potentially at increased risk for infection from contact with blood or other potentially infectious body fluids because there has been a break in the skin's integrity. Patients also may be placed at an increased risk for infection because handwashing will not effectively decrease the bacterial counts on irritated, dry, or cracked skin or dermatic skin because dermatic skin contains high numbers of microorganisms (Larson, 1995).

To prevent the skin from becoming cracked or developing dermatitis, the soap must be thoroughly rinsed off and the skin dried thoroughly. Staff members should try not to use excessive amounts of soap or antimicrobial agents when preparing to wash the hands. Hand creams or lotions can be helpful, but can become contaminated. If lotion is to be used, small, individual-use containers or pump dispensers that will be discarded when empty should be used. Handwashing products that contain iodophor (an antibacterial additive) should be avoided because iodophor dries the skin. Barrier creams and foams are available that help protect the skin. Some products can stay on the skin for 3 to 4 hours during multiple handwashing and thus are like "invisible gloves" (Beaumont, 1997).

Behavioral Aspects of Handwashing

Compliance with handwashing has been a problem for a long time. Home care staff members with cracked skin or dermatitis may avoid handwashing. The following factors may promote the frequency of handwashing (Larson, 1996):

- informing staff members of the infection rate(s) and presence of multidrug-resistant microorganisms
- observing handwashing technique during competence assessment activities
- having the home care organization provide handwashing supplies and not making the staff responsible for providing their own handwashing supplies
- championing and promoting handwashing practices
- involving staff in planning for handwashing education

National Infection Control Week is observed during October of each year. This may be a good opportunity to promote handwashing by providing buttons, posters, inservice education, or written information about handwashing to home care staff, patients, and families.

Handwashing Supplies Needed by Home Care Staff

Handwashing supplies may be brought to the patient's home by home care staff members, or, if appropriate, the patient's handwashing supplies may be used. Staff members providing direct, hands-on patient care activities should have the following supplies:

- plain soap and antimicrobial soap or antimicrobial soap only
- waterless handwashing product
- individual-use towelettes containing detergent
- paper towels
- skin lotion (optional)

Staff members who do not provide hands-on patient care (e.g., chaplain, social worker, or dietitian) and do not reasonably anticipate patient contact should have a waterless handwashing product in their possession during home visits if the patient is being maintained on standard precautions.

Using the Patient's Handwashing Supplies

When washing the hands in the patient's home, home care staff members should bring their own handwashing supplies. The patient's liquid soap may be used if the dispenser appears to be clean and the home environment is clean. The patient's bar soap should not be used if it has been resting in a pool of accumulated water. When drying the hands, staff members may use either their own paper towels or the patient's paper towels. The patient's cloth towels may be used if they are clean and have not been used previously by anyone in the home. The hand-drying materials should not be placed in an area near the sink, where they could become contaminated by splashes of water. Hand drying is also an integral part of cleaning the hands. The friction of hand drying can remove many bacteria by rubbing away transient microorganisms and dead skin cells, and it can remove bacteria from deeper skin layers.

How To Wash the Hands

1. Wet the hands under running water and apply a small amount (dime to quarter size) of liquid soap to the hands.
2. Rub the hands together vigorously for a minimum of 10 to 15 seconds. If the hands are visibly soiled, a longer handwashing time may be needed. Be sure to scrub between fingers and around the tops and palms of the hands, especially around nail beds.
3. Rinse the hands under running water to remove residual soap.
4. Dry the hands with a clean, disposable (or single-use) towel.
5. Discard the used towel in a trash container.

Staff members should consider using hand lotion to prevent chapping of the hands. If lotions are used, liquids or tubes that can be squirted are recommended, so that the hands do not have direct contact with the container spout. Direct contact with the spout could contaminate the lotion inside the container. Staff members should never use jars or containers into which the hands must be dipped.

Alternative Handwashing Technique using a Waterless Handwashing Product

Premoistened towelettes or waterless handwashing products should not be used as a substitute for washing hands with soap and running water. The hands should be washed as soon as possible after a home care visit when clean, running water is not available in the patient's home.

1. If the hands are visibly soiled with dirt, clean them with an individual-use towelette.
2. Apply an antimicrobial hand rinse or foam all over both hands.
3. Rub the hands vigorously for about 30 seconds until they are dry.
4. Wash the hands with soap and running water as soon after as feasible.

If all hand surfaces are not covered with the solution as a result of poor technique or not using sufficient amounts of solution, the hands can still be contaminated. Premoistened cleansing towelettes or hand rinses alone do not effectively clean the hands and should never be used in place of handwashing.

ASSESSMENT OF THE PATIENT AND HOME ENVIRONMENT

During the initial assessment and on an ongoing basis thereafter, the patient should be assessed for factors that may predispose him or her to infection (see Chapter 2). These factors include immunization status, past and present infectious diseases, age, nutritional status, immune status, substance abuse, financial resources available to purchase needed medication, equipment and supplies, motivation to learn, learning needs, mental status, and overall physical condition. Patients at high risk for infection should be encouraged to receive the pneumococcal and influenza vaccines unless contraindicated by their physician. The findings of the initial and ongoing assessments should be incorporated into a plan of care.

The home environment should be assessed on admission not only for safety issues, but also from an infection control perspective. Potential infection risks in the home environment include general cleanliness, refrigeration, health status of other individuals residing in the home (e.g., immunization status and presence of infectious diseases), availability of running water, utility systems (e.g., electricity for refrigeration), heat and air conditioning (so that equipment and supplies can be stored under proper temperature and humidity conditions), availability of toilet facilities, and the presence of pets and pests. Even in the 1990s, some home environments still have dirt floors, and no running water or toilet facilities. Frequently, the home care organization must do the best it can to work within the home situation that its staff members must face. For example, some home care organizations must bring water to the patient's home to bathe the patient because running water to the home is not available. During each staff member's initial home visit, the handwashing facilities should be identified so that appropriate handwashing can be performed.

Pets (e.g., dogs and cats) and pests (e.g., rodents and cockroaches) present another infection control concern over which the home care organization does not have direct control. Although there are situations in which the home environment is infested with roaches and rodents, these are not usually disease vectors. The infection risk related to this unpleasant and distasteful situation may be more perceived than actual, although no data on this subject exist. In these circumstances, the home care staff should educate the patient and family in general principles of hygiene and cleanliness and provide reinforcement and guidance whenever possible.

In setting up for patient care activities, and to the best of the home care staff member's abilities, the patient's direct care environment (not the entire home) should be cleaned or, if necessary, barriers should be used to maintain the area as clean as possible (refer to Chapter 6 for additional information about the staff's use of barriers in the home). When invasive procedures are performed in an unsanitary environment, efforts must be made to provide the care in as safe a manner as possible.

WOUND CARE

The types of wounds that are typically cared for in the home include infected surgical wounds, infected decubiti, and wounds whose healing is slow or difficult. Surgical wounds seal quickly, and unless they are left open, do not heal, or have adjacent drains, there is minimal risk for contamination. When performing wound care in the home, the staff member may have to adapt patient care practices to determine which technique, clean or sterile, is appropriate.

Clean Technique versus Sterile Technique

The term *clean technique* refers to the strategies used in patient care to reduce the overall number of microorganisms or to prevent or reduce the transmission of microorganisms from one person to another or from one place to another. Clean technique involves meticulous handwashing with plain soap, using barriers, and maintaining a clean environment. Barriers involve using no-touch dressing technique to avoid contamination of sterile supplies, wearing sterile gloves to apply a sterile dressing, or wearing personal protective equipment, such as a gown and gloves, to avoid direct contact with infectious materials (refer to Chapter 6 for additional information about personal protective equipment). Other components of clean technique include maintaining a clean environment and using a detergent to remove soil and a disinfectant agent to clean up a spill of blood or other potentially infectious material (DeCastro, Fauerbach, & Masters, 1996).

The term *aseptic technique* or *sterile technique* refers to strategies used in patient care to render and maintain objects and areas maximally free from microorganisms. Sterile technique involves meticulous handwashing with antimicrobial soap, using barriers, and maintaining a clean environment (DeCastro et al., 1996; refer to Chapter 4 for additional information about how to prepare a patient's skin for an invasive procedure). When sterile technique is used in the home, a sterile field should be established to prevent the transmission of microorganisms from the environment or from the staff member to the patient. This involves using a sterile barrier or drape and, at minimum, wearing sterile gloves. Additional attire, such as a sterile gown or mask, should be worn if appropriate. For example, if a peripherally inserted central catheter is being placed in the home, maximum barrier protection should be used, which includes using a mask, sterile gown, sterile gloves, and large sterile drape. As is the case for clean technique in the home, maintaining a clean environment is not within the direct control of the home care organization, but to the best of the home care staff member's abilities the immediate environment in which care is provided should be maintained as clean as possible. When a procedure is performed in the home that requires sterile technique, if possible, door(s) to the room where the procedure is being performed should be closed to reduce potential airborne transmission of microorganisms, and other family members or visitors should be asked to leave the room unless they are needed as assistants in the procedure. Of course, it is the family members' home, and if they want to remain in the room during a sterile procedure, it is not within the home care organization's ultimate control to prevent them. In addition to general housecleaning, maintaining a clean environment includes using a detergent to remove soil and a disinfectant agent to clean up a spill of blood or other potentially infectious material. Equipment that is used in procedures requiring sterile technique should be maintained as sterile or discarded after one-time use.

Wound Care Procedures

Various dressing techniques and wound care procedures may be performed in the home setting. Frequently, staff members do not perform wound care each time it must be performed, and dressing changes are delegated to the patient or family member. Either clean technique or sterile technique may be used to perform wound care. Sterile technique should be used when the wound is a new surgical wound (Garofalo, 1996), when the wound is open, when the staff member must handle a sterile drain site or system, or when required by the physician's orders. Regardless of the technique used, the actual wound itself should never be touched with any item that is not sterile. Home care staff members should not touch an open or fresh wound directly unless they are wearing sterile gloves or are using no-touch technique. When the wound has sealed, wound care may be performed without the use of gloves as long as the hands are freshly washed (Garner, 1986). When wounds are measured in the home with nonsterile measuring devices, special care should be taken to avoid touching the wound directly. When dressings are removed, nonsterile, Latex examination gloves may be worn when there is no direct touching of the wound itself, and a new dressing may be applied with either new, sterile gloves or nonsterile gloves using no-touch technique. In cleaning the wound directly, however, sterile gloves are recommended. Dressings over closed wounds should be removed or changed if they are wet or if the patient has signs or symptoms suggestive of infection (e.g., fever or unusual wound pain). When the dressing is removed, the wound should be evaluated for signs of infection and if necessary the physician should be contacted. Any purulent drainage should be reported to the physician and a culture and smear for Gram's stain obtained if ordered.

Home care staff members and the patient and family members should wash their hands before and after taking care of a wound. Patients with wound or skin infections should be placed on contact precautions (Garner, 1996; refer to Chapter 7 for additional information about contact precautions and Chapter 8 for information about storing wound care supplies in the home).

Irrigating Solution Maintenance

Currently, there are no home care industry standards that prescribe a specific time frame for which an irrigating solution, such as normal saline or sterile water, may be used after it is opened. Thus current practice varies from daily, to weekly, to monthly, to when the container is empty. Although it is preferable to have some policy setting some time limit, the contamination of irrigation fluid is not dependent on time. It is an event-related risk that depends on how the solution and its container are handled. If the inside of the container or the fluid is contaminated, the container and fluid should be discarded immediately. If the container is handled carefully and contamination does not occur, the fluid will probably remain sterile. To address this issue, the home care organization should incorporate some common sense strategies to avoid arbitrary discarding of irrigation fluid, which increases the cost of care.

- There should be more than one size container of irrigating solution available to staff, if possible. The nurse selecting the solution should select a quantity (e.g., 150 mL versus 500 mL) that will be used in a reasonable number of visits or period of time.
- The current date should be placed on the label when the container is opened.
- The solution should be handled in a manner to avoid contamination of the fluid itself as well as the inside of the neck of the bottle and the inside of

the top of the cap (the cap should always be laid face up when the fluid is being used).
- The cap should be replaced as soon as possible after use to avoid potential risk of contamination.

The irrigating solution should be stored in a safe place that minimizes tampering by a family member who has not been trained in its use or by a child or confused adult. The home care staff member will have to judge the safest approach to storage. In addition, the home care staff member can place a piece of tape over the bottle cap to detect whether the bottle has been opened since the last visit.

Before the irrigation solution is used, it should be carefully inspected for foreign material, damage, leaking, mold, or fungus. If any of these problems is identified, the irrigation solution should be immediately discarded. If the home care organization determines that an arbitrary date for discard is prudent, a time from 1 week to 1 month may be selected. Without specific data, it is impossible to know what time frame is safe or necessary.

Preparing Irrigating Solutions in the Home

Most home care organizations provide the patient with commercially prepared, sterile irrigating solutions for their use. If a patient cannot afford to purchase the commercially prepared products, however, the patient or family member in the home can prepare sterile water as follows (Garofalo, 1996):

1. Place a small (quart-size or smaller), closeable glass jar and its lid into a pan of boiling water.
2. Submerge the jar and lid, and boil the jar and the lid for 10 minutes.
3. Fill a separate pan with a sufficient amount of distilled water to fill the jar of water.
4. Boil the distilled water for 10 minutes.
5. Remove the jar and the lid from the pan, being careful not to touch the top of the jar or the inside of the lid (tongs or pick-ups may be used), and allow them to cool.
6. Pour the boiled distilled water into the jar, close tightly, and store.

The patient or family member can prepare 0.9% normal saline by following these steps (Garofalo, 1996):

1. Place a small (quart-size or smaller), closeable glass jar and its lid into a pan of boiling water.
2. Submerge the jar and lid, and boil the jar and the lid for 10 minutes.
3. Fill a separate pan with approximately 1 quart of distilled water and add 1½ tsp of salt.
4. Boil the salt water for 10 minutes.
5. Remove the jar and the lid from the pan, being careful not to touch the top of the jar or the inside of the lid (tongs or pick-ups may be used), and allow them to cool.
6. Pour the boiled salt water into the jar, shake well, and store.

If a family member prepares the normal saline or sterile water, a new mixture should be prepared daily. The patient and family should be instructed never to pour any leftover solution back into the container.

Patient Education Related to Wound Care

Patient and family education related to infection control and wound care should include handwashing, clean technique versus sterile technique, proper storage and set-up of equipment and supplies, the time frame for disposing of irrigation solutions, wound care procedure, wound assessment, signs and symptoms of a localized or systemic infection, and the disposal of soiled dressings.

REUSING EQUIPMENT IN THE HOME

Items that directly or indirectly contact mucous membranes of the respiratory or urinary tract are considered semicritical items (see Chapter 8). According to Spaulding's classification system for cleaning and disinfecting medical equipment (Spaulding, 1968), semicritical items should be sterilized or subjected to high-level disinfection before reuse. In the home environment, however, it is not possible to sterilize equipment or perform high-level disinfection. Many patients being cared for at home are chronically ill and do not have the financial resources to use a new sterile item, such as a tracheal suction catheter or intermittent urethral catheter, each time. For many years, these catheters have been safely reused without reports of infectious complications. As in most home care situations, scientific data are not available to support this practice, but reuse of tracheal suction catheters and intermittent urethral catheters after meticulous cleaning and disinfection is acceptable for most (not all) patients.

Each patient and situation must be evaluated for the potential risk versus cost of using disposable catheters.

URINARY TRACT CARE

Catheter-related urinary tract infection is the most common nosocomial infection (Jarvis et al., 1998). Anecdotal evidence and minimal data suggest that this may be a common site of home care-acquired infection as well. Although not all catheter-associated urinary tract infections can be prevented, proper placement and management of the indwelling catheter can contribute to prevention of associated infections. Long-term indwelling catheterization, which is usually more prevalent in home care patients than intermittent or condom catheterization, is generally associated with a higher urinary tract infection rate. The incidence of infection in acute care is directly related to the duration of catheterization. For example, data show that 50% of patients develop a urinary tract infection by day 15 of catheterization and that almost 100% of patients develop a urinary tract infection by the first month (Kunin, 1987). The risk of acquiring a urinary tract infection depends on the method and duration of catheterization, the quality of catheter care, and host susceptibility. Host factors that increase the risk for a urinary tract infection include advanced age, female gender, general debilitation, meatal colonization by urinary pathogens, and incontinence. Catheter-associated urinary tract infections are caused by various pathogens, including *Escherichia coli*, *Candida albicans*, enterococci, and various species of *Klebsiella*, *Proteus*, *Pseudomonas*, *Enterobacter*, and *Serratia*. Many of these microorganisms are part of the patient's normal bowel flora, but they also can be acquired by cross-contamination from staff members or by exposure to contaminated solutions or nonsterile equipment (Wong, 1983). Whether from endogenous or exogenous sources, infecting microorganisms gain access to the urinary tract by several routes. Microorganisms that inhabit the distal urethra can be directly introduced into the bladder when the catheter is inserted. With indwelling catheters, infecting microorganisms can migrate to the bladder along the outside of the catheter or along the inside lumen of the catheter if the collection bag or catheter drainage tube junction has been contaminated.

One of the most important strategies to prevent a urinary tract infection is to limit the use of urinary catheters and the number of days they are in place, thereby reducing the exposure risk. If possible, alternative techniques of urinary drainage should be considered before an indwelling urethral catheter is inserted, such as a condom catheter for a male patient. The physician will determine other alternatives of urinary drainage, such as intermittent urethral catheterization, with input from the home care staff member.

Indwelling Catheter Insertion and Replacement

In many patients it is difficult to avoid long-term urinary catheterization. In these home care patients, it has become routine to change the catheter and drainage system arbitrarily every 30 days. This practice has been supported by the Health Care Financing Administration (HCFA), which reimburses Medicare-certified home health agencies for the skilled nursing services of insertion, sterile irrigation, and replacement of catheters as well as care of suprapubic catheters and, in selected patients, urethral catheters. The frequency of catheter-related services that is considered reasonable and necessary is as follows: "Absent any complications, Foley catheters generally require skilled care once approximately every 30 days, and silicone catheters generally require skilled care once every 60 to 90 days" (HCFA, 1996, pp. 14-14–14-15). Therefore, most Medicare-certified home health agencies replace the patient's Foley catheter at 30-day intervals because it is considered a billable skilled nursing visit rather than based on a clinical need to have the catheter replaced. Reconsideration should be given to this practice because data demonstrate that this intervention is not necessary.

Indwelling catheters should not be changed at arbitrary fixed intervals (Wong, 1983) in the absence of leakage, malfunction, or palpable concretions in the catheter lumen. Indications for the replacement of an indwelling catheter include catheter damage or leakage, an obstruction that is not relieved by irrigation, and physician's orders. Insertion or replacement of an indwelling catheter should be performed using aseptic technique, sterile equipment, and as small a catheter as possible, consistent with good drainage, to minimize urethral trauma.

Catheter Maintenance

Handwashing should be performed immediately before and after any manipulation of the catheter site or apparatus. As much as possible, a closed urinary catheter system should be maintained. The catheter and drainage tube should not be disconnected unless the catheter must be irrigated, the catheter tubing and bag must be changed for routine maintenance, or the patient was using a temporary leg bag. If the system must be disconnected, the catheter-tubing junction should be disinfected with 70% isopropyl alcohol or povidone-iodine solution. The urinary collection system should be kept below the level of the bladder to prevent a reflux of urine into the bladder, and the tubing should be kept free from kinks. The collection bag should be emptied on a regular basis using a separate collection container. The draining spigot on the collection bag should not come in direct contact with the urine collection container. After use, the urine collection container should be cleaned and disinfected with a bleach solution or sprayed with a commercial disinfectant, with the sprayed solution remaining on the container for the time recommended by the manufacturer. Indwelling catheters should be properly secured after insertion to prevent movement and urethral traction.

Meatal Care

Performing routine meatal care in patients, by cleaning with povidone-iodine twice a day and cleansing daily with soap and water, does not reduce the risk of catheter-related urinary tract infection (Wong, 1983). Meatal care and cleansing in the perineal area should be performed with soap and water during bathing and care of the incontinent patient. In females, cleansing should be performed by wiping from the front to the back.

Indwelling Catheter Irrigation

The home care, indwelling catheters may require frequent irrigation as a result of obstructions caused by clots or mucus or other causes. Routine irrigation should be avoided, however, because it interrupts a sterile system and increases the risk for contamination and infection. When intermittent catheter irrigation must be performed, the catheter-tubing junction should be disinfected before disconnection and the catheter should be irrigated using aseptic technique. If the catheter becomes obstructed and can be kept open only by frequent irrigation, the catheter should be changed if it is likely that the catheter itself is contributing to the obstruction (e.g., by formation of concretions) (Wong, 1983).

Intermittent Catheterization

For patients with certain types of bladder-emptying dysfunction, such as those caused by spinal cord injuries or other neurological disorders, intermittent catheterization is commonly used. Clean technique is considered adequate for intermittent catheterization in the home setting (Garofalo, 1996). Although there are no reported data on the frequency of infection related to this practice, anecdotal experience appears to indicate it is safe. The intermittent urethral catheter may be reused as long as the cleaning and disinfection process is performed effectively and does not change the structural integrity or function of the urethral catheter.

Cleaning and Disinfecting Intermittent Urethral Catheters

Urethral catheters for intermittent catheterization used by a single patient may be reused after cleaning and disinfection. Methods used by home care organizations include either boiling or microwaving the catheter. When the boiling method is used (Garofalo, 1996), the catheter is cleaned with soap and tap water, rinsed with tap water, boiled for 15 minutes, dried on a clean towel or paper towels, and allowed to cool before use or stored in a clean, closeable container or a new plastic bag. When the microwaving method is used (Garofalo, 1996), the catheter is cleaned with soap and tap water on the inside and outside, rinsed with tap water on the inside and outside, placed in a bowl of water and microwaved on high for 15 minutes, dried on a clean towel or paper towels, and allowed to cool prior to use or stored in a clean, closeable container or a new plastic bag.

Cleaning and Disinfecting Urine Collection Tubing and Bags

Several methods may be used to clean and disinfect the urine collection system. One method is as follows:

1. Drain the urine from the bag and rinse the tubing and bag with tap water until clear.
2. With a catheter tip syringe, clean the tubing and bag with soapy water and rinse with tap water until clear.
3. With a catheter tip syringe, instill either 1:3 white vinegar solution or a bleach solution of 1 teaspoon bleach to 1 pint of water.

4. Soak for 30 minutes.
5. Empty the collection system and allow the tubing and bag to air dry.
6. Cover the ends aseptically, such as with a gauze pad, and store in a clean, dry place until used.

The tubing must be completely filled with the selected disinfectant for it to be properly disinfected. When the tubing is submerged, caution should be used to avoid getting air bubbles trapped in it.

Specimen Collection

If small volumes of urine are needed for laboratory analysis, the distal end of the catheter, or preferably the sampling port if present, should be used to obtain the specimen. If the catheter-tubing junction must be disconnected, it should be disinfected before disconnection with a 70% isopropyl alcohol preparation pad. If the sampling port is used, it should be cleansed with a 70% isopropyl alcohol preparation pad and the urine aspirated through a sterile needle and syringe. Larger volumes of urine should be obtained aseptically from the drainage bag.

Patient Education for Prevention of a Urinary Tract Infection

Patient and family education specifically related to infection control and prevention of a urinary tract infection should include handwashing; indwelling, condom, or suprapubic catheter care and maintenance; drainage bag emptying procedures; cleaning and disinfecting procedures for catheter care equipment and supplies; and signs and symptoms of a urinary tract infection.

RESPIRATORY THERAPY AND INFECTION CONTROL

Mechanically Assisted Ventilation

Pneumonia is the second most common type of nosocomial infection in the United States and is associated with substantial morbidity and mortality (Tablan, Anderson, Arden, Breiman, Butler, & McNeil, 1994). Although patients receiving mechanically assisted ventilation do not represent a major proportion of patients who receive home care, they are at highest risk for acquiring pneumonia because mechanical ventilation alters first-line patient defenses. In fact, patients receiving continuous, mechanically assisted ventilation have 6 to 21 times the risk for acquiring pneumonia compared with patients not receiving ventilatory support (Tablan et al., 1994). Other risk factors for pneumonia include host factors (extremes of age and severe underlying conditions, including immunosuppression), factors that enhance colonization of the oropharynx and/or stomach by microorganisms (e.g., administration of antimicrobials, underlying chronic lung disease, or coma), and conditions favoring aspiration or reflux (e.g., insertion of a nasogastric tube or supine position). Most bacterial pneumonias occur by aspiration of bacteria colonizing the oropharynx or upper gastrointestinal tract. Bacteria can invade the lower respiratory tract by aspiration of oropharyngeal organisms, inhalation of aerosols containing bacteria, or, less frequently, hematogenous spread from a distant body site (Tablan et al., 1994).

Breathing Circuits

A breach of the breathing circuit occurs anytime the ventilator is disconnected from the patient's tracheostomy tube for suctioning, to change the ventilator circuit, or to empty condensate that accumulates in the ventilator circuit. Each time the circuit is breached, the patient is placed at risk for infection. Therefore, the Centers for Disease Control and Prevention (CDC) recommends that the breathing circuit, including the tubing and exhalation valve and the attached bubbling or wick humidifier, of a ventilator that is being used on an individual patient should not be changed more frequently than every 48 hours. The maximum time that a circuit can be safely left unchanged on a patient has not been determined, however (Tablan et al., 1994). The American Association of Respiratory Care's clinical practice guideline on long-term mechanical ventilation in the home recommends that the ventilator circuits not be changed more often than once each week (American Association of Respiratory Care, 1995). The condensate that collects in the tubing of a mechanical ventilator should be periodically drained and discarded, with precautions being taken not to allow condensate to drain toward the patient. The internal machinery of mechanical ventilators used for respiratory therapy is not considered an important source of bacterial contamination of inhaled gas, and therefore routine sterilization or high-level disinfection of the internal machinery is not necessary (Tablan et al., 1994).

Suctioning of Respiratory Tract Secretions

Removal of tracheal secretions by gentle suctioning using aseptic technique to reduce cross-contamination from contaminated respiratory therapy equipment or contaminated or colonized staff member hands has traditionally been used to help prevent pneumonia in patients. In home care, practices that may be different from those in other care settings are the reuse of tracheal suction catheters and the use of clean versus sterile technique. The tracheal suction catheter may be reused as long as the cleaning and disinfection process is effective and does not change the structural integrity or function of the catheter. Obviously, the main patient care concern is infection from the introduction of bacteria into the lungs, which could lead to pneumonia. In day-to-day practice, some home care organizations use a new sterile suction catheter each time the patient is suctioned. Some home care organizations rinse the catheter after suctioning, store it a manner to keep it dry and avoid contamination, and replace it with a new, sterile catheter every 8 to 24 hours. Other home care organizations soak or disinfect the catheters at the end of the day, rinse them, and then reuse them. If a patient is an infant, is immunocompromised, or develops a respiratory infection, use of a new sterile suction catheter for each suctioning while maintaining sterile technique is recommended. In most other cases, clean technique is acceptable, although the care of each patient must be evaluated individually. It should be the mutual decision of the home care organization and the patient's physician to determine whether clean or sterile technique will be used and the frequency with which a new suction catheter will be replaced.

The CDC does not have a recommendation for use of sterile rather than clean gloves; minimally, nonsterile gloves should be worn by home care staff when suctioning a patient's respiratory secretions (Tablan et al., 1994). If sterile technique is used to suction the patient and a new sterile suction catheter is used for each episode of suctioning, sterile gloves should be worn. Tap water (Garofalo, 1996) or 3% hydrogen peroxide may be suctioned through the suction catheter to remove secretions if the catheter is going to be used again to suction the patient.

Cleaning and Disinfecting Tracheal Suction Catheters

If it is the home care organization's and physician's mutual decision to reuse tracheal suction catheters, the catheters must be cleaned and disinfected between uses. Various methods are described in the literature to clean and disinfect tracheal suction catheters between uses (Garofalo, 1996). One of two methods may be used for disinfecting tracheal suction catheters. The first method of disinfection involves soaking the tracheal suction catheter in 3% hydrogen peroxide, and the other involves boiling the catheter. Hydrogen peroxide may lose its disinfectant capabilities if it is exposed to air and light for an extended period of time. Therefore, if hydrogen peroxide is poured into a container, it should be changed daily.

When the hydrogen peroxide soaking method is used, the tracheal suction catheter should be:

1. cleaned with soap and tap water
2. rinsed with tap water
3. flushed with 3% hydrogen peroxide
4. placed in a container of 3% hydrogen peroxide to soak for a minimum of 20 minutes
5. rinsed and flushed with sterile water before use
6. stored in a clean, closeable jar that has been boiled, or in a new plastic bag

The suction tubing must be completely filled with hydrogen peroxide to disinfect all internal and external surfaces for proper (complete) disinfection. When the suction tubing is submerged in the hydrogen peroxide, caution should be used to avoid getting air bubbles trapped in the tubing.

When the boiling method is used, the tracheal suction catheter should be:

1. cleaned with soap and tap water
2. boiled in water for 10 minutes
3. dried on a clean towel or paper towels and allowed to cool before use
4. stored in a clean, closeable jar that has been boiled, or in a new plastic bag

Cleaning and Disinfecting the Inner Tracheal Cannula

One of two methods may be used for disinfecting the inner tracheal cannula. The first method involves soaking the inner tracheal cannula in 3% hydrogen peroxide, and the other involves boiling the inner tracheal cannula. When the hydrogen peroxide soaking method is used, the inner cannula should be:

1. cleaned with soap and cold water and friction (if there is a build-up of mucous inside the inner can-

nula, 3% hydrogen peroxide may be used to remove crusted exudate)
2. soaked in 3% hydrogen peroxide or 70% isopropyl alcohol for 20 minutes
3. rinsed with sterile water or tap water, with care taken to ensure that all hydrogen peroxide or alcohol has been removed
4. allowed to air dry on a clean towel or paper towels
5. stored in a clean, closeable jar that has been boiled, or in a new plastic bag

When the boiling method is used, the inner cannula is:

1. cleaned with soap and cold water and friction (if there is a build-up of mucous inside the inner cannula, 3% hydrogen peroxide may be used to remove crusted exudate)
2. rinsed with tap water
3. boiled for 10 minutes
4. allowed to air dry on a clean towel or paper towels and allowed to cool before use
5. stored in a clean, closeable jar that has been boiled or in a new plastic bag

The frequency with which the inner cannula is cleaned and tracheostomy stoma site care provided should be according to the organization's policies and procedures or the physician's orders, but minimally it should be frequently enough to keep the skin clean and dry and to prevent excoriation around the stoma. The outer tracheal cannula should be changed regularly to prevent tissue granulation around the stoma and infection. The frequency of tracheostomy tube changes (inner and outer cannulas) should be according to the physician's orders or every week to every month. When a tracheostomy tube is changed, aseptic technique should be used and the tube replaced with a new disposable tracheostomy tube (sterile from the manufacturer), or a reusable tracheostomy tube that has undergone sterilization or high-level disinfection (Tablan et al., 1994).

Cleaning and Disinfecting Respiratory Equipment and Supplies

Devices used on the respiratory tract for respiratory therapy (e.g., nebulizers) are potential reservoirs and vehicles for infectious microorganisms. Proper cleaning and disinfection of reusable equipment are important components of a home care program to reduce infections associated with respiratory therapy equipment. All respiratory equipment and devices must be cleaned before disinfection. Once the equipment is cleaned and disinfected, care must be taken not to contaminate the equipment in the process of rinsing, drying, and packaging.

A suction collection canister should be emptied and cleaned with soap and water on a daily basis. The suction cannula, tubing, and glass and plastic containers should be disinfected once a week or more often using a 1:3 vinegar solution or a 1:10 bleach solution (Feenan & Voutroubek, 1997). Low-flow oxygen systems without humidifiers do not present a clinically important risk for infection and do not need to be routinely replaced. High-flow systems that employ heated humidifiers or aerosol generators, however, especially when applied to patients with artificial airways, should be cleaned and disinfected on a regular basis. There currently are no definitive studies regarding the frequency of tubing changes at home (American Association of Respiratory Care, 1992). Respiratory equipment tubing, such as for oxygen therapy, should be cleaned or replaced and the cannula changed or replaced when it is visibly contaminated. To clean the tubing or cannula, 1 teaspoon of white vinegar should be added to each quart of water or saline. The tubing must be completely filled with the vinegar solution to be properly disinfected. When the tubing is submerged, caution should be used to avoid trapping air bubbles in it.

Other Measures To Prevent Respiratory Infection

Traditional preventive measures for pneumonia include decreasing the risk of aspiration, preventing cross-contamination or colonization via hands of home care staff members, appropriate disinfection of respiratory therapy devices, and education of staff members, patients, and family members. Regardless of whether gloves are worn, the hands should be washed after contact with mucous membranes, respiratory secretions, or objects contaminated with respiratory secretions and both before and after contact with a patient who has a tracheostomy tube in place and before and after contact with any other respiratory device that is used on the patient. Gloves should be worn when respiratory secretions or objects contaminated with respiratory secretions are handled.

Gloves should be changed and hands washed after contact with a patient, after respiratory secretions or objects contaminated with secretions from one patient are handled and before contact with another object or environmental surface, and between contacts with a contaminated body site and the respiratory tract of, or respiratory device on, the same patient. A gown should be worn if soiling with respiratory secretions from the patient is anticipated, and the gown should be changed after contact (Tablan et al., 1994; refer to Chapter 6 for additional information about when personal protective equipment should be worn in the home).

Measures should be taken to prevent a respiratory infection caused by aspiration in patients receiving enteral therapy. These measures include elevating the head of the bed to 30° to 45° for patients at high risk for aspiration pneumonia (e.g., patients receiving mechanically assisted ventilation), verifying the appropriate placement of the enteral feeding tube, and assessing the patient's intestinal motility by auscultating for bowel sounds and measuring residual gastric volume or abdominal girth and, with a physician's order, adjusting the rate and volume of the enteral feeding to avoid reflux aspiration.

Patient Education for the Prevention of a Respiratory Tract Infection

Patient and family education related to infection control and the prevention of a respiratory tract infection should include handwashing, use of personal protective equipment, tracheostomy care, suctioning procedures, cleaning and disinfecting procedures for respiratory care equipment and supplies, and signs and symptoms of a respiratory infection.

ENTERAL THERAPY

Enteral feedings may be a source of infection from contaminated enteral formula. Enteral nutrition may be administered as either an intermittent or a continuous feeding. Intermittent feedings may be administered as a bolus, rapidly infused via a syringe, or given as a continuous slow feeding via gravity or an infusion pump. Unopened enteral therapy formula may be stored at room temperature in the home. When formulas are reconstituted or diluted, the label instructions for preparation, storage, and stability should be closely followed. Most reconstituted or diluted formulas should be covered, refrigerated, and used within 24 to 48 hours (or as instructed on the product label) from the time when the container was opened. Expiration dates should always be checked before the container is opened and the formula is administered to the patient. Refrigerated formula should sit at room temperature for 30 minutes before administration because enteral feedings should be given at room temperature to avoid abdominal cramping and discomfort. During the 24-hour interval for intermittent feeding and before new formula is added, the enteral feeding bag and tubing should be rinsed with tap water until clean. Newly prepared enteral feeding formula should not be added to the bag of existing enteral feeding that has been hanging. This practice of "topping off" the bag with new feeding formula is not recommended because the new formula may become contaminated if it is mixed with old formula that has been left hanging for too long and has bacterial growth. During the feeding, the bag and tubing should be checked intermittently for foreign matter, mold, and leakage.

Cleaning Enteral Feeding Equipment and Supplies

Proper handling and cleaning of enteral formula, equipment, and supplies using clean technique are important in reducing the risk of formula contamination. Equipment used to prepare the enteral feeding should be washed in a dishwasher or cleaned with hot water and soap. If a blender is used to prepare the enteral feeding solution, all washable components should be washed in a dishwasher or cleaned with hot water and soap. Blender parts that contain electrical components and cannot be placed in the dishwasher or submerged in water should be hand-washed with hot water and soap. Enteral feeding bags and tubing should not be used for more than 24 hours before they are either discarded or washed thoroughly with soap and water, drained, and allowed to air dry.

Patient Education Related to Enteral Therapy

Patient and family education related to infection control and enteral therapy should include handwashing, clean technique, set-up and administration, formula hang time, infusion method, proper storage, cleaning and disinfecting procedures for enteral therapy equipment and supplies, signs and symptoms of a local infection at the gastrostomy tube site or indications of contaminated formula (e.g., diarrhea or vomiting) mouth care, assessment of residual feedings, assessment of feeding tube placement, gastrostomy tube site care (if applicable), and prevention of aspiration pneumonia.

REFERENCES

American Association of Respiratory Care. (1992, August). AARC clinical practice guideline: Oxygen therapy in the home or extended care facility. *Respiratory Care, 37*, 918–922.

American Association of Respiratory Care. (1995). AARC clinical practice guideline: Long-term invasive mechanical ventilation in the home. *Respiratory Care, 40*, 1313–1320.

Beaumont, E. (1997, December). Technology scorecard: Focus on infection control. *American Journal of Nursing, 97*, 51–54.

DeCastro, M.M., Fauerbach, L., & Masters, L. (1996). Aseptic techniques. In R. Olmsted (Ed.), *APIC infection control and applied epidemiology: Principles and practice* (pp. 20-1–20-4). Washington, DC: Association for Professionals in Infection Control and Epidemiology, Inc.

Feenan, L., & Voutroubek, W.L. (1997). Alterations in respiratory functions. In W. Voutroubek & J. Townsend (Eds.), Pediatric home care (pp. 59–94). Gaithersburg, MD: Aspen Publishers, Inc.

Garner, J. (1986, March). CDC guideline for prevention of surgical wound infections, 1985 (revised). *Infection Control, 7*, 193–200.

Garner, J., & Favero, M. (1986, June). CDC guideline for handwashing and hospital environmental control, 1985. *American Journal of Infection Control, 14*, 110–129.

Garner, J.S. (1996). Guideline for isolation precautions in hospitals. *Infection Control and Hospital Epidemiology, 17*, 53–80.

Garofalo, K. (1996). Home health. In R. Olmsted (Ed.), *APIC infection control and applied epidemiology: Principles and practice* (pp. 90-6–90-7). Washington, DC: Association for Professionals in Infection Control and Epidemiology, Inc.

Health Care Financing Administration. (1996, April). *Medicare home health agency manual* (rev. ed.). Washington, DC: U.S. Government Printing Office. Transmittal No. 277.

Jarvis, W., Gaynes, R., Horan, T., Alonso-Echanove, J., Emori, T., Fridkin, S., Lawton, R., Richards, M., Wright, G., Culver, D., Abshire, J., Henderson, T., Peavy, G., Toslon, J., & Wages, J. (1998). National Nosocomial Infections Surveillance (NNIS) system report: Data summary from October 1986–April 1988, issued June 1988. *American Journal of Infection Control, 26*, 522–533.

Kunin, C.M. (1987). *Detection, prevention and management of urinary tract infections* (4th ed.). Philadelphia: Lea & Febiger.

Larson, E.L. (1995). APIC guideline for handwashing and hand antisepsis in health care settings. *American Journal of Infection Control, 23*, 251–269.

Larson, E. (1996). Hand washing and skin preparation for invasive procedures. In R. Olmsted (Ed.), *APIC infection control and applied epidemiology: Principles and practice* (pp. 19-1–19-7). Washington, DC: Association for Professionals in Infection Control and Epidemiology, Inc.

Spaulding, E.H. (1968). Chemical disinfection of medical and surgical materials. In C.A. Lawrence & S.S. Block (Eds.), *Disinfection, sterilization, and preservation* (pp. 517–531). Philadelphia: Lea & Febiger.

Tablan, O.C., Anderson, L.J., Arden, N.H., Breiman, R.F., Butler, J.C., & McNeil, M.M. (1994). Guideline for prevention of nosocomial pneumonia. *American Journal of Infection Control, 22*, 247–292.

Wong, E.S. (1983). Guideline for prevention of catheter-associated urinary tract infections. *American Journal of Infection Control, 11*, 28–31.

CHAPTER 4

Infection Control in Home Infusion Therapy

OVERVIEW

The economic pressures to reduce health care costs have contributed to the growth of the home infusion therapy industry. In home infusion, venous access devices are used to administer intravenous (IV) fluids, medications, blood and blood products, and total parenteral nutrition (TPN). The use of IV access devices, however, may be complicated by infection that may be either systemic or local. Systemic infection includes bloodstream infection, septic thrombophlebitis, and endocarditis. If an IV catheter becomes colonized by pathogenic organisms, these organisms can be spread through the bloodstream and cause infections at distant sites (e.g., endocarditis). Local infections related to IV devices include exit site infections (related to percutaneously placed catheters), pocket infections (related to implanted IV access devices), and tunnel infections (related to surgically placed central venous catheters). Local site infections may lead to bloodstream infections.

Catheter-related infections in hospitalized patients, especially catheter-related bloodstream infections, are of great concern. They have been associated with increased morbidity, mortality rates of 10% to 20%, prolonged hospital stays, and increased medical costs (Pittet, Tarara, & Wenzel, 1994). Each year there are an estimated 200,000 nosocomial bloodstream infections, with infection rates being higher among patients with IV access devices than among patients without these devices (Pearson, 1996). The incidence of home care-acquired catheter-related bloodstream infections is not known, however. As home infusion therapy expands to provide more skilled care to increasingly ill patients, it is imperative that surveillance for local and systemic IV-related infections be conducted. In addition, risk reduction efforts must be undertaken to ensure that home infusion therapy is provided in a safe manner that is also cost effective.

The organisms that cause hospital-acquired IV-related infections have changed in the past decade. In the 1980s there was a predominance of Gram-negative bacilli, such as *Enterobacter* and *Pseudomonas* species. Fungal bloodstream infections were seen in the severely ill patient with many risk factors, including immunosuppression. In the 1990s, however, there has been a shift in the etiology of nosocomial bloodstream infections from Gram-negative to Gram-positive organisms. The most frequently isolated pathogens in catheter-related infections are coagulase-negative staphylococci, particularly *Staphylococcus epidermidis*, and these account for an estimated 28% of all nosocomial bloodstream infections (Banerjee et al., 1991; Schaberg, Culver, & Gaynes, 1991). The prevalence of coagulase-negative staphylococci in these infections is important in that it indicates that the hands of staff members and the flora of patients' skin are likely to be the predominant sources of pathogens for most catheter-related infections (Pearson, 1996). This is an important factor for those involved in home infusion therapy. Although there are no current data on the epidemiology of IV-related infections in home care, the risk related to these skin organisms must be noted. Policies and procedures must be designed and implemented to control this known risk.

There is also an increase in the incidence of enterococci in hospital-acquired infections, including IV-related infections. It was previously assumed that enterococcal infections were endogenous. The emergence of vancomycin-resistant enterococci (VRE) demonstrates that enterococci can also be transmitted from patient to patient. Policies and procedures for the care of patients colonized or infected with VRE should be incorporated into the home care organization's isolation plan (Centers for Disease Control and Prevention [CDC], 1995). Nosocomial bloodstream infections caused by various fungi have also increased in the past decade, with *Candida* species, particularly *C. albicans*, accounting for more than 75% of all nosocomial fungal infections reported (Beck-Sagué & Jarvis, 1993). Candidemia has traditionally been thought of as resulting from the endogenous flora of colonized patients, but recent studies among hospitalized patients have shown that exogenous sources of infection may be due to administration of contaminated fluids, use of contaminated equipment, and cross-contamination via staff members' colonized hands (Pearson, 1996). Gram-negative microorganisms account for the majority of catheter-related infections associated with the use of intrinsically contaminated IV fluids (Maki, Rhame, Mackel, & Bennett, 1976).

CAUSES OF IV CATHETER–RELATED INFECTIONS

The causes and sources of IV catheter-related infections are both intrinsic and extrinsic. An IV catheter may be seeded and colonized if bacteria or fungi travel through the bloodstream from another site of infection or colonization within the patient. This can lead to a catheter-related bloodstream infection. Host factors such as immunosuppressive diseases (e.g., leukemia) or treatments (e.g., chemotherapy) can increase the intrinsic risk for infection.

Based on scientific evidence, however, experts agree that most catheter-related infections result from the migration of microorganisms on the skin (e.g., *S. epidermidis*) around the catheter insertion site into the catheter's insertion tract. This migration can eventually lead to colonization of the catheter tip as well (Snydman, Pober, Murray, Gorbea, Majka, & Perry, 1982). Figure 4–1 shows potential sources for contamination of IV access devices. The catheter hub may also be an important source of contamination leading to the colonization of catheters, particularly long-term central venous catheters (Linares, Sitges-Serra, Garau, Perez, & Martin, 1985; Salzman, Isenberg, Shapiro, Lipsitz, & Rubin, 1993). Another source of extrinsic infection is

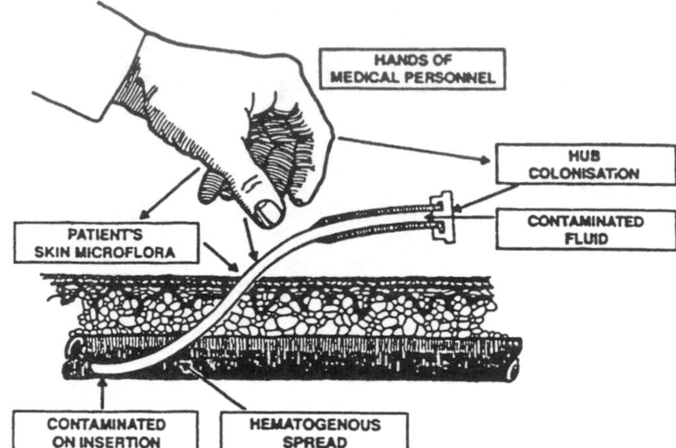

Figure 4–1 Potential Sources of Contamination of IV Access Devices. *Source:* Reprinted with permission from M.J. Pearson, Guideline for the Prevention of Intravascular-related Infections, *American Journal of Infection Control,* pp. 262–293, © 1996, Mosby-Year Book, Inc.

the contamination of the catheter at the time of insertion. This risk seems to be greater in catheters placed during an emergency. In the hospital setting, the CDC recommends that catheters be replaced within 24 hours to remove the potential risk for infection (Pearson, 1996). Contaminated IV fluid is also a risk for bloodstream infection, but it should be rare.

TYPES OF IV CATHETERS AND DEVICES

Peripheral IV Catheters

A peripheral IV catheter is 3 inches or less in length and in adults is inserted into a vein of the forearm or hand. Peripheral IV catheters have rarely been associated with bloodstream infections (Pearson, 1996). This low frequency of bloodstream infections may be due to the short period of time that a peripheral IV catheter is in place. Phlebitis is an inflammation of the vein caused by a chemical or mechanical process rather than an infectious process and is the most important complication associated with the use of a peripheral IV catheter. Exhibit 4–1 lists the risk factors associated with infusion-related phlebitis for patients with a peripheral IV catheter.

Midline Catheter

A midline catheter is 3 to 8 inches long and is a peripheral catheter that is inserted via the antecubital fossa into the proximal basilic or cephalic vein or the

Exhibit 4–1 Factors Associated with Infusion-Related Phlebitis among Patients with Peripheral Venous Catheters

Catheter material
Catheter size
Size of catheter insertion
Experience of person inserting catheter
Duration of catheterization
Composition of infusate
Frequency of dressing change
Catheter-related infections
Skin preparation
Host factors
Emergency department insertion

Source: Reprinted with permission from M.J. Pearson, Guideline for the Prevention of Intravascular-related Infections. *American Journal of Infection Control,* pp. 262–293, © 1996, Mosby-Year Book, Inc.

distal subclavian vein, but the catheter tip does not enter a central vein. The tip of the midline catheter resides below the axilla and is not to be inserted more than $1\frac{1}{2}$ inches above or below the antecubital fossa. A midline catheter should be considered when the duration of IV therapy is expected to be longer than 6 days. Midline catheters appear to have lower rates of phlebitis than short-line peripheral IV catheters and lower cost and rates of infection than central venous catheters (Pearson, 1996).

Central Venous Catheters

Nontunneled Central Venous Catheters

Percutaneously inserted, nontunneled, central venous catheters are used in the home setting, but they are not cared for as often as tunneled central venous catheters or implanted ports. Central venous catheters account for an estimated 90% of all nosocomial catheter-related bloodstream infections (Maki, 1992). Among the factors that influence the risk of infection associated with the use of a central venous catheter are the number of catheter lumens and the site at which the catheter is inserted. Other risk factors for catheter-related infections include repeated catheterization, the presence of an infectious focus elsewhere in the body, exposure of the catheter to bacteremia, absence of systemic antimicrobial therapy, the duration of catheterization, the type of dressing, and the experience of the personnel inserting the device (Pearson, 1996).

Peripherally Inserted Central Catheters

A peripherally inserted central catheter (PICC) may be placed in the home setting by competent nursing staff members. A PICC is inserted in the antecubital space via the cephalic or basilic vein with the catheter inserted into the superior vena cava. The advantages of inserting a PICC over other catheters are that PICCs cost less than other central venous catheters, are easier to maintain than short-line peripheral venous catheters (e.g., less frequent site rotation, infiltration, and phlebitis), have been associated with fewer mechanical complications (e.g., thrombosis, hemothorax, etc.), and have a lower rate of infection than that associated with other nontunneled central venous catheters. The lower rates of infection observed with PICCs may be partially accounted for by the use of the antecubital fossa as the insertion site. This area is usually less colonized, less oily, and less moist than skin on the chest and neck. The optimal length of time for a PICC line to remain in place is not known, but data have shown that PICCs have been used successfully for extended periods, in some cases longer than 300 days (Merrill, Peatross, Grossman, Sullivan, & Harker, 1994; Raad et al., 1993).

Tunneled Central Venous Catheters

Tunneled central venous catheters most commonly include the Hickman, Broviac, Groshong, and Quinton catheters. These catheters are surgically implanted and are used to provide IV access to patients who require prolonged infusion therapy (e.g., chemotherapy, TPN, and hemodialysis). In contrast to nontunneled central venous catheters, tunneled catheters have a Dacron cuff just inside the exit site. This cuff prevents the spread of microorganisms into the tunneled catheter tract by stimulating growth of the surrounding tissue, sealing the catheter tract, and providing a natural anchor for the catheter. Tunneling of central venous catheters also serves to prevent dislodgment of the catheter, reduce the incidence of catheter-related bloodstream infection by increasing the distance between the sites where the catheter exits the skin and where it enters the subclavian vein, and protect the catheter from potentially contaminated sites, such as tracheostomies (Pearson, 1996). According to the CDC, the rates of infection with the use of tunneled catheters have been significantly lower than those reported with the use of nontunneled central venous catheters, but recent studies (Andrivet et al., 1994; Raad et al., 1993) have found no significant difference in the rates of infection among tunneled and nontunneled catheters.

Implanted Ports

An implanted IV access device or port is tunneled beneath the skin, but has a subcutaneous port or reservoir with a self-sealing septum that is accessed by a noncoring needle punctured through intact skin. An implanted port may be placed centrally or peripherally and be accessed via the anterior chest wall or on the patient's forearm just below the antecubital fossa. Implanted ports are low maintenance and generally not visible. According to the CDC, implanted ports have the lowest reported rates of catheter-related bloodstream infections among tunneled and nontunneled venous access devices used for long-term vascular access (Pearson, 1996). The rate of infection may be lower because the catheter is placed below the skin level with no opening for the introduction of microorganisms.

PREVENTING CATHETER-RELATED INFECTIONS

Strict adherence to handwashing and aseptic technique is the most important activity that can be undertaken by home care staff members to prevent a catheter-related infection. Other measures taken by staff members that may reduce the risk of catheter-related infection include the following:

- selecting an appropriate catheter insertion site
- selecting an appropriate type of catheter
- using barrier precautions during catheter insertion
- replacing IV access devices
- replacing administration sets
- replacing IV fluids at appropriate intervals
- maintaining appropriate catheter site care
- avoiding the use of in-line filters for infection control purposes only
- ensuring that only experienced staff members insert and maintain catheters
- safely using an appropriate flush solution

SELECTING AN APPROPRIATE CATHETER INSERTION SITE

Several factors should be assessed when the staff member is determining the site of any peripheral IV catheter placement, including the patient's age, condition, and diagnosis; vein size and location; and the type and duration of infusion therapy.

Peripheral Venous Access Site Selection

The vein selected for infusion therapy must be of sufficient size to accommodate the gauge and length of the IV catheter to be inserted. The site at which a catheter is placed has been shown to influence the subsequent risk of catheter-related infection. In pediatric patients, peripheral catheters should be inserted into a scalp, hand, or foot site instead of a leg or arm or the antecubital fossa. In adults, inserting a peripheral catheter in a lower extremity poses a greater risk of phlebitis than an upper extremity, and upper extremity sites differ in their risk for phlebitis (Pearson, 1996). In adults, hand vein insertions have a lower risk of phlebitis than upper arm or wrist vein insertions. Therefore, peripheral IV catheters should be inserted in the distal areas of the upper extremities, and subsequent catheter insertions should be made proximal to the previous catheter insertion site. If a medication has infiltrated or extravasated and the IV catheter cannot be inserted proximal to the previous insertion site, the patient's opposite upper extremity should be used for insertion of a new peripheral IV catheter. Veins at areas of flexion, sclerotic veins, or injured veins should be avoided unless areas of flexion can be immobilized to reduce the risk of mechanical phlebitis. Veins in the antecubital fossa should not be used for inserting short-line peripheral venous catheters and should be reserved for the insertion of a midline catheter, PICC, or a stainless steel needle for the purpose of obtaining a laboratory specimen. Patients who have undergone a mastectomy or axillary node dissection should not have peripheral venous catheters inserted into the affected arm unless prior approval is obtained from the physician.

Midline Venous Access Site Selection

Appropriate veins for the insertion of a midline catheter include the basilic and cephalic veins. The site selected for the insertion of a midline catheter should be no more than 1 to 1.5 inches above or below the antecubital fossa. Midline catheters should not be used for routine blood drawing unless there is no other accessible access site. Blood pressure cuffs and tourniquets should not be applied to the arm in which a midline catheter has been placed. If a medication has infiltrated or extravasated, the patient's opposite extremity should be used for insertion of a new midline catheter. Patients who have undergone a mastectomy or axillary node dissection should not have a midline catheter inserted into the affected arm unless prior approval is obtained from the physician. Home infusion therapies that should not be administered via a midline catheter include continuous vesicant chemotherapy, TPN formulated for central vein administration, solutions or other medications that have a pH less than 5 or greater than 9, and solutions or medications that have a serum osmolality greater than 500 mOsm/L (Intravenous Nurses Society, 1998).

PICC Site Selection

Appropriate veins for the insertion of a PICC include the basilic and cephalic veins at the antecubital fossa. Patients who have undergone a mastectomy or axillary node dissection should not have a PICC inserted into the affected arm unless prior approval is obtained from the physician. Once a PICC is inserted, the affected extremity should not have blood pressure cuffs or tourniquets applied.

SELECTING AN APPROPRIATE TYPE OF CATHETER

Catheters that may be inserted by a home care nurse include a short-line peripheral venous catheter, a midline catheter, and a PICC. The selection should be on an individual patient basis with consideration of the lowest relative risk of complications (infectious and noninfectious) and the lowest cost for the anticipated type and duration of home infusion therapy. The peripheral venous catheter selected should be of the smallest gauge to maintain adequate perfusion and of the shortest length to administer the prescribed infusion therapy. Stainless steel needles should only be used for short-term therapy or for the administration of a single dose of a nonvesicant medication or fluid. Stainless steel needles should be used with caution because of the high incidence of infiltration into the subcutaneous tissues that can occur during infusion of a fluid that is a vesicant agent. According to the CDC, peripheral venous catheters made of Teflon or polyurethane appear to be associated with fewer infectious complications than catheters made of polyvinyl chloride or polyethylene. Stainless steel needles, used in lieu of a synthetic catheter for peripheral venous access, appear to have the same rate of infectious complications as Teflon catheters (Pearson, 1996).

The type of catheter selected for the insertion of a midline catheter or PICC should be based on the staff member's knowledge of and compliance with the techniques required for insertion, potential complications, the prescribed therapy, and the manufacturer's guidelines. The length of the catheter selected should be appropriate to the size of the patient, so that the integrity of the catheter tip does not need to be altered.

The CDC has not made a recommendation supporting or rejecting the use of antimicrobial- or antiseptic-impregnated peripheral venous catheters. The CDC does recommend, however, a silver-impregnated collagen cuff or an antimicrobial- or antiseptic-impregnated central venous catheter in adults. This recommendation is based on the observation and reporting of unacceptably high rates of infection in catheters without this feature, even after full adherence to other infection control measures (Pearson, 1996).

CATHETER INSERTION

Good handwashing before and attention to aseptic technique during the insertion of any IV catheter provides adequate protection against infection transmission. Insertion of a PICC carries a greater risk of infection, however. According to the CDC, the risk of infection depends on the magnitude of barrier protection used during catheter insertion and not on the sterility of the surrounding environment (Pearson, 1996). Therefore, when PICCs are inserted in the home setting, maximal barrier precautions should be used to reduce the chance of catheter contamination and a subsequent catheter-related bloodstream infection. This includes the wearing of sterile gloves, sterile gown, and a mask by the nurse inserting the PICC, any assistants in the procedure, and the patient; in addition, a large sterile drape should be used. Non-Latex or Latex gloves should be worn when an IV access device is inserted or when the dressing on an IV access device is changed, as required by the Occupational Safety and Health Administration (OSHA) bloodborne pathogen regulations (OSHA, 1991). Either sterile gloves or nonsterile clean gloves and no-touch technique may be used during the dressing changes on an IV access device.

REPLACING IV ACCESS DEVICES

In adults, peripheral venous catheters, not peripherally placed heparin locks used for intermittent infusions, should be replaced every 48 to 72 hours to reduce the risk of phlebitis and catheter-related infections, as well as to reduce the patient's discomfort associated with phlebitis. In adults, peripheral venous catheters used as heparin locks for intermittent infusions should be replaced every 96 hours or every 4 days (Pearson, 1996). In adults, if a peripheral venous catheter has been inserted under emergency conditions, where breaks in aseptic technique are likely to have occurred, a new catheter should be inserted at a new site within 24 hours. In pediatric patients, there are insufficient data to formulate a recommendation for the frequency with which peripheral venous catheters should be replaced or whether catheters inserted under emergency conditions should be replaced (Pearson, 1996). The risk and benefits of replacing an IV access device within the above time frame to reduce infectious complications should be weighed against the risk of mechanical complications and the availability of alternative sites. Peripheral venous catheters in both adult and pediatric patients should be removed when the patient develops signs of phlebitis (i.e., warmth, tenderness, erythema, and palpable venous cord) at the insertion site, and any IV access device should be removed as soon as its use is no longer clinically indicated.

Studies of short peripheral venous catheters have shown that the incidence of thrombophlebitis and bacterial colonization of catheters increases dramatically when catheters are left in place more than 72 hours (Pearson, 1996). The optimal dwell time for a midline catheter or PICC is not known, nor is the time frame known for the frequency of replacing the needles used to access implanted ports. The CDC has no recommendations for this practice. The Intravenous Nursing Standards of Practice recommend a maximum dwell time of 4 weeks for midline catheters (Intravenous Nurses Society, 1998). Dwell times longer than 4 weeks for midline catheters should be based on the length of remaining therapy, the patient's peripheral venous access status, the patient's condition, the condition of the vein in which the catheter is placed, and the skin's integrity (Intravenous Nurses Society, 1998). When a catheter is removed, pressure should be applied to the insertion site with a dry, sterile dressing. When a midline catheter, PICC, or nontunneled central venous catheter is removed, an antiseptic ointment should be applied to the catheter site to occlude the skin tract and prevent an air embolism. The cannula should be inspected to detect any changes in the integrity of the catheter, with appropriate follow-up actions being taken if damage is noted. If a catheter defect is noted, the manufacturer and the Food and Drug Administration (FDA) should be notified, as should the patient's physician.

When a catheter is replaced, only one catheter should be used for each cannulation attempt. Once the catheter has been inserted, all junctions between the administration set and add-on devices should be secured to prevent the separation of the IV system and the risk of infection.

REPLACING ADMINISTRATION SETS

The administration set includes the area from the spike of the tubing entering the fluid container to the hub of the vascular device. IV tubing, including piggyback tubing, should be replaced no more frequently than at 72-hour intervals unless clinically indicated or contamination occurs. Tubing used to administer blood, blood products, or lipid emulsions must be replaced within 24 hours of initiating the infusion because blood, blood products, and lipid emulsions are more likely than other parenteral fluids to support microbial growth if contaminated. The CDC does not have any recommendations for the time frame in which IV tubing used for intermittent infusions, such as IV antibiotics, should be replaced. The Intravenous Nursing Standards of Practice recommend, however, that primary intermittent administration sets be changed every 24 hours and immediately when contamination is suspected or when the integrity of the product has been compromised (Intravenous Nurses Society, 1998).

Piggyback systems pose a risk for contamination of the venous fluid if the needle entering the rubber membrane of the injection port is partially exposed to air or comes in direct contact with the tape used to affix the needle to the port. Therefore, when piggyback systems are used to administer medication, the staff member, patient, or family member should take extra precautions to ensure that the needle is completely enclosed with the "Y" portion of the IV tubing and that the tape used to secure the needle does not touch contaminate the needle and potentially the IV fluids.

Add-on devices, such as extension loops, solid catheter caps, injection and access ports, needles or needleless systems, and extensions sets, increase the potential for infection as a result of the increased manipulation and/or the risk of separation, which can increase risk of contamination. When an add-on device is used, it should be of a Luer lock configuration. Add-on devices should be changed when the administration set is changed, when the catheter is changed, if contamination occurs, or whenever the integrity of either product is compromised. If short extension tubing is directly connected to the IV tubing and a peripheral venous catheter, the extension tubing should be considered a portion of the catheter and replaced when the peripheral venous catheter is replaced (Pearson, 1996).

REPLACING IV FLUIDS

In the early 1970s, there was a nationwide epidemic of nosocomial bloodstream infections that was traced to the intrinsic contamination of IV fluid during manufacturing and transport by infectious agents that were present in the system before it was used (Maki et al., 1976). These outbreaks resulted in the CDC recommending that IV fluids and administration sets be replaced every 24 hours (Maki, Goldmann, & Rhame, 1973). Since that time, studies have shown that endemic bloodstream infections in hospitals due to in-use contamination of IV fluids are a rare complication and that extrinsic contamination or contamination introduced into the system during use of IV fluids is infrequent and sporadic. Even with heavily manipulated lines (e.g., central venous catheters) or TPN fluids, the rate of in-use contamination appears to be low (Pearson, 1996). For that reason, the CDC does not recommend a specific time frame in which IV fluids, including non–lipid-containing parenteral nutrition fluids, need to be replaced. Infusions of lipid-containing parenteral nutrition fluids (e.g., 3-in-1 solutions) must be completed within 24 hours of hanging the fluid. When lipid emulsions are given alone, the lipid infusion must be completed within 12 hours of hanging the emulsion (Pearson, 1996).

CATHETER SITE CARE

Skin cleansing and antisepsis of the catheter insertion site are among the most important measures for preventing catheter-related infection. Before a peripheral venous catheter, midline catheter, or PICC is inserted, the skin should be cleansed with an appropriate antiseptic, which may be 70% alcohol, 10% povidone-iodine, or a 2% tincture of iodine. Single-unit containers or packets are recommended. If the skin is visibly dirty, it must be cleaned with soap and water before the antiseptic solution is applied. Otherwise, the antiseptic solution may not be effective. If 10% povidone-iodine is used to clean the skin, the povidone-iodine should be allowed time to dry and not be wiped off with a 70% isopropyl alcohol preparation pad because this negates the effect of the povidone-iodine. If the patient is allergic to povidone-iodine, 70% isopropyl alcohol should be used. When 70% isopropyl alcohol is used, it should be applied with friction for a minimum of 30 seconds or until the last isopropyl preparation pad is visually clean (Intravenous Nurses Society, 1998). The antiseptic should be applied at the site and wiped outward in a circular motion. The antiseptic should remain on the insertion site for the appropriate length of time and be allowed to air dry. Excess antiseptic should not be wiped off. When the skin is prepared for the insertion of a peripheral IV catheter, an area 2 to 4 inches in diameter is generally considered safe and acceptable. When tincture of iodine is used for skin antisepsis before catheter insertion, it should be removed with alcohol because it may cause skin irritation. Studies of antiseptic skin preparations have shown that tincture of iodine and chlorhexidine in ethyl alcohol are superior to povidone-iodine in reducing the incidence of catheter-related infection for patients receiving TPN (Pearson, 1996). The catheter insertion site should not be palpated after the skin has been cleansed with the antiseptic unless the staff member is wearing sterile gloves.

Applying an organic solvent, such as acetone or ether, to "defat" the skin or remove skin lipids, has been a common procedure during routine dressing changes. According to the CDC, these agents do not appear either to add additional protection against skin colonization or to decrease significantly the incidence of catheter-related infection (Maki & McCormack, 1987). Therefore, organic solvents (e.g., acetone or ether) should not be applied to the skin before the insertion of catheters used for parenteral nutrition and during dressing changes. The use of organic solvents can also increase local inflammation and cause patient discomfort (Pearson, 1996).

If excess hair needs to be removed from the skin before insertion of a catheter, the hair should be removed by clipping with scissors. Shaving with a razor is not recommended because it may cause microabrasions that can damage skin integrity, which can increase colonization and the risk of infection. Removing the hair by using a depilatory is not recommended because of the potential for an allergic reaction. Electric razors should not be used unless they are effective and preserve the skin's integrity. Electric devices that are the property of the home care organization may be used only if it is possible to change or disinfect the heads of the devices between uses (Intravenous Nurses Society, 1998).

Topical antimicrobial ointments have routinely been applied to the catheter site at the time of catheter insertion or during routine dressing changes to reduce microbial contamination of catheter insertion sites. Studies of this practice in preventing catheter-related infections have yielded contradictory findings, however. Therefore, the CDC does not recommend applying topical antimicrobial ointment to the insertion site of a peripheral venous catheter or central venous catheter. For a central venous catheter used for hemodialysis, however, use of povidone-iodine ointment at the catheter insertion site during each dressing change is recommended (Levin, Mason, Jindal, Fong, & Goldstein, 1991; Pearson, 1996).

A sterile gauze dressing or transparent dressing may be used to cover the catheter site. In home care, transparent, semipermeable, polyurethane dressings should be considered over gauze and tape dressings because transparent dressings reliably secure the catheter, permit continuous visual inspection of the catheter site, permit patients to bathe and shower without saturating the dressing, and require less frequent changes, thus saving staff members' valuable time.

If a gauze dressing is used, adhesive material should be placed around all edges to secure the dressing. A nonocclusive type of dressing, such as a self-adhesive bandage, should not be used in lieu of a gauze dressing. Gauze dressings are not recommended when there is a risk of contamination from secretions or external moisture and bacteria. When a transparent dressing is placed over a gauze dressing, it is considered a gauze dressing and should be changed every 48 hours. The CDC does not have a recommendation for the frequency of routine replacement of transparent dressings used on central venous catheter sites (Pearson, 1996). It is a frequent home care practice, however, to change a transparent dressing every 7 days and to change a gauze dressing every 48 hours. Catheter site dressings should be replaced more frequently, when a catheter is replaced; when the dressing becomes damp, loosened, or soiled; when the patient is undergoing hemodialysis (the dressing should be replaced at each hemodialysis session); when inspection of the site is necessary; or if the patient is diaphoretic.

Touch contamination of the catheter insertion site should be avoided when the dressing is replaced. The catheter site should be inspected visually and palpated for tenderness through the intact dressing by the home care staff member during each home visit and on an ongoing basis by the patient or caregiver. If there is tenderness, fever without an obvious source, or symptoms of a local or bloodstream infection, the dressing should be removed and the site directly inspected (Pearson, 1996).

Injection port(s) should be cleaned with 70% alcohol or povidone-iodine before the system is accessed (Pearson, 1996). The injection cap should be changed when the catheter dressing is changed (or every 7 days at a minimum), any time the injection port is removed from the catheter, if residual blood remains in the injection port, or whenever contamination occurs. Injection ports on peripheral venous catheters should be changed when the catheter is replaced. Injection ports should be of a Leur lock design or of a configuration to prevent separation of the IV system (Intravenous Nurses Society, 1998).

FILTERS

In-line filters may be perceived to reduce the incidence of infusion-related phlebitis, but there are no data to support their efficacy in preventing infections associated with IV access devices and infusion systems. Infusate-related bloodstream infections rarely occur, and filtration in the pharmacy before use is a more practical and less costly strategy to remove most particulates. In-line filters may become blocked, especially with certain solutions (e.g., lipids), and consequently can require increased catheter manipulations. Therefore, the CDC does not recommend the routine use of in-line filters for infection control purposes (Pearson, 1996). In-line filters should be used, however, to administer medications to remove particulate matter that could result in an obstruction to the vascular or pulmonary system. The FDA issued a safety alert regarding the hazards of precipitation associated with the administration of TPN. The FDA safety alert suggests that a filter be used when either central or peripheral nutrition is infused. A

1.2-μm air-eliminating filter should be used for lipid-containing admixtures, and a 0.22-μm air-eliminating filter should be used for non–lipid-containing admixtures (FDA, 1994). Particulate matter filters should be used when medications are prepared for administration. Infusions that should be filtered during administration include blood and blood products, TPN formulas, lipids, and substances that are infused via the epidural or intrathecal route (Intravenous Nurses Society, 1998).

FLUSH SOLUTIONS, ANTICOAGULANTS, AND OTHER IV ADDITIVES

Solutions that are used to flush IV access devices are used to prevent thrombosis rather than infection. Fibrin deposits and thrombi in catheters, however, may serve as a central point for microbial colonization of the IV access device. Catheter thrombosis appears to be one of the most important factors associated with infection of central venous catheters and implanted ports. Thus the use of anticoagulants (e.g., heparin) or thrombolytic agents may have a role in the prevention of catheter-related bloodstream infection. Studies suggest that 0.9% saline solution is just as effective as heparin in maintaining catheter patency and reducing phlebitis in peripheral catheters (Pearson, 1996). The routine use of heparin to maintain catheter patency, even at doses as low as 250 to 500 U/day, has been associated with thrombocytopenia and thromboembolic and hemorrhagic complications.

Indwelling central venous catheters (e.g., Hickman and Broviac catheters) should be routinely flushed with an anticoagulant. Groshong catheters may be flushed with normal saline only and may not require routine flushing with an anticoagulant. A peripheral venous heparin lock should be routinely flushed with a 0.9% saline solution. A peripheral venous heparin lock in a neonate or infant should be routinely flushed with a preservative-free 0.9% saline solution. Consideration may be given to the use of a heparin flush solution in low doses (1 to 10 units of preservative-free heparin to 1 mL of preservative-free normal saline) in neonates and infants because of their tiny veins and the small-gauge cannula used. If the heparin lock is used for obtaining blood specimens, a dilute heparin flush solution (10 U/mL) should be used for routine flushing of the heparin lock. If blood has been withdrawn from the catheter, the catheter should be flushed with 0.9% saline in sufficient amounts to remove residual blood from the catheter's lumen(s) before final flushing with the appropriate solution.

The volume of the flush solution also is a consideration in maintaining catheter patency. The flush volume should be equal to two times the volume capacity of the catheter and add-on devices. For example, if the volume of a peripheral venous catheter and the extension loop is 1.5 mL, the minimum amount needed to flush the catheter is 3 mL. The amount of heparin and the frequency of the flush should not alter the patient's clotting time. During and after the administration of the flush, positive pressure must be maintained to prevent reflux of blood into the catheter lumen. If resistance is met during the attempt to flush the catheter, no further flushing attempts should be made because this could result in a clot dislodging into the vascular system or catheter rupture.

NEEDLELESS INFUSION SYSTEMS

Needleless infusion systems were introduced to reduce the number of injuries related to sharps and the risk of staff members acquiring a bloodborne infection. Data on the use of needleless infusion systems are too limited, however, to assess the potential risk of contamination of the catheter and infusate and subsequent catheter-related infection. There have been two reported outbreaks of bloodstream infections in patients at home receiving TPN via a central venous catheter using a needleless infusion system (Danzig et al., 1995; Kellerman et al., 1996). The CDC, however, has not issued recommendations for the use, maintenance, or frequency of replacement of needleless IV devices in any setting.

CULTURING FOR SUSPECTED INFUSION-RELATED INFECTIONS

Primary bloodstream infection (directly related to the IV catheter, access device, or fluid) may occur in home infusion therapy patients. In addition to sampling for blood cultures, the IV fluid or IV catheter may be cultured to determine the cause of the bloodstream infection. If the catheter is suspected as the source of infection, blood cultures should be obtained through the catheter as well as via a peripheral site. Before a cannula is removed for culture, the surrounding skin should be cleaned with 70% isopropyl alcohol and allowed to air dry. If purulent drainage is present, the skin should be cultured before the skin is cleaned. The semiquantitative culturing technique is the recommended method for culturing. The hospital microbiology laboratory should have a procedure to perform and interpret these types of cultures (Maki, Weise, & Sarafin, 1977).

When an infusate is suspected of being contaminated, the infusion should be discontinued immediately. The IV bag and tubing should be removed at the IV hub, and the entire set should be returned to the pharmacy. A sample of the IV fluid is not sufficient for culture to determine whether the fluid was contaminated. The pharmacy should record the type of fluid, additives, and lot numbers (fluid, additives, and tubing) before sending the IV set and fluid to the microbiology laboratory for culture. The microbiology laboratory should have a procedure to culture IV fluid for suspected contamination. If intrinsic contamination is strongly suspected and/or documented, the FDA and the manufacturer should be notified.

ADMINISTRATION OF TPN

Catheter-related bloodstream infection is one of the most important complications of TPN. Because TPN solutions commonly contain dextrose, amino acids, or lipid emulsions, they are more likely than conventional IV fluids to support growth of certain microbial species if they become contaminated. Three-in-one TPN solutions, however, which combine glucose, amino acids, lipid emulsion, and additives in single- or multi-liter administration bags, do not appear to support greater microbial growth than non–lipid-containing TPN fluids and may be changed safely at 24-hour intervals (Goldmann, Martin, & Worthington, 1973). Most infections that occur during the administration of TPN result from contamination of the catheter and not from contamination of the fluids (Maki, 1976). Risk factors associated with the development of catheter-related infections are listed in Exhibit 4–2. In addition, rigorous aseptic nursing care has been shown to reduce greatly the incidence of TPN-related infection.

Single-lumen catheters used for parenteral nutrition should never be used for other purposes, such as administration of medication or obtaining a blood sample. When a multilumen catheter is used, one port should be designated for the administration of parenteral nutrition (Pearson, 1996).

Exhibit 4–2 Risk Factors Associated with Development of Catheter-Related Infections during TPN Therapy

- Catheter site colonization
- Method and site of catheter insertion
- Experience of staff member inserting catheter
- Use of TPN line for purposes other than administration of TPN fluids
- Breaks in protocol for aseptic maintenance of the infusion system
- Use of triple-lumen catheters

Source: Reprinted with permission from M.J. Pearson, Guideline for the Prevention of Intravascular-related Infections, *American Journal of Infection Control,* pp. 262–293, © 1996, Mosby-Year Book, Inc.

PEDIATRIC PATIENTS

As in adults, most catheter-related bloodstream infections in pediatric patients are caused by staphylococci, with *Staphylococcus epidermidis* being the most common species. Other species of Gram-positive cocci and fungi are the next most frequently isolated pathogens, with *Malassezia furfur* being an especially common pathogen in neonates receiving IV lipid emulsions.

Phlebitis, extravasation, and catheter colonization may be associated with the use of peripheral venous access devices in all patients, but extravasation is the most common complication in children. The use of a central venous catheter (e.g., a Hickman or Broviac catheter or an implanted port) has become more common in treating children with chronic medical conditions, especially malignancies. The Broviac catheter, rather than the Hickman catheter, is preferred in children because of its smaller catheter diameter. If a patient is 4 years of age or older and needs long-term (greater than 30 days) vascular access, a PICC, tunneled central venous catheter, or implanted port is recommended (Pearson, 1996). For patients younger than 4 years who need long-term vascular access, an implanted port is recommended because an external central venous catheter segment may be contiguous with the diaper area and thus may be easily contaminated. Implanted ports have also been shown to have a longer survival time and fewer infectious complications than other tunneled catheters. A single-lumen central venous catheter is recommended unless multiple ports are essential for the management of the patient (Pearson, 1996).

MISCELLANEOUS INFUSION ROUTES

Epidural Catheter, Port, or Pump

An epidural catheter may be used to administer analgesics or low-dose anesthetics. The epidural catheter is placed in the epidural space on either a short-term or a long-term basis. When a permanent catheter is placed, it is tunneled subcutaneously from the lumbar region and exits into the flank area. Epidural devices and administration sets must be clearly labeled to distinguish them from other catheter sets. A mask and sterile gloves must be worn when catheter care and maintenance procedures are performed. Epidural infusions given on a continuous basis should be administered via an electronic infusion device. Before any medication is infused via the epidural catheter, the site should be aspirated with a syringe to make sure that spinal fluid is not aspirated. If spinal fluid is aspirated, the physician should be contacted and no medications administered. Medication infused into the epidural catheter must be preservative free and administered through a 0.2-μm filter without surfactant. Alcohol should not be used to clean the exit site or to clean the injection port before the epidural catheter is accessed because of the potential for the alcohol to enter the epidural space via the catheter and cause nerve damage (Intravenous Nurses Society, 1998).

Intrathecal Catheter, Port, or Pump

Intrathecal catheters are used to administer certain antineoplastic agents, antibiotics, analgesics, and low-dose anesthetic agents. Intrathecal catheters and administration sets must be clearly labeled to distinguish them from other catheter sets. Intrathecal catheters may be attached to an internal port or pump. Only noncoring needles should be used to access the intrathecal pump or port, with the manufacturer's guidelines being followed for accessing, filling, and refilling. A mask and sterile gloves must be worn when catheter care and maintenance procedures are performed. Before any medication is infused via the intrathecal catheter, the site should be aspirated with a syringe to make sure that spinal fluid or blood is not aspirated. If spinal fluid or blood is aspirated, the physician should be contacted and no medications administered. When an intrathecal catheter is attached to an implanted pump, the manufacturer's guidelines should be followed regarding aspiration. Medication infused into the intrathecal catheter must be preservative free and administered through a 0.2-μm filter without surfactant. Alcohol should not be used to clean the exit site or to clean the access site port before the intrathecal catheter is accessed because of the potential for the alcohol to enter the intrathecal space via the catheter and cause nerve damage (Intravenous Nurses Society, 1998).

Ventricular Reservoir

The ventricular reservoir is surgically implanted under the scalp with the catheter entering the lateral ventricle through a burr hole placed in the skull. Ventricular reservoirs are used to administer antineoplastic agents, antibiotics, and analgesic agents. A mask and sterile gloves must be worn when catheter care and maintenance procedures are performed. Before any medication is infused via the ventricular reservoir, the site should be aspirated with a syringe to make sure that spinal fluid is not aspirated. If spinal fluid is aspirated, the physician should be contacted and no medications administered. When an intrathecal catheter is attached to an implanted pump, the manufacturer's guidelines should be followed regarding aspiration. Alcohol should not be used to clean the exit site before the ventricular reservoir is accessed because of the potential for the alcohol to enter the central nervous system (Intravenous Nurses Society, 1998).

Hemodialysis Catheter

Approximately 150,000 patients undergo maintenance hemodialysis each year for chronic renal failure. Central venous catheters have gained popularity as a convenient, rapid way of establishing temporary vascular hemodialysis access (until placement or maturation of a permanent arteriovenous fistula) or permanent access for patients without alternative vascular access. Catheter-related bloodstream infections in hemodialysis patients, as in other patient populations, are caused most frequently by *S. epidermidis*. Because of their high rates of colonization with *S. aureus*, however, hemodialysis patients have a greater proportion of catheter-related bloodstream infection due to *S. aureus* than other patient populations. In some studies, as many as 50% to 62% of hemodialysis patients have been found to be carriers of *S. aureus* (Yu et al., 1986).

Therefore, skin antisepsis is a crucial component of home care for the prevention of hemodialysis catheter-associated infections.

According to the CDC, subclavian hemodialysis catheters have been associated with a bloodstream infection rate that exceeds the rates reported for virtually all other subclavian catheters for alternative forms of hemodialysis vascular access. The hemodialysis catheters used also may be complicated by bacterial endocarditis, septic pulmonary emboli, or thrombosis (e.g., venous thrombosis and catheter occlusion). The causes of the increased rate of infection experienced with the central venous catheter used for hemodialysis are not known, but it is thought that manipulations and dressing changes of dialysis catheters by inadequately trained personnel, duration of catheterization, mean number of hemodialysis sessions, and cutdown insertion of the catheter may increase the risk of catheter-related infection among hemodialysis patients. Other potential causes of hemodialysis catheter contamination include penetration of organisms from the skin as a result of the pulsating action of the dialysis pump, manipulation of catheter connections by medical personnel with contaminated hands, leakage of contaminated hemodialysis fluid into the blood compartment, and administration of contaminated blood or other solutions through the catheter during the dialysis session. For these reasons, manipulation of the hemodialysis catheter, including dressing changes, should be restricted to staff members trained in hemodialysis catheter care and maintenance (Vanderweghem et al., 1986).

The CDC recommends that a cuffed central venous catheter should be selected for hemodialysis if the period of temporary access is expected to be a minimum of 1 month. Hemodialysis catheters should be used solely for hemodialysis and not for other purposes (e.g., administration of fluids, blood or blood products, or parenteral nutrition) and should only be used for other purposes (e.g., obtaining a blood specimen) when there are no alternative vascular access sites (Pearson, 1996).

BLOOD STORAGE FOR HOME TRANSFUSIONS

Blood Storage during Transport

Maintaining the appropriate blood or blood product temperature is essential in controlling bacterial growth and preventing hemolysis when the blood is to be administered in the home. When blood and blood products that are to be administered in the home are transported, the blood storage and transportation time should be kept to a minimum, and the blood should be transported directly from the blood center to the patient's home for administration. The blood should be placed in a sealed plastic bag and then placed in an impervious, clean, thermally insulated cooler for transport. The blood should be stored with wet ice or a coolant that maintains a temperature of 1° to 10°C or 33° to 50°F. Fresh-frozen plasma should be stored at 1° to 6°C or 33.0° to 42.8°F. Blood must be protected against direct exposure to ice packs or other coolant sources. Platelets and thawed fresh-frozen plasma should be stored at room temperature, which should not exceed 37°C, in an impervious, clean, thermally insulated cooler without coolants and without exposure to temperature extremes. Temperature-sensitive monitor tags or monitors may be placed on the blood bag to ensure that the blood has been maintained at the proper temperature during transport and before administration (Fridey, Kasparin, & Issitt, 1994).

Blood Storage in the Patient's Home

In the patient's home, if more than 1 unit of blood will be transfused, the unused component(s) should remain in the insulated cooler until transfused into the patient. The blood or blood products should not be stored in the patient's refrigerator or freezer because temperatures may vary. If the ice melts or the temperature-sensitive monitors do not display a temperature reading that is within acceptable temperature limits, the blood center should be contacted for further instructions.

INFECTION CONTROL IN PHARMACEUTICAL SERVICES

Pharmacy Sterile Compounding Requirements

The American Society of Hospital Pharmacists (ASHP, now known as the American Society of Health-System Pharmacists) and the U.S. Pharmacopeia (USP) both publish guidelines for sterile compounding (ASHP, 1993; USP, 1996). It is noteworthy that both organizations consider compounding sterile pharmaceuticals for the home setting riskier than compounding pharmaceuticals for hospital use. The reason for designating a higher risk level is that pharmaceuticals prepared for home use are generally compounded in larger quantities and stored over a longer period of time than drugs dispensed in the hospital.

At this time, the Joint Commission on Accreditation of Healthcare Organizations' home pharmaceutical standards and most state boards of pharmacy do not require home care pharmacies to adhere to the ASHP and USP guidelines regarding sterile compounding. With the exception of a few states, such as New Jersey, the minimally acceptable standard for compounding is a class 100 laminar flow hood placed within a functionally separate area of the pharmacy.

Pharmacy Facilities

Each home care pharmacy should have a designated area for preparing compounded sterile parenteral products that has been designed to avoid unnecessary traffic and airflow disturbances. This area should be large enough to accommodate a laminar flow hood and to provide for the proper storage of medications and supplies under appropriate conditions of temperature, moisture, sanitation, and ventilation. The warehouse and other pharmacy storage areas where ingredients are stored should be monitored to ensure that the temperature, moisture, and ventilation levels remain within manufacturer, USP, and state and federal requirements. Drugs and supplies should be stored on shelves above the floor to avoid contamination and to allow for cleaning of the floor. The floors should be made of a nonporous, washable material to permit daily cleaning. A refrigerator should be in close proximity to the compounding room. The compounding area should be cleaned and disinfected at regular intervals as defined in the pharmacy's policies and procedures. Standard cleaning supplies may be used for this purpose, or cleaning cloths that do not shed lint may be ordered from clean room supply vendors. There should also be a handwashing sink with hot and cold running water that is conveniently located near the compounding area but not within it.

Minimally, the pharmacy should contain a class 100 laminar flow hood. The USP and ASHP guidelines for sterile compounding also recommend that the laminar flow hood be contained in a class 10,000 clean room. Laminar flow hoods generate a great deal of heat. Therefore, the design of the compounding area air conditioning system must account for this extra heat, or the room may be subject to high temperatures. The laminar flow hood should be allowed to remain on continuously. If the laminar flow hood is turned off between compounding sessions, the internal surfaces of the laminar flow hood should be disinfected before use, and when it is turned on again it should be allowed to run long enough (e.g., 30 to 60 minutes) to allow for complete purging of the room air from the hood before it is used again. The external surfaces of the laminar flow hood and other hard, nonporous horizontal surfaces within the compounding area should be cleaned with a germicidal disinfectant weekly and after any unanticipated event that could potentially contaminate the surfaces. Walls should be cleaned on a monthly basis, and spot cleaning of splashes or spills should be ongoing.

Smoking, eating, or drinking should never be permitted in the compounding area. Products and supplies used in preparing sterile products should be removed from their shipping containers in an area away from the compounding area. Packaging material, such as plastic wrapping, light-resistant pouches, and syringe packaging used to retain the sterility or stability of the product, is an exception and may be stored in the compounding area.

Storage

All products should be stored according to the manufacturer's recommendations. The pharmacy must be able to accommodate products that require freezing, refrigeration, or controlled room temperature. All containers of parenteral fluid and additives must be checked for visible turbidity, leaks, cracks, or particulate matter before use, and the manufacturer's expiration date must be checked. Products that have exceeded their expiration dates should be discarded or returned. Single-dose vials for parenteral additives or medications are preferred over multidose vials whenever possible. If multidose vials are used, the vials should be refrigerated after opening if recommended by the manufacturer.

Pharmacy Compounding Garb

The USP and ASHP guidelines recommend that pharmacists and technicians wear clean clothing covers that generate a low level of particulates (e.g., cover gowns or surgical scrubs), cover their heads and facial hair with surgical head covers or hoods, wear surgical face masks, and wear clean Latex gloves during compounding (ASHP, 1993; USP, 1996). The Joint Commission home pharmaceutical standards do not have any specific requirements regarding compounding garb, nor do most state boards of pharmacies.

Thorough handwashing with an antiseptic handwashing product (see Chapter 3) is one of the most important steps a pharmacist and technician can take to control contamination and potential infection. Touch contamination is the most frequent potential source of contamination of sterile products. Jewelry should not be worn during compounding. Pharmacists' and technicians' cleanliness and technique are more important than the design of the clean room itself in ensuring that a sterile product is produced.

Aseptic Technique

Before sterile pharmaceuticals are compounded, the interior of the laminar flow hood should be cleaned using a two-step process. The hood should be cleaned with sterile water and lint-free wipes; the direction of wiping should always be toward the airflow. For example, a horizontal laminar flow hood should be cleaned starting at the top of the hood; then, the rear should be cleaned moving toward the front of the hood in a side-to-side motion. The sides can then be cleaned starting at the back and moving toward the front in a side-to-side motion. The horizontal work surface should be cleaned using the same technique. Cleaning the hood in a front-to-back motion introduces dirty air into the hood and should never be done. Once cleaning is complete, the process should be repeated with 70% isopropyl alcohol. Cleaning the laminar flow hood initially with sterile water is important to remove any dextrose residue from the hood. If dextrose residue is wetted with isopropyl alcohol, it forms a hard, sticky substance that is difficult to remove.

Only materials essential for sterile compounding should be placed in the laminar flow hood. These materials should be unpackaged outside the hood and, if the clean room is a class 10,000 room, outside the room itself. It is recommended that all products be wiped with 70% isopropyl alcohol before being placed in the hood. Products that have been unwrapped and stored on shelves or in the refrigerator should be wiped with 70% isopropyl before being placed in the hood. Materials should be arranged in the hood to ensure that airflow is not blocked. Vials and bottles should be placed about $1\frac{1}{2}$ diameters from each other in the hood (the larger the bottles, the farther apart they should be).

Rubber injection ports on vials, bags, and bottles should be disinfected with 70% isopropyl alcohol before being punctured with a needle. There are three generally acceptable methods to accomplish this task:

1. The traditional method of using individual alcohol preparation pads can be used, but this is time consuming because of the number of pads used. In addition, the rubber diaphragm often becomes contaminated with cotton fibers.
2. Injection ports can be sprayed using a spray bottle of 70% isopropyl alcohol.
3. The rubber diaphragm can be dipped in a small, clean tray containing 70% isopropyl alcohol.

Regardless of the method used, the alcohol should be allowed to dry before the diaphragm is pierced. Aseptic technique should be used to avoid touch contamination of syringes, needles, rubber diaphragms, tubing, and so forth.

If compounding is interrupted and gloved hands are removed from the laminar flow hood for any significant length of time, the gloves should be removed and discarded. The hands should be washed again before work resumes in the hood.

Bulk solutions, such as sterile water for injection, should be labeled with the date and time they were placed in the laminar flow hood. The manufacturer's directions should be followed to establish an appropriate hang time. Generally, this is 24 to 72 hours but is dependent on the stability of the medication. Dispensing syringes used to inject bulk fluids should also be labeled with the date and time they were placed in the laminar flow hood. Dispensing syringes generally should not be used for more than 24 hours. The frequency with which the needle or dispensing pin on the syringe should be changed is based on factors such as time and the number of punctures made (dulling of needles). Also, the needles should be changed between drugs to avoid cross-contamination. If the spike or other sterile area of the syringe is contaminated through touch or contact with any other object, it must be discarded. Pumps and other equipment used for compounding should be cleaned regularly with an appropriate disinfectant.

Pharmacy Quality Control

The temperature of the refrigerator and freezer should be monitored on a daily basis on days when the pharmacy is in use and documented in a refrigerator temperature control log. A refrigerator's temperature must be in the range of 2° to 8°C or 35° to 46°F, and the freezer's temperature must be less than –20°C or 4°F. If the temperatures of the refrigerator and freezer are not within the required ranges, the pharmacist should be notified and appropriate follow-up actions taken. A penny placed on a cup of frozen water may also serve as a means to check the freezer's temperature. If during temperature monitoring the penny is found to have sunk to the bottom of the cup, the freezer has lost power, and the items inside have thawed. If this occurs, the pharmacist should be notified for appropriate follow-up actions to be taken. The refrigerator used to store medications should be cleaned on a monthly basis.

All laminar flow hoods should be certified by Federal Standard 209B for operational efficiency at least every 6 months or when the laminar flow is relocated to ensure operational efficiency and integrity. All maintenance and certifications must be documented. Prefilters in the laminar flow hood should be replaced on a regular basis as defined by the manufacturer's requirements.

The CDC does not recommend routine sterility testing for infusion admixtures prepared in hospital pharmacies. Rather, infection control experts support monitoring through a prospective surveillance program. Identification of potential bloodstream infections on patients receiving home infusion therapy may lead to the identification of contaminated fluids.

The USP and ASHP recommend the following methods for monitoring the sterility of the finished product:

- *End product testing*: This method involves testing a statistically significant sample of either an aliquot or an entire unit of product for microbial growth. This can be done using a number of commercially available kits or by sending the sample to a laboratory. The advantage of end product testing is that it is relatively easy to accomplish. There are a number of disadvantages, however; for example, the aliquot method of sampling may never produce a statistically significant sample, testing an entire unit either results in waste or introduces even more contamination risk, and results take up to 10 days, by which time the patient has probably already used the contaminated product. The ASHP sterile product compounding guidelines recommend statistically significant end product testing (ASHP, 1993). The Joint Commission home pharmaceutical standards only require this type of testing if sterile products are made from nonsterile ingredients.
- *Process validation testing (PVT)*: This method does not test end products but rather involves intensive testing of operator technique using a sterile broth that is more subject to contamination than most actual pharmaceutical products. PVT therefore tests whether a particular individual can consistently produce sterile products under actual operating conditions. A number of commercially available kits may be used to conduct PVT. PVT may be used to meet Joint Commission home pharmaceutical standard requirements regarding assessment of the competency of compounding staff.
- *Limulus amoebocyte lysate (LAL) testing*: LAL is an extract of the blood of the horseshoe crab. It is sensitive to miniscule levels of pyrogens and is thus a relatively quick (about 1 hour) and accurate test of end product sterility. Implementing LAL testing is within the scope of the typical home infusion therapy organization, but it is expensive and time consuming. This type of testing should be implemented if a provider consistently produces sterile end products from nonsterile components.

Quality control to ensure sterility of IV admixture products for home infusion therapy is difficult. Some pharmacies have routinely taken samples of IV fluids and cultured them to determine sterility, but this approach does not allow for an adequate sampling of fluid and is not recommended for use. Because the competence of the pharmacist or technician is critical to the safe compounding of IV admixtures, PVT can be used as part of a quality control program.

Environmental Testing

The USP and ASHP guidelines both recommend various levels of environmental testing in the clean room area. This involves testing the air within the laminar flow hood and the clean room as well as various surfaces in the room. There are a number of commercial products available for this purpose, ranging from simple test kits to sophisticated air samplers. The Joint Commission does not have any requirements regarding environmental testing, although it may be indicated in the intensive analysis of recurring infections.

Expiration Dating

All pharmacy-prepared sterile products should bear an appropriate expiration date. The expiration date should consider the drug's stability and other factors that may affect sterility, such as components used, type of container, type of use, and storage. Appropriate references, such as the *Handbook on Injectable Drugs*, should be consulted (Trissel, 1996). Freezing of drugs should be avoided whenever possible in the home care setting. Maintaining frozen drugs during transport and shipping is difficult. In addition, providing frozen drugs requires that the patient remember to thaw the medication several hours before use.

Storage and Transport of Parenteral Medications

Once parenteral products have been prepared, they should be held in a refrigerator until they are placed in a clean, insulated cooler for delivery. Food or laboratory specimens should not be stored in the same refrigerator as medication.

Medication Storage during Transport

Medications that have been compounded by the pharmacy, such as IV antibiotics, compounded analgesic suppositories, IV admixtures, and TPN formulas, should be kept refrigerated during transport to the patient's home and before administration. During transport of compounded medications that will be administered in the home, medications that require refrigeration should be placed in a sealed plastic bag and then placed in an impervious, clean, thermally insulated cooler. During transport, the medication or TPN solution should be stored with reusable ice blocks that maintain a temperature of 2° to 8°C or 35° to 46°F (USP, 1996). Other drugs that are being delivered to the patient's home that are not compounded, such as heparin or saline flushes, should be placed in an appropriate container to prevent product contamination during transport.

Medication Storage in the Patient's Home

The length of time that compounded medication or TPN solution may be refrigerated is based on the stability of the admixed components. When the medication or TPN is refrigerated in the home, it should be stored in a separate area of the refrigerator, if possible. The compounded medication and or TPN solution needs to remain refrigerated until it is taken out to warm to room temperature just before administration. TPN solutions should be removed from the refrigerator about 1 hour before infusion. If the medication is stored frozen, it should be thawed in the refrigerator and not left out on the patient's kitchen counter for several hours at room temperature. If the medication must be refrigerated and the patient does not have a refrigerator, the home care organization may provide a refrigerator on a temporary basis, or the patient must gain access to a refrigerator (e.g., in a neighbor's kitchen). The temperature in the patient's refrigerator does not have to be monitored or checked with a thermometer, but the refrigerator should maintain the medications cold. Medications and TPN solutions must not be used beyond their expiration date. When new medications are delivered to the patient, they should be rotated in the refrigerator to ensure that the patient uses the older medications first.

Preparation of Parenteral Medication in the Home

Whenever possible, parenteral fluids should be admixed in the pharmacy in a laminar flow hood using aseptic technique (Pearson, 1996). Medications should only be prepared in the patient's home when the stability of the drug requires it. The only drugs that should be mixed in the home are those drugs with a stability of less than 24 hours after reconstitution or drugs whose dosage changes so frequently that preparing them in the pharmacy is not possible. If a medication must be mixed in the home, appropriate aseptic technique must be used. The nurse should select a clean, low-traffic area for medication preparation. Medications prepared in the home should be used immediately. Nurses should avoid preparing several doses of medication for the patient's later use, if possible.

The rubber diaphragm of multidose vials must be cleaned with 70% isopropyl alcohol before a device is inserted into the vial. Each time a multidose vial is accessed, a sterile device must be used before the rubber diaphragm is penetrated, and touch contamination of the device must be avoided. There is no recommendation for the arbitrary discard of multidose vials. A number of experimental studies of contamination of multidose vials have been conducted (Cornish & Montgomery, 1996). Based on these studies, the risk of bacterial growth after contamination appears to be minimal. Safe practice recommends that multidose vials should be thrown out if contamination is suspected or visible and when the manufacturer's expiration date is reached.

Nursing Care and Administration of Parenteral Medications

Insertion and maintenance of IV access devices by inexperienced or incompetent staff may increase the risk of catheter colonization and catheter-related bloodstream infection (Pearson, 1996). Many home care organizations have established a core group of clinicians responsible for providing care to patients receiving infusion therapy at home. To reduce catheter-related infections and overall costs, only home care staff members specially trained in or designated with the responsibility for insertion and maintenance of IV access devices should provide infusion therapy for home care patients. Continuing education should be provided to ensure that knowledge related to parenteral therapy is maintained. Competency skills should be monitored at least annually and when new drug therapies or equipment are introduced.

Nursing policies and procedures for home infusion therapy should emphasize methods to prevent catheter-related infection. Patient assessment for signs and symptoms of potential infection should be performed during every visit and should include evaluation for systemic infection, such as fever, chills, and change in mental status, as well as evaluation for local site infection, such as redness, pain, swelling, and tenderness at the IV insertion site. Family members and patients should also be taught to observe and report both local and systemic signs and symptoms of infection related to IV therapy. If family members and patients are administering IV therapy, they must be well trained. Their understanding and competence should be verified on initiation of IV therapy and during the course of therapy.

When parenteral medications are given in the home, the medication label must be verified before the medication is administered to the patient. Each label should contain the patient's name (additional identifiers, including a medical record number, may be included), type of IV solution and additives, dose, date and time of compounding, expiration date, prescribed administration regimen, and storage requirements. In addition, ASHP recommends that the label include the identification of the person who compounded the medication, batch numbers (if appropriate), and control or lot numbers of fluids and additives (ASHP, 1993). The nurse administering the medication must check the label to ensure that it matches the medication orders for the patient. Before administering any IV fluid or medication, the nurse should inspect the fluid for particulate matter and check the container for cracks, leaks, or punctures. If the fluid's appearance is questionable or the container's integrity is compromised, the solution or medication should be returned to the pharmacy. Appendix 4–A contains a summary of the CDC's guidelines for the prevention of IV access device–related infections.

REFERENCES

American Society of Hospital Pharmacists. (1993). ASHP technical assistance bulletin on quality assurance for pharmacy prepared sterile products. *American Journal of Hospital Pharmacists, 50*, 2386–2397.

Andrivet, P., Bacquer, A., Ngoc, C.V., Ferme, C., Letinier, J.Y., Gautier, H., Gallet, C.B., & Brun-Buisson, C. (1994). Lack of clinical benefit from subcutaneous tunnel insertion of central venous catheters in immunocompromised patients. *Clinical Infectious Diseases, 18*, 199–206.

Banerjee, S.N., Emori, T.G., Culver, D.H., Gaynes, R.P., Jarvis, W.R., Horan, T., Edwards, J.R., Tolson, J., Henderson, T., & Martone, W.J. (1991). Secular trends in nosocomial primary bloodstream infections in the United States, 1980–1989. National Nosocomial Infections Surveillance system. Hospital infections. *American Journal of Medicine, 16*, 86S–89S.

Beck-Sagué, C.M., & Jarvis, W.R. (1993). Secular trends in the epidemiology of nosocomial fungal infections in the United States, 1980–1990. *Journal of Infectious Diseases, 167*, 1247–1251.

Centers for Disease Control and Prevention. (1995). Recommendations for preventing the spread of vancomycin resistance: Recommendations of the Hospital Infection Control Practices Advisory Committee (HICPAC). *American Journal of Infection Control, 23*, 87–94.

Cornish, L., & Montgomery, P. (1996). Pharmacy. In R. Olmstead (Ed.), *Infection control and applied epidemiology: Principles and practice* (pp. 113-1–113-6). St. Louis: Mosby.

Danzig, L.E., Short, L.J., Collins, K., Mahoney, M., Sepe, S., Bland, L., & Jarvis, W.R. (1995). Bloodstream infections associated with a needleless intravenous infusion system in patients receiving home infusion therapy. *Journal of the American Medical Association, 273*, 1862–1864.

Food and Drug Administration (FDA). (1994). *FDA safety alert: Hazards of precipitation associated with parenteral nutrition*. Rockville, MD: Department of Health and Human Services.

Fridey, J., Kasparin, C., & Issitt, L. (Eds.). (1994). *Out-of-hospital transfusion therapy.* Bethesda, MD: American Association of Blood Banks.

Goldmann, D.A., Martin, W.T., & Worthington, J.W. (1973). Growth of bacteria and fungi in total parenteral nutrition. *American Journal of Surgery, 126*, 314–318.

Intravenous Nurses Society. (January/February, 1998). Revised intravenous nursing standards of practice. *Journal of Intravenous Nursing, 21*(suppl.).

Kellerman, S., Shay, D., Howard, J., Goes, C., Feusner, J., Rosenberg, J., Vugia, P., & Jarvis, W. (1996). Bloodstream infections in home infusion patients: The influence of race and needleless intravascular access devices. *Journal of Pediatrics, 129*, 711–717.

Levin, A., Mason, A.J., Jindal, K.K., Fong, I.W., & Goldstein, M.B. (1991). Prevention of hemodialysis subclavian vein catheter infections by topical povidone-iodine. *Kidney International, 40*, 934–938.

Linares, J., Sitges-Serra, A., Garau, J., Perez, J.L., & Martin, R. (1985). Pathogenesis of catheter sepsis: A prospective study with quantitative and semiquantitative cultures of catheter hub and segments. *Journal of Clinical Microbiology, 21*, 357–360.

Maki, D.G. (1976). Sepsis arising from extrinsic contamination of the infusion and measures for control. In I. Phillips, P.D. Meers, & P.F. D'Arcy (Eds.), *Microbiological hazards of infusion therapy* (pp. 99–143). Lancaster, England: MTP.

Maki, D.G. & Mermel, L. (1998). Infections due to infusion therapy. In J.V. Bennett & P.S. Brachman (Eds.), *Hospital Infections* (pp. 689–724). (4th ed.). Philadelphia: Lippincott-Raven Publishers.

Maki, D.G., Goldmann, D.A., & Rhame, F.S. (1973). Infection control in intravenous therapy. *Annals of Internal Medicine, 79*, 867–887.

Maki, D.G., & McCormack, K.N. (1987). Defatting catheter insertion sites in total parenteral nutrition is no value as an infection control measure. *American Journal of Medicine, 83*, 833–840.

Maki, D.G., Rhame, F.S., Mackel, D.C., & Bennett, J.V. (1976). Nationwide epidemic of septicemia caused by contaminated intravenous products. *American Journal of Medicine, 60*, 471–485.

Maki, D., Weise, C., & Sarafin, H. (1977). A semiquantitative culture method for identifying intravenous-catheter-related infection. *New England Journal of Medicine, 9*, 1305–1309.

Merrill, S., Peatross, B., Grossman, M., Sullivan, J., Harker, W. (1994). Peripherally inserted central venous catheters: Low-risk alternatives for ongoing venous access. *Western Journal of Medicine, 160*, 25–30.

Occupational Safety and Health Association. (1991). Occupational exposure to bloodborne pathogens: Final Rule. 29 CFR 1910.1030. *Federal Register, 56*, 64003–64282.

Pearson, M.J. (1996). Guideline for the prevention of intravascular-related infections. *American Journal of Infection Control, 24*, 262–293.

Pittet, D., Tarara, D., & Wenzel, R.P. (1994). Nosocomial bloodstream infection in critically ill patients: Excess length of stay, extra costs, and attributable mortality. *Journal of the American Medical Association, 271*, 1958–1601.

Raad, I., Davis, S., Becker, M., Hohn, D., Houston, D., Umphrey, J., & Bodey, J. (1993). Low infection rate and long durability of nontunneled Silastic catheters. A safe and cost-effective alternative for long-term venous access. *Archives of Internal Medicine, 153*, 1791–1796.

Salzman, M.B., Isenberg, H.D., Shapiro, J.F., Lipsitz, P.J., & Rubin, L.G. (1993). A prospective study of the catheter hub as the portal of entry for microorganisms causing catheter-related sepsis in neonates. *Journal of Infectious Diseases, 167*, 487–490.

Schaberg, D., Culver, D., & Gaynes, R. (1991, September 16). Major trends in the microbial etiology of nosocomial infection. *American Journal of Medicine, 91*, 72S–75S.

Snydman, D.R, Pober, B.R., Murray, S.A., Gorbea, H.F., Majka, J.A., & Perry, L.K. (1982). Predictive value of surveillance skin cultures in total parenteral nutrition–related infection. Prospective epidemiologic study using semiquantitative cultures. *Lancet, 2*, 1385–1388.

Trissel, LA. (1996). *Handbook on injectable drugs* (9th ed.). Bethesda, MD: American Society of Health Systems Pharmacists.

U.S. Pharmacopeia. (1996). *The U.S. pharmacopeia* (23rd rev.). Rockville, MD: U.S. Pharmacopeia Convention.

Vanherwegham, J., Dhaene, M., Goldman, M., Stolear, J., Sabot, J., Waterlot, Y., Serruys, E., Thayse, C. (1986). Infections associated with subclavian dialysis catheters: The key role of nurse training. *Nephron 42*, 116–119.

Yu, V., Goetz, A., Wagener, M., Smith, P., Rihs, J., Hanchett, J., & Zuravleff, J. (1986). Staphylococcus aureus nasal carriage and infection in patients on hemodialysis: Efficacy of antibiotic prophylaxis. *New England Journal of Medicine, 10*, 91–96.

APPENDIX 4–A

Summary of the CDC's Guidelines for the Prevention of IV Access Device–Related Infections

Source: Adapted with permission from M.J. Pearson, Guideline for the Prevention of Intravascular-related Infections. *American Journal of Infection Control,* Vol. 24, pp. 262–293, © 1996, Mosby-Year Book, Inc..

Device	Replacement and Relocation of Device	Replacement of Catheter Site Dressing	Replacement of Administration Sets	Hang Time for Parenteral Fluids	Insertion Technique
Peripheral venous catheters	In adults, replace catheter and rotate site every 48 to 72 hours. Replace catheter at a different site within 24 hours.	Replace dressing when catheter is replaced or when dressing becomes damp, loosened, or soiled. Replace dressings more frequently in diaphoretic patients.	Replace IV tubing, including piggyback tubing and stopcocks, no more frequently than at 72-hour intervals unless clinically indicated.	No recommendation for hang time of IV fluids, including non–lipid-containing parenteral nutrition fluids.	Clean
	In adults, replace heparin locks every 96 hours. In pediatric patients, no recommendation for removal of catheters inserted under emergency conditions.	In patients who have large, bulky dressings that prevent palpation or direct visualization of catheter insertion site, remove dressing daily, visually inspect catheter site, and apply new dressing.	Replace tubing used to administer blood, blood products, or lipid emulsions within 24 hours of initiating infusion. No recommendation for replacement of tubing used for intermittent infusions. Consider short extension tubing connected to device as portion of device. Replace such extension tubing when device is changed.	Complete infusion of lipid-containing parenteral nutrition fluids (e.g., 3-in-1 solutions) within 24 hours of hanging. When lipid emulsions are given alone, complete infusion within 12 hours of hanging.	
Midline catheters	No recommendation for frequency of catheter replacement.	No recommendation for frequency of routine replacement of catheter site dressings.	Replace IV tubing, including piggyback tubing and stopcocks, no more frequently than at 72-hour intervals.	No recommendation for hang time of IV fluids, including non–lipid-containing parenteral nutrition fluids.	Sterile
		Replace dressing when catheter is replaced; when dressing becomes damp, loosened, or soiled; or when inspection of site is necessary. Replace dressings more frequently in diaphoretic patients.	Replace tubing used to administer blood, blood products, or lipid emulsions within 24 hours of initiating infusion.	Complete infusions of lipid-containing parenteral nutrition fluids (e.g., 3-in-1 solutions) within 24 hours of hanging. When lipid emulsions are given alone, complete infusion within 12 hours of hanging.	

PICCs	No recommendation for frequency of catheter replacement.	No recommendation for frequency of routine replacement of catheter site dressing.	Replace IV tubing, including piggyback tubing and stopcocks, no more frequently than at 72-hour intervals.	No recommendation for hang time of IV fluids, including non–lipid-containing parenteral nutrition fluids.	Sterile
		Replace dressing when catheter is replaced; when dressing becomes damp, loosened, or soiled; or when inspection of site is necessary.	Replace tubing used to administer blood products or lipid emulsions within 24 hours of initiating infusion.	Complete infusion of lipid-containing parenteral nutrition fluids (e.g., 3-in-1 solutions) within 24 hours of hanging. When lipid emulsions are given alone, complete infusion within 12 hours of hanging.	
Central venous catheters (includes nontunneled, tunneled, and totally implanted devices)	Do not routinely replace nontunneled (percutaneously inserted) catheters either by rotating insertion site or use of guidewire.	No recommendation for routine replacement of catheter site dressings. Replace dressing when catheter is replaced; when dressing becomes damp, loosened, or soiled; or when inspection of site is necessary.	Replace IV tubing, including piggyback tubing and stopcocks, no more frequently than at 72-hour intervals.	No recommendation for hang time of IV fluids, including non–lipid-containing parenteral nutrition fluids.	Sterile (in acute care or outpatient settings; not suitable for home environment)
	No recommendation for frequency of replacement of tunneled catheters, totally implantable devices (i.e., ports), or needles used to access them.		Replace tubing used to administer blood, blood products, or lipid emulsions within 24 hours of initiating infusion.	Complete infusion of lipid-containing parenteral nutrition fluids (e.g., 3-in-1 solutions) within 24 hours of hanging.	
				When lipid emulsions are given alone, complete infusion within 12 hours of hanging.	

CHAPTER 5

Infection Control in Pediatrics, Pets, and Preparation of Food

INFECTION CONTROL FOR PEDIATRIC PATIENTS

Keeping a child's environment clean and orderly is important for a child's health, safety, and emotional well-being. One of the most important steps in reducing the number of infectious agents, and therefore the spread of disease, is the thorough cleaning of surfaces that could pose a risk to children or staff members. Surfaces considered most likely to be contaminated are those with which children are likely to have close contact. These include toys that children put in their mouths, crib rails, and surfaces that are likely to become contaminated, such as diaper changing areas. Routine cleaning with soap and water is the most useful method for removing infectious agents from surfaces. A good mechanical scrubbing with soap and water will reduce the numbers of infectious agents from the surface. Surfaces that infants and young toddlers are likely to touch or mouth, such as crib rails, should be washed with soap and water and disinfected with a nontoxic disinfectant, such as a bleach solution, on a regular basis and if visibly soiled. Disinfectants that contain phenol should not be used for cleaning toys or other items with which an infant may have contact because phenol is a neurotoxin that can be adsorbed through the skin. After being drenched, soaked, or sprayed with the disinfectant for up to 10 minutes, surfaces that are likely to be mouthed should be thoroughly wiped with a fresh towel. Items that can be washed in a dishwasher or the hot water cycle of a washing machine do not have to be disinfected because these machines use water that is hot enough for a long enough period of time to kill most infectious agents (Centers for Disease Control and Prevention [CDC], 1996a).

Diapering a Child

Two different diaper changing methods may be used to minimize the risk of transmitting infection. One method involves the use of gloves, and the other does not. Gloves should be worn when the person changing the diapers has severe dermatitis or hand abrasions with open sores or when the child has severe diaper rash or dermatitis (CDC, 1996b). The recommended procedure outlined in Exhibit 5–1 contains additional steps to be included when gloves are used. The use of gloves is a matter of personal preference; some staff members prefer to avoid direct contact with fecal matter.

Cleaning and Disinfecting Diaper Changing Areas

Diaper changing areas should be used only for changing diapers. Work surfaces should be smooth, nonabsorbent, and easy to clean, and they should have a raised edge, a low "fence" around the area, or a buckle to prevent the child from falling off the changing area. Areas that come in close contact with children during play, such as couches and floor areas where children play, should not be used to change diapers. Diaper changing areas should be cleaned and disinfected on a regular basis and when soiled as follows:

1. Wipe the surface with a premoistened disposable towelette.
2. Dry the surface with a paper towel.

Exhibit 5–1 Changing a Diaper

1. Place the needed supplies (diapers, wipes, ointment), and if necessary a change of clothes, within reach.
2. Place the child on the diapering surface.
3. Remove the child's clothes and soiled diaper.
4. Clean the child's bottom with a premoistened disposable towelette. If the child is female, remember to wipe from front to back.
5. Place the soiled towelette inside the disposable diaper or in a trash receptacle if cloth diapers are used.
6. Place the disposable diaper in a trash receptacle, or place the soiled reusable diaper in the designated diaper pail.
7. If you are wearing gloves, remove and dispose of the gloves in a trash receptacle.
8. Wipe your hands with a premoistened towelette.
9. Diaper and dress the child.
10. Return the child to a safe area. *Never* leave a child alone on the diapering surface.
11. Clean and disinfect the diapering area.
12. Wash your hands with soap and running water.

Source: Adapted from *The ABC's of Safe and Healthy Child Care,* the Centers for Disease Control and Prevention, 1996.

3. Thoroughly wet the surface with a commercially prepared disinfectant spray or bleach and water solution.
4. Allow the spray to air dry; do not wipe off.

Cleaning and Disinfecting Clothing and Linen

Clothing soiled with bulk fecal material should be washed after the stool is emptied into the toilet, which should be done slowly to avoid splashing. Children's sheets, pillowcases, blankets, and crib mattress pads should be washed weekly and when soiled or wet. If the crib sheet and mattress pad become wet, the crib mattress should be cleaned and disinfected.

Cleaning and Disinfecting "Potty Training" Equipment

If a potty chair is used for toilet training, it should only be used in a bathroom area and, if possible, out of the child's direct reach of the toilet. After the child uses the potty chair, it should be emptied into the toilet, with care being taken not to splash or touch the water in the toilet. It should then be rinsed with water and the water poured into the toilet. The chair is not to be rinsed under the faucet of a sink used for food preparation. Finally, the chair should be cleaned and disinfected.

Washing and Disinfecting Toys

If a child has a communicable disease and is on transmission-based precautions and there are other children in the home, toys should be cleaned with mild soap and tap water and disinfected with alcohol, a 1:10 bleach solution, or a general household disinfectant. Nonwashable toys, such as cloth dolls, should not be shared with other children in the home if the patient is on precautions other than standard precautions. Toys such as blocks, dolls, tricycles, trucks, and other similar toys that are used by older children and not put into their mouths should be cleaned with soap and water on a regular basis and when obviously soiled. No disinfection is required. Hard plastic toys that are washed in a dishwasher or cloth toys that are washed in the hot water cycle of a washing machine do not need additional disinfection (CDC, 1996c). To hand wash and disinfect a hard plastic toy or pacifier:

1. Scrub in warm, soapy water. If necessary, use a brush to reach into crevices.
2. Rinse under running hot tap water.
3. Immerse in a mild bleach solution and allow to soak in the solution for 10 minutes.
4. Remove from the bleach solution and rinse well in cool water.
5. Air dry.

Preparing Infants' Bottles

Two different methods can be used to clean infant bottles, nipples, and bottle collars. Most infant bottles and nipples only need to be cleaned with hot soap and water. The aseptic sterilization method is required only when ordered by the physician and noted on the patient's plan of care.

If the bottles, nipples, and bottle collars are to be cleaned with soap and water, the following method should be followed:

1. Rinse the bottles, nipples, and bottle collars under hot running water.
2. Squeeze a small amount of liquid detergent into each bottle.
3. Scrub the inside of the bottle with a brush, ideally a brush that is designed for scrubbing infant bottles.
4. Rinse under running hot water.

5. Place the bottles upside-down on a clean towel to dry or place on a rack designed for air drying infant bottles.
6. Place a small amount of liquid detergent on a sponge, towel, or (ideally) a brush designed to clean infant bottle nipples and collars.
7. Rinse the nipples and bottle collars under running hot water and allow to air dry.

Bottles, nipples, and bottle collars washed in the hot water cycle of a dishwasher do not need additional disinfection.

If the physician recommends that the bottles be sterilized, the following procedure may be followed:

1. Place all bottles, nipples, and bottle collars in a deep pan.
2. Cover with tap water and boil for 10 minutes.
3. Remove with tongs and place on a clean towel, with the open ends of the bottles, nipples, and bottle collars facing down.

If disposable bottle liners are used, only the nipples and bottle collars need to be sterilized because the manufacturer sterilizes the plastic bottle liners.

Preparing Infant Formula

Staff should always wash their hands before preparing an infant's formula. The formula may be prepared in bottles that have been either washed in hot water and soap or aseptically sterilized. Unless otherwise noted on the plan of care, the formula should be prepared using bottles that have been cleaned with soap and water. If concentrated liquid or powdered formula will be used, the following method of preparation is recommended:

1. Boil the water to be used for mixing for at least 5 minutes and let it cool.
2. Mix the boiled water with the concentrated liquid or powdered formula according to the instructions on the formula label.
3. If applicable, place a disposable bottle liner inside the plastic bottle and mix.
4. Place the nipple on the bottle and cover with the bottle collar. If plastic covers are available, place a cover over the nipple and snap it onto the collar.
5. Cover the formula and store in the refrigerator.

Terminal Sterilization

Another technique that can be used to prepare infant formula is called terminal sterilization, but this sterilization technique is used only for concentrated formulas (a formula that is premixed and is not diluted with water):

1. Prepare the formula in clean bottles according to the instructions on the label.
2. Place the nipples upside-down on the bottle tops and cover with disks, or put the nipples on upright and cover the nipples with nipple covers.
3. Loosely screw the bottle collars onto the bottles.
4. Using a rack in a large pot or sterilizer, place the bottles in 2 inches of water.
5. Bring the water to a boil, cover, and boil briskly for 10 minutes.
6. Remove the pot or sterilizer from the heat and let it stand until cool for about 1 hour before removing the lid.
7. Tighten the bottle collars and, if possible, cover with plastic bottle covers.
8. Place the bottles in the refrigerator.

Formula and Breast Milk Storage

Formula made from ready-to-use or concentrated liquid should be used within 48 hours, and formula made from powder should be used within 24 hours. The staff member may prepare enough formula for one feeding or for 24 hours. If formula is made for one feeding, it should be cooled before feeding the infant. If the infant does not drink all the formula or expressed breast milk in the bottle, the leftover amount should not be placed back in the refrigerator for use at the next feeding. It should be poured down the drain and the bottle and nipple rinsed out with hot water and stored until washed. When the infant is old enough to eat solid food, the infant food should be poured into a small bowl because the infant should not be fed directly from the infant food jar.

If the staff member will accompany the child out of the home for an extended period of time (e.g., to attend a physician's office visit), an extra bottle of formula or expressed breast milk may need to be taken along to feed the infant. The formula or expressed breast milk should not be left out at room temperature or above 40°F for more than 2 hours. If a longer time before feeding is anticipated, the bottle should be stored on ice or placed in a container with an ice pack. During transport in the summer months, the bottle should be stored in the air-conditioned portion of the vehicle if possible to delay ice melting.

Expressed breast milk should be placed in a container that is marked with the date and a notation of any medications taken by the mother. Breast milk may be stored in the refrigerator for up to 8 days at 32°F to 39°F with no increase in harmful bacteria. It may be kept in the freezer at 0°F or –18°C or below for up to 6 months. In a separate-door freezer, it can be stored for 3 to 4 months (La Leche League International, 1997).

Thawing Frozen Breast Milk

Frozen breast milk should be thawed in the refrigerator or by submersion of the container in warm water. Breast milk should never be thawed in a microwave oven, in a pan of boiling water, or by allowing it to stand at room temperature (La Leche League International, 1997). Once the milk has thawed, the container should be gently shaken to blend any fat that has separated.

ESTABLISHING A PET THERAPY PROGRAM

Many home care programs, especially those that provide hospice services, are establishing pet therapy programs. In a pet therapy program, a home care staff member or volunteer takes animals, such as dogs, cats, and rabbits, to the patient's home for a visit. Studies have shown that pets can help a sick person feel psychologically and even physically better. If the home care program is considering establishing a pet therapy program, with common sense and some precautions the benefits usually outweigh the risks. Reptiles such as snakes, lizards, and turtles should not be used for pet therapy because reptiles are carriers of *Salmonella* organisms. Exotic pets such as monkeys and ferrets should not be used for pet therapy because, aside from rabies, little is known about the risk of infections from these animals (CDC, 1998b). Table 5–1 gives additional information about infections that are carried by animals and can be transmitted to humans.

Several simple precautions are all that is needed in handling pets or other animals. The following guidelines should be followed when a pet therapy program is established:

- Animals should have current immunizations as recommended by the American Veterinary Medical Association and be on flea, tick, and worm control programs. Proof of immunizations should be available.
- Animals should be free of any signs or symptoms of infections at the time of each visit.
- Animals must be clean and well groomed and have their nails clipped or blunted at the time of the visit.
- Animals should be checked for aggression and tolerance with various patients and their behavior monitored.
- All animals should be kept on a leash and be friendly toward children.
- A home care staff member or volunteer should always be present with the animal, especially when children play with the animal.
- A veterinarian should evaluate animals with skin rashes. If a fungus or ringworm caused the animal's rash, the animal should be temporarily removed from the pet therapy program until all lesions are healed.

Table 5–1 Diseases Carried by Animals

Disease	*Infective Agent*	*Transmission*	*Symptoms*
Bartonellosis	Bacteria	Cat scratch	Skin lesions
Campylobacteriosis	Bacteria	Animal stool	Diarrhea/blood infection
Cryptosporidiosis	Parasite	Animal stool	Severe diarrhea
Rabies	Virus	Saliva	Hyperexcitability, fever, paralysis, convulsions, tetany, respiratory paralysis
Ringworm	Fungus	Animal skin	Rash, itching, flaky patches of baldness
Salmonellosis	Bacteria	Animal stool	Diarrhea/blood infection
Toxoplasmosis	Parasite	Cat stool	Brain infection*

* Infants infected before birth can be born retarded or with serious mental or physical problems.

Source: Adapted from *MMWR Recommendations and Reports: Preview, Opportunistic Infections and Your Pets, A Guide for People with HIV Infection,* the Centers for Disease Control and Prevention, Office of Communication. Division of Media Relations, 1998.

- Hands should be washed with soap and running water after handling the animal or anything that had contact with the animal.

PREPARING THE PATIENT'S MEALS

Overview of Foodborne Illnesses

According to the CDC, up to 6 million cases of foodborne disease are reported each year in the United States, and these diseases account for approximately 9,000 deaths annually. Only about 400 to 500 foodborne disease outbreaks are reported each year, however (CDC, 1995). When a group of people develop the same illness after ingesting the same food, this is considered a foodborne disease outbreak. Most cases of foodborne disease are single cases not associated with a recognized outbreak. Not all outbreaks or diseases are equally likely to be reported because most cases of foodborne diseases are sporadic and because many times, when individuals develop gastrointestinal symptoms, they think that they have the "stomach flu." More than 250 different diseases can be caused by contaminated food or drink.

The great majority of food items that cause foodborne illnesses are raw or undercooked foods of animal origin, such as meat, unpasteurized milk, eggs, cheese, fish, and shellfish. Harmful bacteria also are commonly present in or on soil, pets, insects, rodents, sneezes, coughs, and unwashed hands. These bacteria can cause problems if they come in contact with food and are allowed to grow. Bacteria can grow rapidly on protein-rich foods (e.g., eggs, milk, and meat), which are usually considered perishable.

Foodborne illness is caused by bacteria or by the toxic substances they produce. For example, *Escherichia coli* 0157:H7 is one of hundreds of strains of the bacterium *E. coli*. Although most strains are harmless and live in the intestines of healthy humans and animals, *E. coli* 0157:H7 produces a powerful toxin and can cause severe illness. The most common foodborne diseases are infections caused by bacteria, such as *Salmonella* and *Campylobacter* species, or by the Norwalk family of viruses. Some foodborne illnesses, such as botulism and trichinosis, are becoming less common, whereas others, such as salmonellosis and illnesses caused by contamination with *E. coli* 0157:H7, are becoming more common.

The CDC reports that about 85 percent of all foodborne illnesses are avoidable if appropriate steps are taken and if food is handled properly. Home care staff members can help reduce the hazards of foodborne illness in the patient's home by observing the following simple principles of food safety.

Shopping for the Patient

If the plan of care includes food shopping for the patient, the following are guidelines that should be followed:

- Buy the cold food last, and get it to the patient's home as quickly as possible.
- If other errands need to be performed for the patient, do the grocery shopping last, and never leave perishable food in a hot car.
- Check expiration dates. Buy food only if the "sell-by" or "use-by" date has not expired.
- Buy food in good condition. Make sure that refrigerated food is cold to the touch and that frozen food is rock hard. Canned goods should be free of dents, cracks, or bulging lids, any of which can indicate a serious food poisoning threat.

Food Storage in the Patient's Home

The following are recommended guidelines for storing food in the patient's home:

- Keep the food safe and refrigerated and, if indicated on the plan of care, regularly clean the refrigerator's inside surfaces with hot soapy water.
- Suggest that the patient keep the refrigerator as cold as possible without freezing the milk or lettuce. The refrigerator should be set at 40°F or cooler and the freezer set at 0°F. Freeze fresh meat, poultry, and fish immediately if the patient will not consume them within a few days. If milk spoils in 1 week, the refrigerator is too warm.
- Keep all foods wrapped or in covered containers, and make sure the containers are shut tightly.
- Place leftovers in small containers for quick cooling.
- Remove stuffing from poultry or other stuffed meats, and refrigerate the meat and stuffing in separate containers.
- Do not leave leftovers out for extended periods of time.
- Keep foods purchased frozen in their original wrapping.
- When in doubt, throw it out.

Preparing the Patient's Food

The CDC states that the mishandling of food causes most foodborne illnesses (CDC, 1995). Cross-contamination can occur when bacteria from one source are transferred to another source. Sponges and kitchen towels used for cleaning can harbor bacteria and lead to cross-contamination. Kitchen towels, sponges, and cloths used in meal preparation and cleaning should be washed often. Sponges should be placed in the dishwasher during every load and replaced every few weeks. Cross-contamination can also occur in unexpected places, such as the refrigerator door handle, sink faucet handle, stove knobs, microwave oven handle, highchair, and appliance handles. Grooves in cutting boards can harbor bacteria. Vegetables and salad ingredients should not be cut on a cutting board that was used for raw meat unless the board has been washed with hot soapy water and disinfected with a bleach solution. After contact with meat, poultry, or dairy products, the cutting board can be disinfected with a solution of 2 teaspoons liquid bleach in 1 quart water and rinsed thoroughly. The blender and can opener also should be washed by hand or in the dishwasher each time they are used. The same utensils should not be used to prepare more than one food. For example, one knife should be used to cut up chicken and another one to dice the potatoes. Figure 5–1 shows how cross-contamination can occur.

The following guidelines should be followed in preparing the patient's food:

- Wash hands with running water and soap for 10 to 15 seconds before handling food.
- Keep all food preparation items clean.
- Do not leave food between 40° and 140°F for more than 2 hours, and do not thaw foods between 40° and 140°F (CDC, 1996a).
- Do not eat or taste any food before it is cooked.
- Wear Latex gloves if there are any cuts or sores on the hands.
- Keep raw meat, poultry, and fish and their juices away from other food.
- Marinade meats in the refrigerator and discard any leftover marinade.
- Thaw food in the microwave or refrigerator, not on the kitchen counter, because bacteria can grow in the outside of food before the inside thaws. An alternative is to cook the food while it is still frozen.

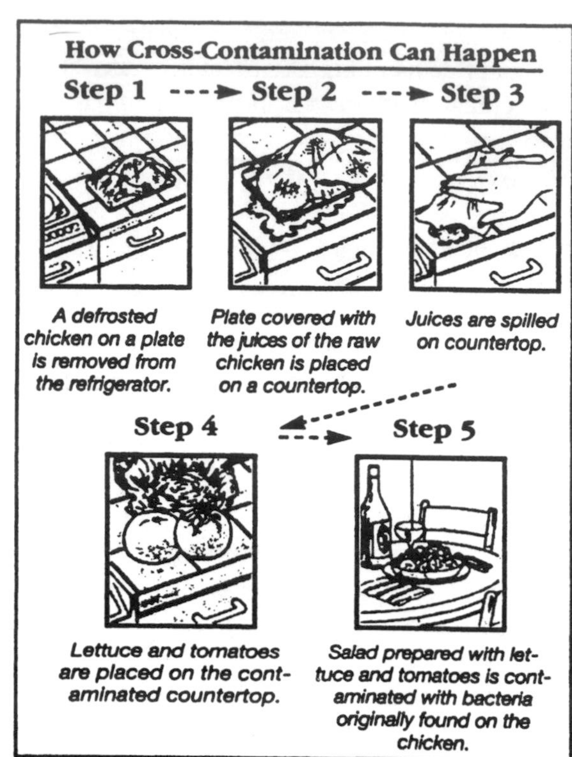

Figure 5–1 Cross-contamination happens when bacteria from one source are transferred to another, usually inadvertently and unknowingly. Here's a step-by-step example.

Courtesy of Reckitt & Coleman, Inc., Wayne, New Jersey.

- Check poultry and seafood for stale odors before cooking.
- Wash all fresh fruits and vegetables with cold water.
- Turn your face away, or cover your mouth and nose with a tissue, if you sneeze or cough when preparing food, and then wash your hands again.
- Keep uncooked meats separate from vegetables and from cooked and ready-to-eat foods.
- Stuff a turkey or chicken just before roasting.
- Do not use cracked eggs.

Cooking and Serving the Patient's Food

These guidelines are recommended for cooking and serving food for a patient:

- Bring sauces, soups, and gravies to a boil. Heat leftovers thoroughly to 165°F.

- Never partially cook meats or casseroles on one day and finish cooking them later.
- Use a meat thermometer, if the patient has one, to check that the meat is cooked all the way through. Beef, veal, and lamb should reach 160°F, pork should reach 160° to 170°F, and poultry should reach 165° to 180°F.
- Roast meat and poultry at an oven temperature of 325°F or higher.
- Visually check that the food is cooked enough or is done. Red meat will be brown or gray inside, poultry juices will be clear, and fish will flake with a fork.
- Cook eggs until the yolk and white are firm, not runny. Scrambled eggs should have a firm texture.
- If a large quantity of food is cooked for the patient to use later, divide large portions into small, shallow containers for refrigeration because this ensures safe, rapid cooling.
- Never leave food that needs to be refrigerated out for more than 2 hours.
- Use clean dishes and utensils to serve the food, not the dishes used to prepare it.
- Serve grilled food on a clean plate, not one that held raw meat, poultry, or fish.

Microwaving the Patient's Food

Microwaving food can leave cold spots in food, where bacteria can survive. The following guidelines will prevent cold spots and ensure that microwaved food is thoroughly cooked:

- Cover the food with a lid or plastic wrap so that steam can aid thorough cooking. Vent the wrap so that it does not touch the food.
- Stir and rotate the food for even cooking. If the microwave does not have a turntable, rotate the dish by hand once or twice during cooking.
- If the microwave cooking instructions require the food to stand for a certain amount of time before eating, make sure that the stand time is observed because this time is needed to complete cooking.
- Insert an oven temperature probe or a meat thermometer into the food at several spots to check that the food is done.
- If the defrost setting is used to microwave food, cook the food immediately after defrosting.

What If the Patient's Power Goes Out?

If the power will be coming back on fairly soon, food can last longer if the refrigerator door is kept shut as much as possible. If the power will be off for an extended period, the food may be taken to a relative's freezer, or some other method should be sought to keep the food frozen, or it will need to be thrown out. Without power, the refrigerator section should keep food cool for 4 to 6 hours, depending on the kitchen temperature. A full, well-functioning freezer unit or upright or chest freezer should keep food frozen for 2 days. A half-full freezer should keep food frozen for 1 day (CDC & U.S. Department of Agriculture [USDA], 1996).

After the power comes back on, food that still contains ice crystals or that feels refrigerator-cold can be refrozen (CDC & USDA, 1996). Any thawed food that has risen to room temperature and remained there for 2 hours or more should be discarded. Any food or drink with a strange color or odor must be discarded immediately.

Immunocompromised Patients

In addition, persons at high risk for infection should avoid soft cheeses such as feta, brie, camembert, blue-veined cheeses, and Mexican-style cheeses. Hard cheeses, processed cheeses, cream cheese, cottage cheese, and yogurt do not need to be avoided. Cold cuts should be thoroughly reheated before eating. Fruit that the patient will eat raw should be peeled after washing (CDC, 1998a).

Health Department Warnings

If the health department issues a warning to boil water, the water should be maintained at a rolling boil for 1 minute to kill *Cryptosporidium parvum* and other organisms. After the boiled water cools, it should be placed in a clean bottle or pitcher with a lid and stored in the refrigerator. This water should be used for drinking, cooking, or making ice. Water bottles and ice trays should be cleaned with soap and water before use. The inside of the bottle or tray should not be touched after cleaning (CDC, 1998c).

REFERENCES

Centers for Disease Control and Prevention. (1998a). Cryptosporidiosis. Atlanta: Author. http://www.cdc.gov/ncidod/dpd/cryto.htm

Centers for Disease Control and Prevention. (1998b). Opportunistic infections and your pets. A guide for people with HIV infection. MMWR recommendations and reports—Preview. Atlanta: Author. http://www.cdc.gov/od/oc/media/pressrel/salmchic.htm

Centers for Disease Control and Prevention. (1998c). Preventing foodborne illness: Listeriosis. Atlanta: Author. http://www.cdc.gov/ncidod/publications/brochures/lister.htm

Centers for Disease Control and Prevention. (1996a). Following protective devices to reduce disease and injury. Cleaning and disinfecting. The ABC's of safe and healthy child care. Atlanta: Author. http://www.cdc.gov/ncidod/hip/practi9.htm

Centers for Disease Control and Prevention. (1996b). Following protective devices to reduce disease and injury. Diapering. The ABC's of safe and healthy child care. Atlanta: Author. http://www.cdc.gov/ncidod/hip/practi7.htm

Centers for Disease Control and Prevention. (1996c). Following protective devices to reduce disease and injury. Washing and disinfecting toys. The ABC's of safe and healthy child care. Atlanta: Author. http://www.cdc.gov/ncidod/hip/practi10.htm

Centers for Disease Control and Prevention. (1995). Food and waterborne bacterial diseases. Atlanta: Author. http://www.cdc.gov/ncidod/foodborn.htm

Centers for Disease Control and Prevention and the U.S. Department of Agriculture Food Safety and Inspection Service. (1996, October). A quick consumer guide to safe food handling (Publication No. 458-014). Atlanta: Author. http://www.cdc.gov/niosh/nasd/nasdhome.html

La Leche League International. (1997). *The womanly art of breastfeeding*. (6th rev. ed.) Shamburg, IL: Author.

CHAPTER 6

Personal Protective Equipment and Staff Supplies

USE OF PERSONAL PROTECTIVE EQUIPMENT

The Occupational Safety and Health Administration (OSHA) codified universal precautions with the Occupational Exposure to Bloodborne Pathogen regulations (OSHA, 1991). These regulations prescribe the use of personal protective equipment for all health care workers when blood and other potentially infectious materials are handled. After the bloodborne pathogen regulations were promulgated in 1991, they were legally challenged, and certain of their provisions were vacated or partially vacated for home care by a decision of the U.S. Circuit Court of Appeals for the Seventh Circuit (*Home Health Services and Staffing Association v. Martin*, 1993). Table 6–1 contains a summary of the effects of the court's decision on the bloodborne pathogen regulations as they relate to home care. One portion of the regulations that was vacated pertains to the use of personal protective equipment. For example, all home care organizations are required to provide or make available personal protective equipment for the home care staff member's use in the home. If the staff member does not properly use the personal protective equipment in his or her possession, however, the home care organization will not receive a citation from OSHA because the home care organization does not have control over the work site: the patient's home. Problems could result from other regulatory or accrediting bodies, however, if staff members are not following the home care organization's policies and procedures. For example, the home care organization could receive a recommendation from the Joint Commission on Accreditation of Healthcare Organizations (if the home care organization is surveyed for accreditation) or a deficiency from a state licensure or Medicare surveyor (if the home care organization is state licensed and/or Medicare certified). A model OSHA exposure control plan for home care is given in Appendix B.

GLOVES

Since the inception of universal precautions, the use of gloves as a protective barrier has increased dramatically. Even so, microbial contamination and the transmission of infections have been reported while a health care worker was wearing gloves. This is because wearing gloves creates a warm, moist environment that supports the growth of microorganisms. Therefore, after gloves are removed, the hands should be washed with soap and water or a waterless handwashing product (Larson, 1995). Gloves should never be considered a substitute for handwashing; rather, they should be used as an adjunct to handwashing.

Types of Gloves

Disposable gloves are made from different types of materials: natural rubber (e.g., Latex) or synthetic materials (e.g., vinyl). Clean, nonsterile, intact, disposable Latex gloves of appropriate size and quality for the home care procedure to be performed should be available for each staff member. Should a home care staff member exhibit an allergy to standard powdered Latex gloves, other types of gloves must be made available by the home care organization. Generally, nonsterile examination gloves are worn, but sterile gloves should be worn when a procedure requires that a field be with-

Table 6–1 Effect of Court Decision on OSHA Bloodborne Pathogen Regulations

Regulation	*OSHA Requirement*	*Final Status*
§1910.1030(c)(1) and (2)	Exposure control plan and determination	In effect, but should be modified to delete site-specific requirements and to include a statement that employer will not be responsible for site-specific activities beyond its control
§1910.1030(d)(1)	Universal precautions shall be observed	Vacated, except for inclusion in training program
§1910.1030(d)(2)(i)	Use of engineering and work practice controls	Vacated
§1910.1030(d)(2)(i)	Use of personal protective equipment (PPE)	Vacated
§1910.1030(d)(2)(ii)	Examination, maintenance, or replacement of engineering controls	Vacated
§1910.1030(d)(2)(iii)	Provision of handwashing facilities	Vacated
§1910.1030(d)(2)(iv)	Provision of hand cleanser or antiseptic towelettes	Vacated
§1910.1030(d)(2)(v)	Ensuring that employees wash hands	Vacated
§1910.1030(d)(2)(vi)	Ensuring that employees wash hands and skin after exposure	Vacated
§1910.1030(d)(2)(vii)	Ensuring that contaminated sharps are not bent, recapped, or removed	Vacated
§1910.1030(d)(2)(viii)	Ensuring that sharps are placed in containers	Vacated
§1910.1030(d)(2)(ix)	Prohibiting eating, drinking, smoking while applying cosmetics or lip balm or handling contact lenses in work area	Vacated
§1910.1030(d)(2)(x)	Prohibiting food and drink from being kept near potentially infectious materials	Vacated because it applies to worksites beyond employer's control
§1910.1030(d)(2)(xi)	Procedures involving blood must be performed in a manner to minimize splashing	Vacated
§1910.1030(d)(2)(xii)	Ensuring that employees do not use mouth pipetting/suctioning of potentially infectious materials	Vacated
§1910.1030(d)(2)(xiii)	Ensuring that potentially infectious materials are placed in a container	Vacated because it applies to worksites beyond employer's control
§1910.1030(d)(2)(xiii)(A)–(C)	Use of labeled, leak-proof containers for shipping or storage	In effect
§1910.1030(d)(2) (xiv)	Decontamination of equipment before serving or shipping	In effect
§1910.1030(d)(3)(i)	Provision of appropriate PPE	In effect
§1910.1030(d)(3)(ii)	Ensuring that employee uses PPE	Vacated
§1910.1030(d)(3)(iii)	Ensuring that PPE is accessible at worksite or issued to employees	In effect
§1910.1030(d)(3)(iv)	Cleaning, laundering, and disposal of PPE	In effect
§1910.1030(d)(3)(v)	Repair and replacement of PPE	Vacated
§1910.1030(d)(3)(vi)	Ensuring immediate removal of penetrated PPE	Vacated

Regulation	*OSHA Requirement*	*Final Status*
§1910.1030(d)(3)(vii)	Removal of PPE before leaving worksite	Vacated
§1910.1030(d)(3)(viii)	Placing PPE in designated area upon removal`	Vacated
§1910.1030(d)(3)(ix)	Use of gloves	Vacated
§1910.1030(d)(3)(x)	Use of masks, eye protection, face shields	Vacated
§1910.1030(d)(3)(xi)	Use of gowns, aprons, other protective clothing	Vacated
§1910.1030(d)(3)(xii)	Use of surgical caps, hoods, shoe covers or boots	Vacated
§1910.1030(d)(4)(i)	Ensuring that worksite is maintained in clean and sanitary condition	Vacated
§1910.1030(d)(4)(ii)(A)–(E)	Cleaning and decontaminating all equipment and environmental work surfaces	Vacated
§1910.1030(d)(4)(iii)(A)(1)	Immediately discarding contaminated sharps in specified containers	Vacated
§1910.1030(d)(4)(iii)(A)(2)	Use of sharps containers	Vacated
§1910.1030(d)(4)(iii)(A)(3)	Requirements for moving sharps containers from area of use	Vacated
§1910.1030(d)(4)(iii)(A)(4)	Prohibition on reusable containers not being opened or cleaned manually	Vacated, to extent that it applies to worksite
§1910.1030(d)(4)(iii)(B)	Placing regulated waste in leak-proof labeled containers	Vacated, to extent that it applies to worksite
§1910.1030(d)(4)(iii)(C)	Disposal of regulated waste in accordance with other regulations	In effect
§1910.1030(d)(4)(iv)(A)(1)–(3)	Use of labeled bags for contaminated laundry at worksite or for transportation	Vacated, to extent that it applies to worksite
§1910.1030(d)(4)(iv)(B)	Ensuring that employees who contact contaminated laundry wear PPE	Vacated
§1910.1030(d)(4)(iv)(C)	Use of labeled bags to transport contaminated laundry	Vacated
§1910.1030(e)	HIV and HBV research laboratories and production facilities	Not applicable
§1910.1030(f)(1)–(6)	HBV vaccinations, postexposure evaluation, follow-up	In effect
§1910.1030(g)(1)	Use of labels and signs to designate regulated waste	Vacated because applicable to worksites outside employer's control
§1910.1030(g)(2)(i)–(ix)	Required training and content of training programs	In effect, unless employer can demonstrate that requirement is worksite related
§1910.1030(h)(1)–(3)	Maintaining medical records of HBV vaccination status and a copy of medical testing results	In effect

Note: The above list is based on an application of the holding in the court case. Individuals should seek legal counsel or contact OSHA for updated status.

Source: Reprinted with permission from James Pyles, *Home Health Services and Staffing Association, Inc., v. Martin,* Court of Appeals No. 92-1482, January 28, 1993, Powers, Pyles, Sutter and Verville, P.C., Washington, District of Columbia.

out pathogens or microorganisms, such as when an indwelling urinary catheter is inserted.

When To Wear Gloves

OSHA (1991) mandates that gloves be worn when there is a reasonable likelihood of hand contact with blood or other potentially infectious material, mucus membranes, or nonintact skin as well as when vascular access procedures are being performed and contaminated items or surfaces are being handled. The term *reasonable likelihood* is open to interpretation and may result in home care organizations having different policies and procedures. The home care organization's bloodborne pathogen exposure control plan should outline when staff members are required to wear gloves. Generally, staff members should wear gloves when:

- handling blood and other potentially infectious materials that are visibly contaminated with blood or when having contact with mucus membranes
- handling or touching contaminated items or surfaces
- performing any invasive procedure, including venous access procedures and heelsticks or fingersticks
- performing wound care
- staff member's hands are chapped, cut, scratched, or abraded
- contamination is likely with uncooperative or combative patients
- touching the patient's abraded or nonintact skin
- providing care for a patient with active bleeding
- handling any drainage collection appliance
- taking a rectal temperature
- shaving a patient with a safety razor
- obtaining laboratory specimens
- entering the room of, and providing care for, a patient colonized or infected with vancomycin-resistant enterococci (VRE) or multidrug-resistant *Staphylococcus aureas*
- there is the possibility of exposure to blood or body fluids

Gloves are not necessary when routine injections are given as long as hand contact with blood or other potentially infectious material is not anticipated. If bleeding is anticipated and the staff member is required to clean the site after the injection, then gloves must be worn. Additionally, if the patient's skin is abraded, gloves must be worn (OSHA, 1992b).

If a home care organization provides maternal and child services, and staff members will be teaching new mothers about breastfeeding and observing or coaching return breastfeeding demonstrations, gloves do not need to be worn because breast milk is not included in OSHA's definition of potentially infectious material. OSHA has determined that gloves should be worn if contact with breast milk will be frequent, such as in milk banking (OSHA, 1992a). The Centers for Disease Control and Prevention's (CDC's) guidelines for isolation precautions recommend, however, that gloves be worn when any body fluid except sweat will be touched (Garner, 1996). Therefore, to follow the CDC's Standard Precautions, gloves should be worn when the staff member will have direct contact with the patient's breast when teaching breastfeeding techniques.

When Gloves Should Be Changed or Removed

Gloves should be changed between tasks and procedures on the same patient, after contact with material that may contain a high concentration of microorganisms (e.g., during changing and cleaning of an incontinent patient's bed or removing an old dressing), and after contact with infective material that may have high concentrations of VRE (e.g., fecal material). Gloves should be removed and changed when the integrity of the gloves is in doubt (e.g., if the gloves are torn or punctured) and between patient care procedures as soon as safety permits. Gloves should be removed as soon after the task is completed as possible to avoid cross-contamination. Hands should not touch potentially contaminated environmental surfaces or items in the patient's room after the gloves are removed, and the hand should be washed to prevent the transfer of microorganisms to others and the environment. Disposable, single-use gloves should not be washed or decontaminated for reuse.

Latex Allergies

Many home care staff members are allergic to Latex gloves. The signs and symptoms of an allergic reaction to Latex gloves and other natural rubber products may include skin rash; hives; nasal, eye, or sinus symptoms; asthma; and (rarely) shock. These allergic reactions are mainly due to the proteins that fasten to the powder used in some Latex gloves, which can cause reactions through contact or breathing. Table 6–2 contains ex-

Table 6–2 Products Containing Latex

Medical Equipment	*Personal Protective Equipment*	*Office Supplies*	*Medical Supplies*
Blood pressure cuffs	Gloves	Adhesive tape	Condom-style urinary collection device
Breathing circuits	Goggles	Erasers	Enema tubing tips
Disposable gloves	Rubber aprons	Rubber bands	Injection ports
IV tubing	Surgical masks		Rubber tops of multidose vials
Oral and nasal airways			Urinary catheters
Stethoscopes			Wound drains
Syringes			
Tourniquets			

Source: Reprinted from *Preventing Allergic Reactions to Natural Rubber Latex in the Workplace,* the Centers for Disease Control and Prevention, National Institute for Occupational Safety and Health Alert, Atlanta, GA, June 1997.

amples of items commonly used in home care that contain Latex. Options with traditional Latex include extra-thin gloves (which allow for more sensitivity in palpation), gloves with texture for handling breakable items, and powder-free gloves to reduce allergic reactions. Nylon or cotton glove liners are available, but because hands perspire when in gloves the protective factor can be lost.

Preventing Allergic Reactions to Latex in the Workplace

Latex allergy may be prevented if the home care organization adopts policies to protect staff members from undue Latex exposure. The goal is to reduce exposure to allergy-causing proteins (antigens). The National Institute for Occupational Safety and Health (NIOSH) recommends that home care organizations take the following steps to protect staff members from Latex exposure and allergy (NIOSH, 1997):

- Provide staff members with non-Latex gloves to use when there is little potential for contact with infectious materials.
- If Latex gloves are chosen for barrier protection, provide reduced-protein, powder-free gloves.
- Provide staff members with education programs and training materials about Latex allergy.
- Periodically screen high-risk staff members for Latex allergy symptoms. Detecting symptoms early and removing symptomatic staff members from Latex exposure are essential for preventing long-term health effects.
- Evaluate current prevention strategies whenever a worker is diagnosed with Latex allergy.

Staff members with ongoing exposure to Latex should take the following steps to protect themselves (NIOSH, 1997):

1. Use non-Latex gloves for activities that are not likely to involve contact with infectious materials.
2. Choose powder-free Latex gloves with a reduced protein content.
3. Do not use oil-based creams or lotions when wearing Latex gloves unless they have been shown to reduce Latex-related problems.
4. Recognize the symptoms of Latex allergy: skin rashes; hives; flushing; itching; nasal, eye, or sinus symptoms; asthma; and shock.
5. Avoid direct contact with Latex gloves and products if symptoms of Latex allergy develop until a physician experienced in treating Latex allergy can be seen.

Consult a physician regarding the following precautions:

1. avoiding contact with Latex gloves and products
2. avoiding areas where the powder from the Latex gloves worn by others might be inhaled
3. telling the home care organization's management about the Latex allergy
4. wearing a medical alert bracelet
5. taking advantage of all Latex allergy education and training provided by the home care organization

MASKS, RESPIRATORY PROTECTION, EYE PROTECTION, AND FACE SHIELDS

Face masks, goggles, and face shields can be used alone or in combination to prevent airborne pathogens that may be encountered during patient care activities from being inhaled or ingested. The type of mask selected depends on the purpose of the mask. For example, if the staff member requires protection against eye, nose, or mouth contamination from splashes, spray, spatter, or droplets of blood or other potentially infectious materials, then a mask should be worn together with protective eye wear. Protective eye wear includes goggles, glasses with solid side shields, and chin-length face shields. Only masks that claim fluid protection should be worn by staff members. If the mask will be worn to protect the staff member from *Mycobacterium tuberculosis*, then a NIOSH-certified N95 respiratory protective device should be worn. If the mask will be worn to protect the staff member against the transmission of large- and small-particle airborne droplets, then a regular surgical mask should be worn. A surgical mask should be worn to protect against large-particle droplets that can be transmitted by close contact (up to 3 feet) with infected patients who are coughing or sneezing.

When To Wear a Mask

The staff member should wear either a surgical mask or a NIOSH-certified N95 respiratory protective device when home care procedures are likely to generate droplets of blood or other body fluids. This includes during patient instruction, demonstration, and/or return demonstration in the home use of aerosolized Pentamidine; during care of patients with a productive cough who cannot or do not appropriately use tissues; and during care of patients diagnosed with pulmonary tuberculosis who have a positive sputum culture. The home care staff member should wear a NIOSH-certified N95 respiratory protective device, the minimally acceptable level of respiratory protection, when entering the home of a patient with suspected or confirmed active pulmonary infection with *Mycobacterium tuberculosis* until the patient is no longer infectious or when caring for such a patient if the patient is not wearing a surgical mask.

N95 respiratory protective devices that are classified as disposable may be reused by the same home care staff member as long as they remain functional (CDC, 1994). The manufacturer's guidelines should be followed for inspecting, cleaning, and maintaining respirators to ensure that the N95 respiratory protective device continues to function properly. Masks and eye protection should be put on before gloving and taken off after contaminated gloves are removed.

Mask Varieties

There are now masks available to meet most home care staff members' needs. For example, masks with a foam liner can prevent eyeglasses from fogging, masks with ties can prevent Latex allergies, masks with no-dye fabrics can prevent allergic reaction, masks with more pleats or an extra fold can prevent nose discomfort, masks with a smooth lining can prevent skin irritation, masks with a metal nosepiece can conform to the face's shape, and masks with extra bacterial filtration can prevent the spread of infectious agents in the staff member's respirations.

Gowns, Aprons, Laboratory Coats, and Other Protective Clothing

Gowns, laboratory coats, aprons, or other similar outer garments appropriate for the activity and amount of fluid that are likely to be encountered should be worn when splashing of clothing or skin with blood or other potentially infectious material is likely to occur during patient care activities. Gowns or plastic aprons should be worn when direct contact with the patient's body fluids and soiling of clothing are likely. Gowns also should be worn when care is provided for a patient infected with epidemiologically important microorganisms (e.g., multidrug-resistant microorganisms) to reduce the transmission of pathogens to other patients. When a gown is worn for this purpose, it should be removed before the staff member leaves the room where the patient resides, and the hands should be washed.

Gowns should be made of or lined with impervious material, should protect all areas of exposed skin, and should prevent soiling of clothing during home care procedures. If a garment becomes soiled with blood or other potentially infectious material, it should be removed immediately or as soon as feasible and the hands washed to prevent the spread of microorganisms. Gowns made of single-layer polyolefin films offer the most protection but are uncomfortable because the fabric does not breathe. Reinforced gowns made of a combination material that includes polyolefin film offer the next best level of protection. Cotton and cotton-polyester blends offer the least protection because they have limited fluid protection.

RESUSCITATION EQUIPMENT

One-way valve pocket masks, resuscitation bags, or other ventilation devices should be made available to minimize the risk of unprotected mouth-to-mouth resuscitation. Each staff member should have one-way valve resuscitation equipment in his or her possession during home visits to use in the resuscitation of patients. Disposable airway devices are preferred and should not be used on more than one patient.

PATIENT TRANSPORT OUTSIDE THE HOME

Patients infected with virulent or epidemiologically important organisms (e.g., multidrug-resistant microorganisms or organisms that require transmission-based precautions) should leave their homes only for essential purposes, such as dialysis, physician office visits, or emergency department visits, to reduce the opportunities for transmission of microorganisms. When the patient must leave the home, it is important that he or she wear a barrier (e.g., a mask or a dressing over a wound) to reduce the spread of infection to others with whom the patient may come in contact. The patient also should be instructed about precautions that he or she can take to prevent the spread of infection. Physician office or emergency department personnel should be notified of the patient's impending arrival and any precautions that they must take to reduce the risk of transmission of microorganisms.

NEEDLESTICK PREVENTION EQUIPMENT DESIGN

Home care staff members, caregivers, and the patient are at risk from needlestick injuries in the home. OSHA estimates that 50 percent of needlesticks can be prevented by the use of resheathing or retracting syringe devices. Other sharps protection devices include retractable needles, devices with needles that are recessed behind protective covers, and needleless intravenous connectors. Wherever possible, these protective devices should be made available to staff members.

REMOVAL OF IMPLANTED PORT ACCESS NEEDLES

Three devices are available to reduce the risk of needlestick injury to home care staff members in removing needles from implanted ports. These devices should be considered for use because hollow-bore needles in direct contact with blood have the greatest risk of transmitting bloodborne pathogens to home care staff members (Hadaway, 1997). One protective device fits over the port. The staff member uses a hemostat to pull the needle up into the device, which contains and disposes of the needle. The second device contains two blades that slide under the needle's wings and the patient's skin. The bottom blade stabilizes the device while the upper blade pulls out the needle. With this device, the needle remains exposed, and so does the staff member. The third device consists of a small plastic box and a lever. The device slides forward so that it is between the needle's wings and the patient's skin. The staff member pushes down on top of the device with the thumb to stabilize it and the port. While pushing down with the thumb, the staff member pulls up with the index and middle fingers to remove the needle from the port, pulls the needle up, and locks it in place. The needle is fully contained inside a plastic cover. The device and needle are then placed in an impervious container for disposal (Carroll, 1998).

STAFF MEMBER ACCESS TO PERSONAL PROTECTIVE EQUIPMENT

If a supply bag is taken into the patient's home during a visit, it is not necessary that every type of personal protective equipment be provided to each individual staff member. What is most important is that the equipment is available to the staff member in the home. For example, on a private duty home care case where there is 24-hour coverage by registered nurses, licensed practical nurses, or licensed vocational nurses for a ventilator-dependent patient, the home care organization may place in the home for all staff's use a box of nonsterile Latex gloves, goggles, gowns, resuscitation equipment, and any other supplies that may be necessary. Personal protective equipment must be available for each staff member when needed. For example, each staff member does not have to be issued his or her own N95 respiratory protective device. As long as the staff member is fitted and provided with an N95 respiratory protective device before making a home visit, that is sufficient.

Many organizations provide each staff member an "OSHA kit," which contains all the personal protective equipment that may be needed during a home visit. The type of personal protective equipment provided to each staff member will vary based on the likelihood of exposure to blood and other potentially infectious body fluids. The risk of occupational exposure is greater for a nurse and home health aide than it is for a social worker or hospice chaplain. If a professional or nonprofessional staff member is expected to perform cardiopulmonary resuscitation (CPR) in the event of cardiopulmonary arrest, then each staff member should have a one-way valve resuscitation mask on his or her person or have access to one in the home. The patient cannot wait while the staff member goes out to the car to get the resuscitation mask. If the staff member is not required to perform CPR according to the home care organization's policies and procedures, a resuscitation mask does not have to be in the home or issued to the staff member. As long as the staff member has immediate access to the necessary supplies during the course of care, that is sufficient.

TRAINING

OSHA requires that the home care organization educate staff members on the location and use of personal protective equipment upon hire and on an annual basis. Refer to Chapter 13, Exhibit 13–5. Table 6–3 provides guidelines as to when gloves and other personal protective equipment should be worn when various home care tasks are performed.

NURSING SUPPLY BAG

A nursing supply bag is not required, although most home care organization staff members who provide intermittent home care services use one. Ideally, the bag should be constructed of a washable fabric and have multiple compartments for the storage of supplies. If

Table 6–3 Staff Member Barrier Requirements

Task	*Gloves*	*Gown or Plastic Apron*	*Mask*	*Goggles*	*One-Way Valve Resuscitation Mask*
Bath	Optional	If soiling is likely			
Blood glucose monitoring	Required				
Changing visibly soiled linens	Required	Required			
Cleaning blood/body fluid spills	Required	If soiling is likely	If splashing is likely	If splashing is likely	
Cleaning incontinent patient	Required	If soiling is likely			
CPR					Required
Inserting peripheral short-line or midline catheter	Required				
Inserting peripherally inserted central catheter	Required				
Ostomy care	Required				
Tracheostomy care	Required	If soiling is likely likely	If splashing is likely	If splashing is likely	
Wound care	Required	Optional		If irrigation is performed	

Note: The type of personal protective equipment needed for a task is based on three criteria: volume of blood or fluids expected, length of time for which exposure is expected, and conditions of the exposure, such as temperature, humidity, and the possibility of unpredictable situations. This information is intended to serve as a guideline only and may not identify all equipment necessary to take care of a home care patient. Each home care situation should be assessed to determine the minimum type of personal protective equipment required. Personal protective equipment generally is not required for patient assessments, feeding the patient, assisting with ambulation, or taking vital signs unless the patient requires transmission-based precautions.

the inside or outside of the bag does become significantly soiled, the bag should be washed in hot soapy water, rinsed, and dried in a dryer. On a regular basis and when soiled, the internal contents should be removed and the inside wiped out with a detergent disinfectant.

Bag Placement in the Home

Currently there is debate in home care over "bag technique" and whether a barrier placed under the supply bag is required. There is no scientific basis for barrier placement, and studies have not shown that a barrier placed under a nursing bag in the home is effective against preventing the transmission of infections; therefore, such a barrier is not required. Common sense and the fundamentals of infection control should prevail. "Although microorganisms are a normal contaminant of walls, floors, and other surfaces, these environmental surfaces are rarely associated with transmission of infections to patient or personnel" (Garner & Favero, 1986, p. 115). The supply bag should be placed on a clean, dry surface away from small children and pets.

If the home environment is heavily infested with insects or rodents, the bag should not be brought into the patient's home. The supplies that will be needed for the home visit can be taken out of the bag and placed in a disposable container, such as a brown paper bag or plastic bag, or carried in a "fanny pack." Once the visit is over, the noncritical supplies can be cleaned and then carried back to the car to be placed inside the nursing bag. The disposable bag that was used to carry the supplies into the patient's home and store them should be discarded.

Bag Placement in the Car

The supplies kept in the staff member's vehicle should be checked on a regular basis to ensure that sterile supplies have not become contaminated and that expiration dates have not passed. Temperature-sensitive supplies, such as digital and glass thermometers, should not be exposed to temperature extremes. Although not a direct infection control issue, if the bag contains epinephrine, a glucometer, or other temperature-sensitive equipment or supplies, they too should not be exposed to temperature extremes. This includes over the weekend, at night, and when the heat or air conditioning is turned off between home visits. If a thermometer is exposed to cold temperature extremes, it should be warmed to room temperature before use.

Bag Technique

As a good infection control measure, staff members should wash their hands before reaching into the bag to obtain any necessary supplies. Reaching into the bag generally signifies the beginning of patient care activities, and the hands should always be washed before patient care is provided. When noncritical equipment is taken out of the bag and used in patient care, it should be cleaned or disinfected, if necessary, before it is returned to the nursing supply bag. Chapter 8 provides additional information about how and when medical equipment such as blood pressure cuffs and stethoscopes should be cleaned. If the patient has equipment in the home that can be used in patient care (e.g., a thermometer), it is preferred that the patient's equipment be used in lieu of the equipment from the nursing supply bag. When reaching into the bag again to obtain additional supplies, the staff member must make certain that gloves that were used to provide patient care are removed. Otherwise, the equipment can become contaminated. Inside the supply bag, semicritical items should be kept covered and critical items should be contained in a sterile wrapper that will prevent contamination.

Bag Contents

Not every staff member must be issued a supply bag, but all staff members should have access to the needed supplies in the home. Most important is that the personal protective equipment and supplies needed to provide patient care are available to the staff when they are needed. As mentioned earlier, home care organizations that provide private duty services may store Latex gloves, plastic aprons, a CPR mask, and handwashing supplies in a box that is kept in the patient's home for staff members' use. Intermittent rehabilitation staff members may use a "fanny pack" to carry handwashing and other needed supplies.

INFECTION CONTROL SUPPLIES

Infection control supplies should be available for home care staff members who are providing direct patient care and for admission staff. Frequently, when a patient is referred to a home care organization, only partial information is received from the referral source, and the admitting staff member may need personal protective equipment that was not anticipated, such as a mask. Infection control supplies may be kept either in a supply bag that is carried from patient home to patient home or left in the patient's home for staff members' use. Staff members who will be visiting patients on standard precautions but do not provide direct hands-on patient care, such as social workers, chaplains, and dietitians, do not have to have in their possession a full complement of infection control supplies. The minimum supplies should include a waterless handwashing product and a towelette, a mask, gloves, and a one-way valve resuscitation mask (if the home care organization requires these staff members to be certified in basic life support). If a patient is on airborne, droplet, or contact precautions, additional personal protective equipment such as a gown, mask, or N95 respiratory protective device should be provided to the staff member or made available in the home.

Exhibit 6–1 lists infection control supplies that should be available to staff who provide direct patient care and staff who go to the patient's home to screen the patient for admission to the home care program.

Exhibit 6–1 Supplies To Be Made Available as Needed to Staff Providing Direct Patient Care and Admission Staff

- Plain soap and antimicrobial soap or antibacterial soap only
- Waterless handwashing product and individual-use towelettes containing detergent to remove gross contamination
- Hand drying supplies
- Lotion (optional)
- One-way valve resuscitation mask (only if staff are required to be CPR certified)
- Nonsterile Latex gloves
- Impermeable gown
- Surgical mask
- NIOSH N95 respiratory protective device
- Goggles
- Blood spill kit
- Sharps container
- Impermeable red container or impervious container labeled as biohazardous to carry laboratory samples
- Red plastic bag or bag labeled as biohazardous
- Sterile gloves for procedures requiring sterile technique
- 70% ethyl alcohol wipes or other disinfectant

REFERENCES

Carroll, O. (1998, April). Reducing the risk of needlestick injury associated with implanted ports. *Home Health Care Nurse, 16*, 225–234.

Centers for Disease Control and Prevention. (1994, October 28). Guidelines for preventing the transmission of *Mycobacterium tuberculosis* in health-care facilities. *Morbidity and Mortality Weekly Report, 43*(RR-13), 1–125.

Garner, J.S. (1996). Guideline for isolation precautions in hospitals. *Infection Control and Hospital Epidemiology, 17*, 53–80.

Garner, J., & Favero, M. (1986, June). CDC guideline for handwashing and hospital environmental control, 1985. *American Journal of Infection Control, 14*, 110–129.

Hadaway, L. (1997). Vascular access in home care: 1997 update. *Infusion, 4*, 27.

Larson, E. (1995). APIC guidelines for handwashing and hand antisepsis in health care settings. *American Journal of Infection Control, 23*, 251–269.

National Institute for Occupational Safety and Health. (1997, June). Preventing allergic reactions to natural rubber latex in the workplace. National Institute for Occupational Safety and Health Alert, Publication No. 97-135. http://www.cdc.gov/niosh/latexalt.html

Occupational Safety and Health Administration. (1991). Occupational exposure to bloodborne pathogens: Final rule. 29 CFR 1910,1030. *Federal Register, 56*, 64003–64282.

Occupational Safety and Health Administration. (1992a, December 14). Breast milk does not constitute occupational exposure as defined by standard. OSHA standards interpretation and compliance letters. http://www.osha-slc.gov/OshDoc/Interp_data/I19921214A.html

Occupational Safety and Health Administration. (1992b, September 1). Using gloves in administering routine injections. OSHA standards interpretation and compliance letters. http://www.osha-slc.gov/OshDoc/Interp_data/I19920901A.html

CHAPTER 7

Isolation Precautions in Home Care

HISTORY OF ISOLATION PRECAUTIONS

The appropriate use of isolation precautions is a key element in infection control. It has become even more important with the rapid emergence of multidrug-resistant microorganisms. Isolation precautions have two primary goals in home care: to prevent the transmission of microorganisms from an infected or colonized patient to other patients via home care staff members, and to protect home care staff from potential exposure to infectious diseases. Although most home care organizations have developed policies and procedures for isolation precautions based on these two goals, there is currently no standardized scheme for the application of these strategies in home care. Consequently, the use of isolation precautions in home care varies widely.

In acute care settings, isolation precautions have been based on guidelines and recommendations from the Centers for Disease Control and Prevention (CDC). Since the CDC published the first isolation manual in 1970, the use of precautions in hospitals has undergone significant changes and evolution. These changes are based on new scientific knowledge as well as newly emerging pathogens and illnesses, including acquired immune deficiency syndrome and the increased prevalence of multidrug-resistant microorganisms. The most recent CDC isolation guideline was published in 1996 (Garner, 1996) and includes even more changes in the recommended approach to isolation.

Throughout the evolution of isolation precautions and even before the publication of the 1970 CDC manual, isolation precautions have been hospital based, with the exception of some public health quarantine measures employed to prevent or limit outbreaks of disease. All the CDC publications have included guidance on issues such as patient placement, use of protective apparel (e.g., gowns, gloves, and masks), care of patient equipment, patient transport, ventilation, linens and laundry, dishes and utensils, and cleaning of the isolation room. Although some of these issues are important in developing isolation policies and procedures in home care (e.g., use of protective apparel), many of them do not have the same relevance (e.g., patient placement) or must be significantly modified for home care.

The application of isolation precautions to prevent the transmission of infectious diseases is based on the principles discussed in Chapter 2. Any tactic or procedure incorporated into an isolation policy should be scientifically based and consider the agent, host, and environment (see Figure 2–2). The chain of infection (see Figure 2–3) should also be considered in developing policies and procedures for home care isolation as well as in making decisions during the course of care because not every individual situation can be covered in a policy or procedure. As demonstrated in the chain of transmission, precautions must be based on the mode of transmission of the infection, the portal of exit from the infected or colonized patient, and the portal of entry for the susceptible host (this may be another patient or a home care staff member). Other factors, including the length of time the patient is contagious and the type of care being provided, should also be considered.

Actions should not be arbitrary, and rituals should be avoided. Scientific knowledge and principles should be applied in assessing the risk of transmission and in taking steps to interrupt the transmission and thus to reduce the risk. For example, hospitals used to use disposable paper trays to provide meals for patients on isolation. Once this practice was examined on its scientific merits and infection control professionals realized that there is no risk of transmission on hospital food trays, the practice was abandoned. In home care, many organizations have abandoned the use of barriers under nursing bags because of a lack of scientific merit.

The early CDC isolation guidelines, before the introduction of Universal Precautions, were developed on these principles and divided into categories of precautions based on the modes of transmission. As discussed in Chapter 2, infectious diseases can be transmitted via several routes: airborne transmission, droplet transmission, direct and indirect contact transmission, common vehicle transmission (e.g., contaminated water and food), and vectorborne transmission (e.g., insects, rodents, etc.). Home care organizations should have policies and procedures for isolation precautions that address airborne, droplet, and contact transmission. The CDC refers to this type of system as transmission-based precautions. The use of transmission-based precautions has evolved since 1985, when Universal Precautions were first introduced. The 1996 CDC Guideline for Isolation Precautions in Hospitals integrated the concepts of Universal Precautions and other systems, such as body substance isolation, that were initiated to reduce exposure to blood and other body secretions, into Standard Precautions.

Many of the items addressed in the CDC's Guideline for Isolation Precautions in Hospitals that refer to patient cohorting, restriction of access and traffic flow, and placing patients in rooms with negative air pressure obviously do not apply to home care. Despite the Guideline's title, the isolation precautions and other strategies that it describes can be adapted and applied to the delivery of home care. The revised isolation system is based on two tiers of precautions. The first tier is Standard Precautions, which apply to all patients, and the second tier is transmission-based precautions, which apply only to patients with confirmed or suspected infection or colonization with certain microorganisms. Whether the transmission-based precautions are used singly or in combination, they are always used in addition to Standard Precautions. Exhibit 7–1 provides a synopsis of the types of precautions that should be taken and the patients requiring such precautions.

STANDARD PRECAUTIONS

Standard Precautions should be utilized for all patients regardless of their diagnosis or presumed infection status, and are considered the primary method of preventing transmission of infection in home care. Standard Precautions apply to blood; all body fluids, secretions, and excretions except sweat, regardless of whether they contain visible blood; nonintact skin; and mucus membranes.

Standard Precautions are designed to reduce the risk of transmission of microorganisms from both recognized and unrecognized sources of infection (Garner, 1996). Table 7–1 provides recommendations for implementing Standard Precautions. Chapter 6 provides additional information about the use of personal protective equipment.

TRANSMISSION-BASED PRECAUTIONS

The three types of transmission-based precautions are Airborne Precautions, Droplet Precautions, and Contact Precautions. Transmission-based precautions should be used in the home when staff are caring for patients with a documented or suspected infection that may be transmitted to others, for patients suspected of being infected, and for patients who are colonized or infected with a highly transmissible or epidemiologically important pathogen. An epidemiologically important pathogen is one that is known to cause serious infection or is difficult to treat; examples are vancomycin-resistant enterococci (VRE) and other multidrug-resistant microorganisms. Epidemiologically important pathogens are usually identified as such by the current infection control literature; state, regional, or national recommendations; the patient's physician; or the infection control department in a hospital. These pathogens are most commonly transmitted by direct or indirect contact, but in some cases there may be risk for droplet transmission.

As previously stated, transmission-based precautions are always used in addition to Standard Precautions to prevent or interrupt the transmission of infection. Some patients may require one or two types of transmission-based precautions in addition to Standard Precautions, depending on the type of infection and the potential modes of transmission. For example, a patient with chickenpox requires both Airborne Precautions (for virus spread via respiratory droplet nuclei) and

Exhibit 7–1 Types of Precautions and Patients Requiring Them

Standard Precautions

Use standard precautions for the care of all patients

Airborne Precautions

In addition to standard precautions, use airborne precautions for patients known or suspected to have serious illnesses transmitted by airborne droplet nuclei:

1. Measles
2. Varicella (including disseminated zoster)*
3. Tuberculosis (active pulmonary or laryngeal)†

Droplet Precautions

In addition to standard precautions, use droplet precautions for patients known or suspected to have serious illnesses transmitted by large particle droplets:

1. Invasive *Hemophilus influenzae* type b disease, including meningitis, pneumonia, epiglottitis, and sepsis
2. Invasive *Neisseria meningitidis* disease, including meningitis, pneumonia, and sepsis
3. Other serious bacterial respiratory infections spread by droplet transmission:
    - Diphtheria (pharyngeal)
    - Mycoplasma pneumonia
    - Pertussis
    - Pneumonic plague
    - Streptococcal (group A) pharyngitis, pneumonia, or scarlet fever in infants and young children
4. Serious viral infections spread by droplet transmission:
    - Adenovirus*
    - Influenza
    - Mumps
    - Parvovirus B19
    - Rubella

Contact Precautions

In addition to standard precautions, use contact precautions for patients known or suspected to have serious illnesses easily transmitted by direct patient contact or by contact with items in the patient's environment:

1. Gastrointestinal, respiratory, skin, or wound infections or colonization with multidrug resistant bacteria judged by the infection control program, based on current state, regional, or national recommendations, to be of special clinical and epidemiologic significance
2. Enteric infections with a low infectious dose or prolonged environmental survival:
    - *Clostridium difficile* infection
    - For diapered or incontinent patients, enterohemorrhagic *Escherichia coli* 0157:H7, *Shigella,* hepatitis A, or rotavirus infection
3. Respiratory syncytial virus, parainfluenza virus, or enteroviral infections in infants and young children
4. Skin infections that are highly contagious or that may occur on dry skin:
    - Diphtheria (cutaneous)
    - Herpes simplex virus (neonatal or mucocutaneous)
    - Impetigo
    - Major (noncontained) abscesses, cellulitis, or decubiti
    - Pediculosis
    - Scabies
    - *Staphylococcus furunculosis* in infants and young children
    - Zoster (disseminated or in the immunocompromised host)*
5. Viral hemorrhagic conjunctivitis
6. Viral hemorrhagic infections (Ebola, Lassa, or Marburg)

* Certain infections require more than one type of precaution.

† See the CDC's *Guidelines for Preventing the Transmission of Tuberculosis in Health-Care Facilities.* http://www.cdc.gov/epo/mmwr/preview/rr4313.html

Source: Reprinted with permission from J.S. Garner, Guideline for Isolation Precautions in Hospitals, *Infection Control and Hospital Epidemiology,* Vol. 17, No. 1, pp. 53–80, © 1996, Slack, Inc.

Table 7–1 Recommendations for Standard Precautions

Activity	*Recommendation*
After touching blood, body fluids, secretions, excretions, contaminated items Immediately after removing gloves Between patient contacts	Handwashing
For touching blood, body fluids, secretions, excretions, contaminated items For touching mucus membranes and nonintact skin	Gloves
During procedures and patient care activities likely to generate splashes or sprays of blood, body fluids, secretions, excretions	Mask, eye protection, face shield
During procedures and patient care activities likely to generate splashes or sprays of blood, body fluids, secretions, excretions	Gown
Handling soiled patient care equipment	Handle in a manner that prevents contamination or transfer of microorganisms to others and environment
Environmental control	Develop procedures for routine care, cleaning, and disinfection of environmental surfaces
Handling linen	Handle in a manner to prevent exposures, contamination, transfer of microorganisms to others and environment
Using sharps	Avoid recapping, bending, breaking, manipulating used needles Place used sharps in puncture-resistant container
Patient resuscitation	Mouthpiece, resuscitation bag, other ventilation devices
Patient placement	If patient contaminates environment or does not maintain appropriate hygiene, maintain patient in separate room, if possible.

Source: Reprinted with permission from J.S. Garner, Guideline for Isolation Precautions in Hospitals, *Infection Control and Hospital Epidemiology*, Vol. 17, No. 1, pp. 53–80, © 1996, Slack, Inc.

Contact Precautions (for virus contained within the skin vesicles).

The information to guide the decision to place a home care patient on transmission-based precautions should be outlined in the patient care policies and procedures and should not depend solely on a physician's order. The need for precautions may be based on the report of the patient's history and current condition from a referral source, the physician's order, or information obtained and/or observations made during the initial assessment or as the result of any assessment made during the course of home care treatment.

At the time of admission to the home care organization, the patient may not have a definitive diagnosis of an infectious disease. The patient may be symptomatic, or the diagnosis may be pending laboratory results. In these cases, the appropriate transmission-based precautions should be initiated based on the staff member's assessment and professional experience or judgment rather than specific data, such as laboratory results. When the patient presents with a clinical syndrome or condition on admission or at any time throughout the course of care, the patient should be treated as if he or she were contagious and placed on the appropriate transmission-based isolation precautions. The CDC recommends this empiric use of precautions to avoid potential exposures or transmission while the confirmation of a diagnosis is pending. Table 7–2 describes situations and clinical syndromes or conditions that warrant the empiric use of isolation precautions.

Airborne Precautions

In addition to Standard Precautions, Airborne Precautions should be used for patients known or suspected to have an infection transmitted by the airborne route via tiny respiratory secretions known as airborne droplet nuclei. Airborne droplet nuclei are small particle

Table 7–2 Clinical Syndromes or Conditions Warranting Additional Empiric Precautions To Prevent Transmission of Epidemiologically Important Pathogens Pending Confirmation of Diagnosis*

Clinical Syndrome or Condition†	*Potential Pathogens‡*	*Empiric Precautions*
Diarrhea		
Acute diarrhea with a likely infectious cause in an incontinent or diapered patient	Enteric pathogens§	Contact
Diarrhea in an adult with a history of recent antibiotic use	*Clostridium difficile*	Contact
Meningitis	*Neisseria meningitidis*	Droplet
Rash or exanthems, generalized, etiology unknown		
Petechial/ecchymotic with fever	*Neisseria meningitidis*	Droplet
Vesicular	Varicella	Airborne and contact
Maculopapular with coryza and fever	Rubeola (measles)	Airborne
Respiratory infections		
Cough, fever, upper lobe pulmonary infiltrate in a patient negative for human immunodeficiency virus (HIV) or a patient at low risk for HIV infection	*Mycobacterium tuberculosis*	Airborne
Cough, fever, pulmonary infiltrate in any lung location in an HIV-infected patient or a patient at high risk for HIV infection	*Mycobacterium tuberculosis*	Airborne
Paroxysmal or severe persistent cough during periods of pertussis activity	*Bordetella pertussis*	Droplet
Respiratory infections, particularly bronchiolitis and croup, in infants and young children	Respiratory syncytial or parainfluenza virus	Contact
Risk of multidrug-resistant microorganisms		
History of infection or colonization with multidrug-resistant organisms‖	Resistant bacteria‖	Contact
Skin, wound, urinary tract infection in a patient with a recent hospital or nursing home stay in a facility where multidrug-resistant organisms are prevalent	Resistant bacteria‖	Contact
Skin or wound infection (abscess or draining wound that cannot be covered)	*Staphylococcus aureus*, group A streptococcus	Contact

* Infection control professionals are encouraged to modify or adapt this information according to local conditions. To ensure that appropriate empiric precautions are implemented always, hospitals must have systems in place to evaluate patients routinely according to these criteria as part of preadmission and admission care.

† Patients with the listed syndromes or conditions may present with atypical signs or symptoms (e.g., pertussis in neonates and adults may not present with paroxysmal or severe cough). The clinician's index of suspicion should be guided by the prevalence of specific conditions in the community as well as clinical judgment.

‡ The pathogens listed are not intended to represent the complete, or even the most likely, diagnoses. Rather, they are possible etiologic agents that require additional precautions beyond standard precautions until they can be ruled out.

§ Enterohemorrhagic *Escherichia coli* 0157:H7, *Shigella* species, hepatitis A, rotavirus.

‖ Resistant bacteria judged by the infection control program, based on current state, regional, or national recommendations, to be of special clinical or epidemiological significance.

Source: Reprinted with permission from J.S. Garner, Guideline for Isolation Precautions in Hospitals, *Infection Control and Hospital Epidemiology*, Vol. 17, No. 1, pp. 53–80, © 1996, Slack, Inc.

residues (5 μm or smaller). Some infectious microorganisms, such as *Mycobacterium tuberculosis*, can be transmitted in evaporated droplets or dust particles. The microorganisms can remain suspended in the air and can be dispersed widely by air currents within a room or over a long distance. Diseases transmitted by the airborne route that require Airborne Precautions include chickenpox (varicella), measles (rubeola), and pulmonary or laryngeal tuberculosis (TB).

Personal Protective Equipment for Airborne Precautions

If the patient is diagnosed or suspected to be actively infected with pulmonary or laryngeal TB, home care staff members entering the patient's home should wear a National Institute for Occupational Safety and Health–certified N95 respiratory protective device as long as the patient's disease is potentially contagious. If the patient is diagnosed or suspected to be infected with an airborne illness other than TB, susceptible staff members who are in contact with the patient should wear a regular surgical mask.

Patient Placement for Airborne Precautions

Most of the infectious diseases that require Airborne Precautions in the hospital, with the notable exception of TB, are childhood illnesses. It may not be possible or necessary to isolate a home care patient with chickenpox or measles in a single room in the home with the door closed. In most cases, the other members of the household are either immune to the illness or have already been exposed. There may be situations, however, where there are other members of the household who may be susceptible and immunocompromised. In these circumstances, it may be necessary for the susceptible individual to be isolated from the patient; this may involve temporary displacement of the susceptible individual from the home. The family should be educated about the contagious nature of the airborne illness and the need to discourage visits during the period when the patient's disease is contagious from friends or family members who may not be immune. Home care staff members may need to use personal protective equipment if they are susceptible, as discussed later.

Patients with pulmonary or laryngeal TB may require more specific placement measures in the home while they are contagious. A patient with contagious pulmonary TB should be instructed to reside in a separate room with the door closed when there are susceptible children present in the home. When the patient does come out of the room, he or she should wear a surgical mask to prevent the microorganisms from being dispersed to susceptible individuals in the home and should maintain distance from others. A patient with contagious pulmonary TB does not need to be isolated or wear a surgical mask if there are only healthy adults present in the home. The patient should also be instructed to cover the mouth and nose with tissue when sneezing or coughing. Patients do not need to wear an N95 respiratory protective device, which is designed to filter the air before it is inhaled by the person wearing the mask. Patients suspected of having or known to have TB should never wear a respirator that has an exhalation valve because the device would provide no barrier to the expulsion of droplet nuclei into the air (CDC, 1994). If there is a ceiling fan or freestanding fan in the patient's room, it should not be used to circulate the air in the room. A patient with TB is usually monitored by a public health agency as well as being under care of a physician. Follow-up of exposures within the household and outside the household is usually part of the public health function. In addition, the public health staff provide information about TB to the patient and family, monitor the patient's compliance with medication, and provide information and guidance about any precautions that need to be taken to prevent exposure of others.

Linen and laundry can be washed with soap and water and do not need any special treatment. Cups and glasses used by the patient should not be shared among family members before being washed. No special treatment of dishes and eating utensils is required. Chapter 8 provides information about handling linen and laundry and cleaning dishes, glasses, cups, and eating utensils.

Home Care Staff Assignments

If possible, assignment of home care staff members who are not immune to the airborne childhood diseases, such as measles (rubeola) and chickenpox (varicella), should be avoided, especially if other immune staff members are available. If a susceptible staff member is assigned to the infected patient or there is someone else in the household who has an airborne illness, the staff member should wear a mask in the home. Persons who are known to be immune to measles and chickenpox do not need to wear a mask. The immune status of all home care staff should be determined at the time of employment.

Airborne Precautions during Patient Transport

If it is medically necessary for a patient with known or suspected pulmonary TB to leave the home while his or her disease is contagious, such as to attend dialysis or for an appointment with the physician, he or she should wear a surgical mask (CDC, 1994). The surgical mask is not necessary for patients on Airborne Precautions for infectious diseases other than TB while they are riding in the car with family members who have already been exposed, and it is not necessary for them to wear a mask when outdoors. Patients should wear a mask, however, whenever they enter a building or closed space where they may come in contact with susceptible people. Every effort should be made to minimize contact with other persons.

If a patient needs to visit the physician's office, he or she should request the last appointment of the day. When the appointment is made, the physician's office staff should be notified that the patient is on Airborne Precautions. If possible, the patient should enter the physician's office through a back entrance to avoid exposing others unnecessarily. The patient should not sit in a general waiting room with others. If the patient must go to an emergency department, the emergency staff should be notified as soon as possible (either before or immediately on arrival) that the patient requires Airborne Precautions so that they can avoid exposure of patients and staff. If transport by ambulance is necessary, the ambulance crew must also be notified before they come into direct contact with the patient.

Duration of Airborne Precautions

The decision about how long the Airborne Precautions must be maintained is dependent on the known period of communicability. For airborne childhood diseases such as chickenpox, the patient's disease is usually contagious for several days before the onset of a rash and until the lesions are crusted over. Appendix 7–A provides a list of diseases requiring transmission-based Airborne Precautions and the duration of precautions.

The length of time that precautions are necessary for pulmonary TB is dependent on the treatment of the infection. Even though most patients' disease is no longer contagious after 2 to 3 weeks of appropriate antitubercular therapy, the decision to discontinue Airborne Precautions is based on laboratory results. This is because some patients may not be compliant and take their medication as prescribed. In addition, there has been a significant increase in TB that is resistant to the usual drugs used to treat the infection (multidrug-resistant TB). Therefore, the CDC recommends that the patient have three negative sputum smears for acid-fast bacilli, obtained on different days, before Airborne Precautions are discontinued (CDC, 1994). This provides more direct evidence that the TB medications have been effective and the patient's disease is no longer contagious.

When the patient is no longer on Airborne Precautions, terminal cleaning of the room where the patient resides is not required (see Chapter 8 for more information about terminal cleaning).

Droplet Precautions

In addition to Standard Precautions, Droplet Precautions should be used for a patient known or suspected to be infected with microorganisms transmitted by large-particle respiratory droplets (5 μm or larger). Large droplets do not remain suspended in the air and do not travel more than 3 feet from the patient. Droplets may be spread to others who are physically close to the patient (closer than 3 feet) as a result of the patient coughing, sneezing, or talking or during clinical procedures such as suctioning.

Diseases or conditions that require Droplet Precautions include invasive *Hemophilus influenzae* type b disease (meningitis, pneumonia, epiglottis, and sepsis) and invasive *Neisseria meningitidis* disease (meningitis, pneumonia, and sepsis). Other serious bacterial respiratory infections spread by droplet transmission include diphtheria (pharyngeal), *Mycoplasma pneumoniae* disease, pertussis, pneumonic plague, and streptococcal pharyngitis, pneumonia, or scarlet fever in infants and young children. Serious viral infections spread by droplet transmission include adenovirus, influenza, mumps, parvovirus B19, and rubella. Infants and children with adenoviral infection require both contact and Droplet Precautions.

Personal Protective Equipment for Droplet Precautions

In addition to Standard Precautions, home care staff members and other individuals who will be within 3 feet of a patient diagnosed with or suspected to have one of the above conditions should wear a surgical mask. Staff members should wear a mask during wound care, bathing, checking vital signs, or auscultating the lungs, for example. A mask does not need to be worn when the staff member will not have close (within 3 feet) physical contact with the patient.

Patient Placement for Droplet Precautions

Patients requiring Droplet Precautions should be placed in a room away from susceptible individuals whenever possible. When a separate room is not possible or when the patient leaves the room, he or she should maintain a distance of at least 3 feet from other family members and visitors at all times to ensure that droplets will not be spread. The patient should be instructed to cover the mouth and nose with tissue when sneezing or coughing and not to share personal items, such as drinking cups. If there is a ceiling fan or other freestanding fan in the patient's room, it should not be used to circulate the air in the room. If follow-up of exposures is necessary, this is usually managed by a public health department (such as would occur with bacterial meningitis) or by the family's physician (as might occur with streptococcal infections). The family should be instructed about the contagious nature of the droplet infection; visits from family members and friends should be discouraged while the patient's or any family members' illness is potentially contagious. Appendix 7–A includes illnesses requiring Droplet Precautions and the duration for which Droplet Precautions should be maintained.

Linen and laundry can be washed with soap and water and do not need any special treatment. Cups and glasses used by the patient should not be shared among family members before being washed. No special treatment of dishes and eating utensils is required. Chapter 8 provides information about handling linen and laundry and cleaning dishes, glasses, cups, and eating utensils.

Droplet Precautions during Patient Transport

If it is medically necessary for an adult patient requiring Droplet Precautions to leave the home while his or her disease is contagious, the patient should wear a surgical mask. This is frequently not possible with small children because a mask may be frightening to them, and in fact a mask may not be necessary. Every effort should be made to minimize close physical contact between the patient and other persons. The surgical mask is not necessary while the patient is riding in the car with family members who have already been exposed, and it is not necessary for the patient to wear a mask when outdoors. The mask should be put on whenever the patient enters a building or closed space where he or she may come in close contact with others. The same directions for notifying other health care providers as described for Airborne Precautions can be followed for Droplet Precautions. When the patient is no longer on Droplet Precautions, terminal cleaning of the room where the patient resided is not required. Chapter 8 provides additional information about cleaning environmental surfaces in the home.

Contact Precautions

In addition to Standard Precautions, Contact Precautions should be used for patients known or suspected to be infected or colonized with epidemiologically important microorganisms that may be transmitted to others by direct or indirect contact. Direct contact involves skin-to-skin contact with the patient, as occurs in the performance of patient care activities that require touching the patient's skin. Indirect contact involves contact with the patient's care items or environmental surfaces in the home that may be contaminated with pathogenic agents. The patient's environment can be an important reservoir of multidrug-resistant microorganisms because patients may shed these organisms onto horizontal surfaces, bedsheets, and the like (Shlaes et al., 1997).

Diseases or conditions that require Contact Precautions include, but are not limited to, the following:

- gastrointestinal, respiratory, skin, or wound infections or colonization with multidrug-resistant bacteria (e.g., methicillin-resistant *Staphylococcus aureus* and VRE)
- enteric infections with a low infectious dose or prolonged environmental survival (e.g., *Clostridium difficile*)
- enterohemorrhagic *Escherichia coli* 0157:H7, shigellosis, hepatitis A, or rotavirus in patients wearing diapers or those who are incontinent
- respiratory syncytial virus, parainfluenza virus, or enteroviral infections in infants and children
- skin infections that are highly contagious or that may occur on dry skin (cutaneous), including:
  - herpes simplex virus (neonatal or mucocutaneous)
  - impetigo
  - major (noncontained) abscesses, cellulitis, or decubiti
  - pediculosis

  - scabies
  - staphylococcal furunculosis in infants and young children
  - herpes zoster (disseminated or in the immunocompromised host)
- viral or hemorrhagic conjunctivitis
- viral hemorrhagic infections (Ebola, Lassa, or Marburg virus)

Patients with varicella (chickenpox) and disseminated herpes zoster require both contact and Airborne Precautions. Infants and children with adenovirus infection require both Contact and Droplet Precautions (Garner, 1996).

The home care organization should minimize the number of staff members assigned to care for patients who are colonized or infected with multidrug-resistant microorganisms. Other strategies to decrease the risk of transmission to other patients should be considered, including the following:

- Schedule the infected patient for the last visit of the day. If this is not possible, avoid scheduling surgical patients or patients with open skin lesions for visits after the infected patient's.
- Leave reusable patient care items, such as blood pressure cuffs and stethoscopes, in the patient's home. If this is not possible, the equipment or items should be cleaned and disinfected before being used on another patient.
- Minimize the number of items that are taken into the patient's home. The nurse's bag may be left in the car and only necessary items carried into the home in a plastic bag that can be disposed of in the patient's home.
- Minimize the amount of patient care supplies that is allowed to accumulate and will have to be disposed of.
- Perform daily cleaning and disinfection of contaminated patient care items, bedside equipment, and frequently touched horizontal surfaces.

Linen and laundry can be washed with soap and water and do not need any special treatment. Cups and glasses used by the patient should not be shared among family members before being cleaned. No special treatment of dishes and eating utensils is required. Chapter 8 presents additional information about cleaning linens, laundry, dishes, glasses, cups, and eating utensils.

Gowns, Gloves, and Handwashing for Contact Precautions

In addition to wearing gloves as outlined under Standard Precautions, staff should wear clean, nonsterile Latex gloves when entering the patient's room if the patient is infected or colonized with a multidrug-resistant microorganism. Otherwise, gloves should be worn for all patient contact. While providing care to a patient, staff should change gloves after contact with the patient (e.g., when bathing the patient, making the bed, or changing a dressing) or after contact with inanimate objects that may have high concentrations of microorganisms (e.g., items contaminated with stool). Staff should remove gloves before leaving the patient's care area and wash their hands immediately with an antimicrobial agent. Hands can become contaminated via glove leaks or during glove removal. Staff should be careful not to touch potentially contaminated environmental surfaces (e.g., a doorknob, sink, or commode) or items in the patient's room after gloves are removed and the hands are washed to prevent the transfer of microorganisms to the patient's environment or to the next patient visited. The main mode of multidrug-resistant *Staphylococcus aureus* transmission is via contaminated hands of health care workers (CDC, 1997).

In addition to wearing a gown as outlined under Standard Precautions (see Table 7–1), staff should wear a clean, nonsterile gown when providing care for a patient requiring Contact Precautions when there is substantial contact with the patient, environmental surfaces, or items in the patient's room or if such contact is anticipated as well as when the patient is incontinent or has diarrhea, an ileostomy, a colostomy, or uncontained wound drainage. The gown should not be worn out of the patient's room. After the gown is removed, the staff member's clothing should not contact potentially contaminated environmental surfaces to prevent the transmission of microorganisms to the environment or the next patient to be visited.

Contact Precautions during Patient Transport

Patients requiring Contact Precautions may need to attend physician appointments or may wish to visit other sites not related to health care. If possible, the colonized or infected site should be covered. If a visit to another health care provider is necessary (e.g., a physician's office or emergency department), staff at the location should be informed of the need for Contact Precautions on the patient's arrival. If the patient must visit the physician's office, the office staff should be asked to schedule the patient as the last visit of the day.

Guidelines for Discontinuing Contact Precautions

The optimal time to discontinue contact isolation precautions for patients with multidrug-resistant microorganisms such as VRE is not known. Because VRE colonization can persist indefinitely, however, stringent criteria might be appropriate, such as VRE-negative results on at least three consecutive cultures (at least 1 week apart) from multiple body sites (stool or rectal area, perineal area, axilla or umbilicus, and wound, Foley catheter, and/or colostomy sites, if present; CDC, 1995). Multidrug-resistant *Staphylococcus aureus* colonization is also frequently persistent. Multiple negative cultures (at least three obtained on separate days) should be obtained before discontinuation of Contact Precautions is considered. Appendix 7–A provides a list of diseases requiring Contact Precautions and the necessary duration of Contact Precautions.

Once a patient is no longer on Contact Precautions, terminal cleaning of the room where the patient resides is not required. Chapter 8 provides information about cleaning environmental surfaces in the home.

GUIDELINES FOR CARE OF THE NEUTROPENIC PATIENT

Patients who are immunocompromised are generally at risk for bacterial, fungal, parasitic, and viral infections from both exogenous and endogenous sources. The neutrophils (polymorphonuclear leukocytes) are the first line of defense against invading microorganisms. The normal neutrophil count is 2,500/mm^3 to 6,000/mm^3 (40 percent to 60 percent of white blood cells). When the neutrophil count is 1,000/mm^3 or lower, the patient is at high risk for infection.

Within the past 10 years, most hospitals have abandoned the category of protective isolation for neutropenic patients. It is not recommended in the CDC guidelines (Garner, 1996) because there is no evidence to demonstrate its benefit. Staff should adhere to Standard Precautions (and, if applicable, transmission-based precautions for specified patients) and pay rigorous attention to handwashing during the care of the neutropenic patient. In addition, patients themselves may take measures to prevent the acquisition of pathogens during temporary periods of neutropenia. These include the following:

- maintaining an optimal nutritional status
- avoiding the cleaning of bird cages and cat litterboxes and avoiding areas containing dog excreta because excreta contain a high level of fungi and bacteria
- maintaining personal hygiene and cleanliness by showering or bathing daily
- preventing injury to the rectal mucosa by avoiding rectal thermometers, rectal suppositories, enemas, and straining at stool
- assessing for signs of infection frequently by taking the temperature at the same time of the day every day, reporting a temperature greater than 100°F, and reporting any signs or symptoms of infection (e.g., cough with or without sputum, fever, burning on urination, urgency or frequency of urination, or cloudy urine)
- using a soft toothbrush and cleaning the mouth and teeth after every meal
- conserving energy and maintaining adequate periods of sleep and rest
- limiting visitors, clearing visitors for communicable diseases, and avoiding crowded places

INFORMING OTHERS OF ISOLATION PRECAUTIONS WHILE MAINTAINING PATIENT CONFIDENTIALITY

During the patient's initial assessment, the admitting staff member will determine whether additional precautions besides Standard Precautions should be taken. If transmission-based precautions need to be implemented, the staff member will initiate the appropriate precautions, include the information in the clinical record and care plan, and inform the supervisory staff and other staff members who will be providing patient care. The supervisor should also ensure that the appropriate personal protective equipment is available to staff members or that a sufficient supply is available in the patient's home for their use.

Some home care organizations place isolation signs in the patient's home. Isolation signs are not necessary, especially for Standard Precautions. If the home care organization determines that there is some benefit to the use of signs, however, they should be labeled in clinical terms and in such a manner that the general public will not know the patient's diagnosis or the specific clinical condition for which the infection control precautions have been instituted. If isolation signs are used, they should state the kind of precautions that are in effect (i.e., Airborne Precautions, Contact Precautions, etc.). It is a breach in confidentiality for a home care staff member to post a sign that states "possible TB," "TB precautions," "stool precautions," "hepatitis precautions," or "open draining wound."

PATIENT AND FAMILY EDUCATION RELATED TO ISOLATION PRECAUTIONS

Patient and family education related to isolation precautions is important to prevent the transmission of microorganisms from an infected or colonized patient to other individuals in the home via family members. All patients and families should receive basic education on Standard Precautions. As applicable, the patient and family should receive education about Airborne, Droplet, or Contact Precautions. The education should address handwashing, mode of transmission of the infection, how long the patient's disease will be contagious, when isolation precautions can be discontinued, when to use personal protective equipment, patient placement in the home, and strategies to prevent the transmission of infection when the patient must leave the home.

REFERENCES

Centers for Disease Control and Prevention. (1994). Guidelines for preventing the transmission of *Mycobacterium tuberculosis* in health-care facilities. *Morbidity and Mortality Weekly Report, 43*(RR-13), 1–125.

Centers for Disease Control and Prevention. (1995). Recommendations for preventing the spread of vancomycin resistance: Recommendations of the Hospital Infection Control Practices Advisory Committee (HICPAC). *American Journal of Infection Control, 23*, 87–94.

Centers for Disease Control and Prevention. (1997, January 21). Methicillin-resistant *Staphylococcus aureus*. http:/www.cdc.gov/ncidod/diseases/hip/mrsa.htm.

Garner, J.S. (1996). Guideline for isolation precautions in hospitals. *Infection Control and Hospital Epidemiology, 17*, 53–80.

Shlaes, D.M., Gerding, D.N., John, J.F., Craig, W.A., Bornsteril, D.L., Duncan, R.A., Eckman, M.R., Farrer, W.E., Greene, W.H., Lorian, V., Levy, S., McGowan, J.E., Paul, S.M., Ruskin, J., Tenover, F.C., & Watanakunakorn, C. (1997). Society for Healthcare Epidemiology of America and Infectious Diseases Society of America Joint Committee on the Prevention of Antimicrobial Resistance: Guidelines for the prevention of antimicrobial resistance in hospitals. *Infection Control and Hospital Epidemiology, 18*, 275–291.

Appendix 7–A

Type and Duration of Precautions Needed for Selected Infections and Conditions

Infection/Condition	Precautions Type*	Precautions Duration†
Abscess		
Draining, major[1]	C	DI
Draining, minor or limited[2]	S	
Acquired immune deficiency syndrome[3]	S	
Actinomycosis	S	
Adenovirus infection, in infants and young children	D, C	DI
Amebiasis	S	
Anthrax		
Cutaneous	S	
Pulmonary	S	
Antibiotic-associated colitis (see *Clostridium difficile*)		
Arthropodborne viral encephalitides (eastern, western, Venezuelan equine encephalomyelitis; St. Louis, California encephalitis)	S[4]	
Arthropodborne viral fevers (dengue, yellow fever, Colorado tick fever)	S[4]	
Ascariasis	S	
Aspergillosis	S	
Babesiosis	S	
Blastomycosis: North American, cutaneous, or pulmonary	S	
Botulism	S	
Bronchiolitis (see respiratory infections in infants and young children)		
Brucellosis (undulant, Malta, Mediterranean fever)	S	
Campylobacter gastroenteritis (see gastroenteritis)		
Candidiasis, all forms including mucocutaneous	S	
Cat-scratch fever (benign inoculation lymphoreticulosis)	S	
Cellulitis, uncontrolled drainage	C	DI

* A, airborne; C, contact; D, droplet; S, standard. When A, C, or D is specified, also use S.

† CN, until off antibiotics and culture is negative; DI, for the duration of illness (with wound lesions, until wound stops draining); U, until time specified (in hours) after initiation of effective therapy; F, see footnote.

1. No dressing or dressing does not contain drainage adequately.
2. Dressing covers and contains drainage adequately.
3. Also see syndromes or conditions listed in Table 2.
4. Install screens in windows and doors in endemic areas.

Source: Reprinted with permission from J.S. Garner, Guideline for Isolation Precautions in Hospitals, *Infection Control and Hospital Epidemiology,* Vol. 17, No. 1, pp. 53–80, © 1996, Slack, Inc.

Infection/Condition	*Precautions*	
	*Type**	*Duration†*
Chancroid (soft chancre)	S	
Chickenpox (varicella; see F[5] for varicella exposure)	A, C	F[5]
Chlamydia trachomatis		
Conjunctivitis	S	
Genital	S	
Respiratory	S	
Cholera (see gastroenteritis)		
Closed cavity infection		
Draining, limited or minor	S	
Not draining	S	
Clostridium		
C. botulinum	S	
C. difficile	C	DI
C. perfringens		
Food poisoning	S	
Gas gangrene	S	
Coccidioidomycosis (valley fever)		
Draining lesions	S	
Pneumonia	S	
Colorado tick fever	S	
Congenital rubella	C	F[6]
Conjunctivitis		
Acute bacterial	S	
Chlamydia spp.	S	
Gonococcal	S	
Acute viral (acute hemorrhagic)	C	DI
Coxsackievirus disease (see enteroviral infections)		
Creutzfeldt-Jakob disease	S[7]	
Croup (see respiratory infections in infants and young children)		
Cryptococcosis	S	
Cryptosporidiosis (see gastroenteritis)		
Cysticercosis	S	
Cytomegalovirus infection, neonatal or immunosuppressed	S	
Decubitus ulcer, infected		
Major[1]	C	DI
Minor or limited[2]	S	
Dengue	S[4]	
Diarrhea, acute infective etiology suspected (see gastroenteritis)		
Diphtheria		
Cutaneous	C	CN[8]
Pharyngeal	D	CN[8]

5. Maintain precautions until all lesions are crusted. The average incubation period for varicella is 10 to 16 days (range, 10 to 21 days). After exposure, use varicella zoster immune globulin (VZIG) when appropriate, and discharge susceptible patients if possible. Place exposed susceptible patients on airborne precautions beginning 10 days after first exposure and continuing until 21 days after last exposure (up to 28 days if VZIG has been given). Susceptible persons should not enter the room of patients on precautions if other immune caregivers are available.
6. Place infant on precautions during any admission until 1 year of age, unless nasopharyngeal and urine cultures are negative for virus after age 3 months.
7. Additional special precautions are necessary for handling and decontamination of blood, body fluids, tissues, and contaminated items from patients with confirmed or suspected disease. See latest College of American Pathologists guidelines or other references.
8. Until two cultures taken at least 24 hours apart are negative.

continues

Appendix 7–A continued

Infection/Condition	*Precautions*	
	*Type**	*Duration†*
Ebola viral hemorrhagic fever	C[9]	DI
Echinococcosis (hydatidosis)	S	
Echovirus (see enteroviral infections)		
Encephalitis or encephalomyelitis (see specific etiologic agents)		
Endometritis	S	
Enterobiasis (pinworm disease, oxyuriasis)	S	
Enterococcus spp. (see multidrug-resistant microorganisms if epidemiologically significant or vancomycin resistant)		
Enterocolitis, *Clostridium difficile*	C	DI
Enteroviral infections		
Adults	S	
Infants and young children	C	DI
Epiglottitis, due to *Haemophilus influenzae*	D	U (24 hours)
Epstein-Barr virus infection including infectious mononucleosis	S	
Erythema infectiosum (also see parvovirus B19)	S	
Escherichia coli gastroenteritis (see gastroenteritis)		
Food poisoning		
Botulism	S	
Clostridium perfringens or *C. welchii*	S	
Staphylococcal	S	
Furunculosis, staphylococcal		
Infants and young children	C	DI
Gangrene (gas gangrene)	S	
Gastroenteritis		
Campylobacter spp.	S[10]	
Cholera	S[10]	
Clostridium difficile	C	DI
Cryptosporidium spp.	S[10]	
Escherichia coli		
Enterohemorrhagic O157:H7	S[10]	
Diapered or incontinent	C	DI
Other species	S[10]	
Giardia lamblia	S[10]	
Rotavirus	S[10]	
Diapered or incontinent	C	DI
Salmonella spp. (including *S. typhi*)	S[10]	
Shigella spp.	S[10]	
Diapered or incontinent	C	DI
Vibrio parahaemolyticus	S[10]	
Viral (if not covered elsewhere)	S[10]	
Yersinia enterocolitica	S[10]	
German measles (see rubella)		
Giardiasis (see gastroenteritis)		
Gonococcal ophthalmia neonatorum (gonorrheal ophthalmia, acute conjunctivitis of newborn)	S	
Gonorrhea	S	
Granuloma inguinale (donovanosis, granuloma venereum)	S	

9. Call the state health department and the Centers for Disease Control and Prevention for specific advice about management of a suspected case. During the 1995 Ebola outbreak in Zaire, interim recommendations were published. Pending a comprehensive review of the epidemiological data from the outbreak and evaluation of the interim recommendations, the 1988 guidelines for management of patients with suspected viral hemorrhagic infections will be reviewed and updated if indicated.
10. Use contact precautions for diapered or incontinent children younger than 6 years of age for the duration of illness.

Infection/Condition	*Precautions*	
	*Type**	*Duration†*
Guillain-Barré syndrome	S	
Hand, foot, and mouth disease (see enteroviral infections)		
Hantavirus pulmonary syndrome	S	
Helicobacter pylori	S	
Hemorrhagic fevers (e.g., Lassa and Ebola)	C[9]	DI
Hepatitis, viral		
Type A	S	
Diapered or incontinent patients	C	F[11]
Type B, HBsAg positive	S	
Type C and other unspecified non-A, non-B	S	
Type E	S	
Herpangina (see enteroviral infections)		
Herpes simplex (Herpesvirus hominis)		
Encephalitis	S	
Neonatal[12] (see F[6] for neonatal exposure)	C	DI
Mucocutaneous, disseminated or primary, severe	C	DI
Mucocutaneous, recurrent (skin, oral, genital)	S	
Herpes zoster (varicella-zoster)		
Localized in immunocompromised patient, or disseminated	A, C	DI[13]
Localized in normal patient	S[13]	
Histoplasmosis	S	
HIV (see human immunodeficiency virus)	S	
Hookworm disease (ancylostomiasis, uncinariasis)	S	
Human immunodeficiency virus (HIV infection)	S	
Impetigo	C	U (24 hours)
Infectious mononucleosis	S	
Influenza	D[14]	DI
Kawasaki syndrome	S	
Lassa fever	C[9]	DI
Legionnaires' disease	S	
Leprosy	S	
Leptospirosis	S	
Lice (pediculosis)	C	U (24 hours)
Listeriosis	S	
Lyme disease	S	
Lymphocytic choriomeningitis	S	
Lymphogranuloma venereum	S	
Malaria	S[4]	
Marburg virus disease	C[9]	DI
Measles (rubeola), all presentations	A	DI
Melioidosis, all forms	S	
Meningitis		
Aseptic (nonbacterial or viral meningitis; also see enteroviral infections)	S	

11. Maintain precautions in infants and children younger than 3 years of age for the duration of hospitalization, in children 3 to 14 years of age until 2 weeks after onset of symptoms, and in others until 1 week after onset of symptoms.
12. For infants delivered vaginally or by cesarean section and if mother has active infection and membranes have been ruptured for more than 4 to 6 hours.
13. Persons susceptible to varicella are also at risk for developing varicella when exposed to patients with herpes zoster lesions; therefore, susceptibles should not enter the room if other immune caregivers are available.
14. The *Guideline for Prevention of Nosocomial Pneumonia* recommends surveillance, vaccination, antiviral agents, and use of private rooms with negative air pressure as much as feasible for patients for whom influenza is suspected or diagnosed. Many hospitals encounter logistic difficulties and physical plant limitations when admitting multiple patients with suspected influenza during community outbreaks. If sufficient private rooms are unavailable, consider cohorting patients, or, at the very least, avoid room sharing with high-risk patients.

continues

Appendix 7–A continued

Infection/Condition	Precautions Type*	Precautions Duration†
Bacterial, Gram-negative enteric, in neonates	S	
Fungal	S	
Haemophilus influenzae, known or suspected	D	U (24 hours)
Listeria monocytogenes	S	
Neisseria meningitidis (meningococcal) known or suspected	D	U (24 hours)
Pneumococcal	S	
Tuberculosis[15]	S	
Other diagnosed bacterial	S	
Meningococcal pneumonia	D	U (24 hours)
Meningococcemia (meningococcal sepsis)	D	U (24 hours)
Molluscum contagiosum	S	
Mucormycosis	S	
Multidrug-resistant microorganisms, infection or colonization[16]		
Gastrointestinal	C	CN
Respiratory	C	CN
Pneumococcal	S	
Skin, wound, or burn	C	CN
Mumps (infectious parotitis)	D	F[17]
Mycobacteria, nontuberculosis (atypical)		
Pulmonary	S	
Wound	S	
Mycoplasma pneumoniae	D	DI
Necrotizing enterocolitis	S	
Nocardiosis, draining lesions or other presentations	S	
Norwalk agent gastroenteritis (see viral gastroenteritis)		
Orf	S	
Parainfluenza virus infection, respiratory in infants and young children	C	DI
Parvovirus B19	D	F[18]
Pediculosis (lice)	C	U (24 hours)
Pertussis (whooping cough)	D	F[19]
Pinworm infection	S	
Plague		
Bubonic	S	
Pneumonic	D	U (72 hours)
Pleurodynia (see enteroviral infections)		
Pneumonia		
Adenovirus	D, C	DI
Bacterial not listed elsewhere (including Gram-negative bacterial)	S	
Burkholderia cepacia in cystic fibrosis (CF) patients, including respiratory tract colonization	S[20]	
Chlamydia	S	
Fungal	S	

15. Patient should be examined for evidence of current (active) pulmonary tuberculosis. If evidence exists, additional precautions are necessary (see tuberculosis).
16. Resistant bacteria judged by the infection control program, based on current state, regional, or national recommendations, to be of special clinical and epidemiologic significance.
17. For 9 days after onset of swelling.
18. Maintain precautions for the duration of hospitalization when chronic disease occurs in an immunodeficient patient. For patients with transient aplastic crisis or red cell crisis, maintain precautions for 7 days.
19. Maintain precautions until 5 days after patient is placed on effective therapy.
20. Avoid cohorting or placement in the same room with a CF patient who is not infected or colonized with *B. cepacia*. Persons with CF who visit or provide care and are not infected or colonized with *B. cepacia* may elect to wear a mask when within 3 feet of a colonized or infected patient.

Infection/Condition	*Precautions* Type*	Duration†
Haemophilus influenzae		
Adults	S	
Infants and children (any age)	D	U (24 hours)
Legionella	S	
Meningococcal	D	U (24 hours)
Multidrug-resistant bacterial (see multidrug-resistant microorganisms)		
Mycoplasma (primary atypical pneumonia)	D	DI
Pneumococcal	S	
Multidrug-resistant (see multidrug-resistant microorganisms)		
Pneumocystis carinii	S[21]	
Pseudomonas cepacia (see *Burkholderia cepacia* under this heading)	S[20]	
Staphylococcus aureus	S	
Streptococcus, group A		
Adults	S	
Infants and young children	D	U (24 hours)
Viral		
Adults	S	
Infants and young children (see respiratory infectious disease, acute)		
Poliomyelitis	S	
Psittacosis (ornithosis)	S	
Q fever	S	
Rabies	S	
Rat-bite fever (*Streptobacillus moniliformis* disease, *Spirillum minus* disease)	S	
Relapsing fever	S	
Resistant bacterial infection or colonization (see multidrug-resistant microorganisms)		
Respiratory infectious disease, acute (if not covered elsewhere)		
Adults	S	
Infants and young children[3]	C	DI
Respiratory syncytial virus infection, in infants, young children, and immunocompromised adults	C	DI
Reye's syndrome	S	
Rheumatic fever	S	
Rickettsial fevers, tickborne (Rocky Mountain spotted fever, tickborne typhus fever)	S	
Rickettsialpox (vesicular rickettsiosis)	S	
Ringworm (dermatophytosis, dermatomycosis, tinea)	S	
Ritter's disease (staphylococcal scalded skin syndrome)	S	
Rocky Mountain spotted fever	S	
Roseola infantum (exanthem subitum)	S	
Rotavirus infection (see gastroenteritis)		
Rubella (German measles; also see congenital rubella)	D	F[22]
Salmonellosis (see gastroenteritis)		
Scabies	C	U (24 hours)
Scalded skin syndrome, staphylococcal (Ritter's disease)	S	
Schistosomiasis (bilharziasis)	S	
Shigellosis (see gastroenteritis)		
Sporotrichosis	S	

21. Avoid placement in the same room with an immunocompromised patient.
22. Until 7 days after onset of rash.

continues

Appendix 7–A continued

Infection/Condition	*Precautions*	
	*Type**	*Duration†*
Spirillum minus disease (rat-bite fever)	S	
Staphylococcal disease (*S. aureus*)		
Skin, wound, or burn		
Major[1]	C	DI
Minor or limited[2]	S	
Enterocolitis	S[10]	
Multidrug-resistant (see multidrug-resistant microorganisms)		
Pneumonia	S	
Scalded skin syndrome	S	
Toxic shock syndrome	S	
Streptobacillus moniliformis disease (rat-bite fever)	S	
Streptococcal disease (group A streptococcus)		
Skin, wound, or burn		
Major[1]	C	U (24 hours)
Minor or limited[2]	S	
Endometritis (puerperal sepsis)	S	
Pharyngitis in infants and young children	D	U (24 hours)
Pneumonia in infants and young children	D	U (24 hours)
Scarlet fever in infants and young children	D	U (24 hours)
Streptococcal disease (group B streptococcus), neonatal	S	
Streptococcal disease (not group A or B) unless covered elsewhere	S	
Multidrug-resistant (see multidrug-resistant microorganisms)		
Strongyloidiasis	S	
Syphilis		
Skin and mucus membrane, including congenital, primary, secondary	S	
Latent (tertiary) and seropositivity without lesions	S	
Tapeworm disease		
Hymenolepis nana	S	
Taenia solium (pork)	S	
Other	S	
Tetanus	S	
Tinea (fungus infection, dermatophytosis, dermatomycosis, ringworm)	S	
Toxoplasmosis	S	
Toxic shock syndrome (staphylococcal disease)	S	
Trachoma, acute	S	
Trench mouth (Vincent's angina)	S	
Trichinosis	S	
Trichomoniasis	S	
Trichuriasis (whipworm disease)	S	
Tuberculosis		
Extrapulmonary, draining lesion (including scrofula)	S	
Extrapulmonary, meningitis[15]	S	
Pulmonary, confirmed or suspected or laryngeal disease	A	F[23]
Skin-test positive with no evidence of current pulmonary disease	S	
Tularemia		
Draining lesion	S	
Pulmonary	S	
Typhoid (*Salmonella typhi*) fever (see gastroenteritis)		
Typhus, endemic and epidemic	S	

23. Discontinue precautions *only* when TB patient is on effective therapy, is improving clinically, and has three consecutive negative sputum smears collected on different days or when TB is ruled out. Also see CDC *Guidelines for Preventing the Transmission of Tuberculosis in Health-Care Facilities.*

Infection/Condition	Precautions	
	*Type**	*Duration†*
Urinary tract infection (including pyelonephritis), with or without urinary catheter	S	
Varicella (chickenpox)	A, C	F[5]
Vibrio parahaemolyticus (see gastroenteritis)		
Vincent's angina (trench mouth)	S	
Viral diseases		
Respiratory (if not covered elsewhere)		
Adults	S	
Infants and young children (see respiratory infectious disease, acute)		
Whooping cough (pertussis)	D	F[19]
Wound infections		
Major[1]	C	DI
Minor or limited[2]	S	
Yersinia enterocolitica gastroenteritis (see gastroenteritis)		
Zoster (varicella-zoster)		
Localized in immunocompromised patient, disseminated	A, C	DI[13]
Localized in normal patient	S[13]	
Zygomycosis (phycomycosis, mucormycosis)	S	

Chapter 8

Cleaning and Disinfecting Patient Care Equipment

Because it is not possible or necessary to sterilize all equipment used in patient care, the home care organization's policies and procedures should identify whether cleaning, disinfecting, or sterilizing an item is needed to decrease the risk of infection. Any microorganism, including bacterial spores, that comes in contact with normally sterile tissue can cause an infection. Therefore, in general all equipment and supplies that will come in contact with normally sterile tissue should be sterile themselves, although there are some exceptions based on a large accumulation of experience without adverse outcomes (e.g., urinary catheters used for self-catheterization). Equipment and supplies that come in contact with mucus membranes must be cleaned and disinfected to kill all microorganisms except resistant bacterial spores. Equipment and supplies that touch intact skin should minimally be clean.

DEFINITION OF TERMS

Cleaning is the physical removal of visible organic material or soil from objects, environmental surfaces, and skin. A detergent or enzymatic product used with water to apply friction can accomplish cleaning. Cleaning will remove most microorganisms but will not destroy them. Decontamination is the use of physical or chemical means to remove, inactivate, or destroy pathogens on a surface or item to the point where the item or surface is no longer capable of transmitting infectious particles and is rendered safe for handling, use, or disposal (Occupational Safety and Health Administration [OSHA], 1991).

A germicide is an agent that destroys microorganisms on both living tissue and inanimate objects, hence the suffix *-cide* to reflect the destruction of microorganisms. There are three types of germicides: antiseptics, disinfectants, and chemical sterilants. An antiseptic is a germicide that eliminates all pathogenic microorganisms, except bacterial spores, from the skin or tissue. Antiseptics should not be used to decontaminate inanimate objects. A disinfectant is a germicide that eliminates all pathogenic microorganisms, except bacterial spores, from inanimate objects. Disinfection is an intermediate process between cleaning and sterilizing an inanimate object. The disinfection process uses chemicals that are stronger than soap and water. Before an item can be disinfected, it must be cleaned because organic matter, such as blood, can neutralize the disinfectant, and the disinfectant may not be able to penetrate the debris and destroy microorganisms.

In home care, disinfection is usually accomplished by soaking, spraying, or drenching an item in liquid chemicals for several minutes (to give the chemical time to kill the microorganisms) or by wet pasteurization (i.e., boiling for up to 30 minutes after detergent cleaning). Commercial products that meet the Environmental Protection Agency's (EPA's) standards for hospital grade germicides may be used for this purpose. One of the most commonly used chemicals for disinfection is a homemade solution of household bleach and water. Bleach is inexpensive and easy to obtain. The solution of bleach and water is easy to mix, is nontoxic, is safe if handled properly, and kills most infectious agents. (Be aware that some infectious agents are not killed by bleach. For example, *Cryptosporidium* species are only killed by ammonia or hydrogen peroxide.) If a commercially prepared disinfectant is used, it should only be used as noted on the label, and the manufacturer's instructions should be followed exactly.

The effectiveness of the disinfection process is determined by the following factors (Rutala, 1996):

- whether the object was cleaned before it was disinfected
- the object's organic load (i.e., the amount of soil and contamination)
- the type and level of microbial contamination
- the type, concentration of, and contact time with the germicide
- the physical configuration of the object
- the temperature and pH of the disinfection process

Sterilization is the complete removal of all forms of microbial life, including bacterial spores. Either physical or chemical processes, such as steam under pressure, dry heat, ethylene oxide gas, or liquid chemicals, accomplish sterilization. The sterilization process is usually not performed in home care either at the office or in the patient's home. Therefore, this chapter focuses primarily on disinfecting medical equipment in home care.

LEVELS OF DISINFECTION

Disinfectants vary in the way they work and in their active ingredients. Not all disinfectants perform in the same manner. For this reason, they are categorized by the level to which they eradicate microorganisms. The three levels of disinfection are low-level, intermediate, or high-level disinfection. High-level disinfection destroys all microorganisms except bacterial spores. Intermediate disinfection destroys *Mycobacterium tuberculosis*, vegetative bacteria, and most fungi and neutralizes most viruses but does not kill bacterial spores. Low-level disinfection destroys most bacteria, some viruses, and some fungi but may not destroy resistant microorganisms (e.g., tubercle bacilli or bacterial spores; Rutala, 1996).

INFECTION RISK CLASSIFICATION SYSTEM

Spaulding (1968) developed a classification system for cleaning, disinfection, and sterilization of medical equipment and supplies. The classification is based on the potential risk of infection identified in the use of the medical equipment and supplies. This potential risk can be classified into three categories of noncritical items, semicritical items, and critical items. Noncritical, semicritical, and critical items that may be used in the home care setting include, but are not limited to, those identified in Table 8–1.

Noncritical items come in contact with intact skin but not mucus membranes. Intact skin serves as an effective barrier to most microorganisms; therefore, sterility is not essential. Except under special circumstances, items that do not ordinarily touch the patient or touch only intact skin are not involved in disease transmission and generally do not necessitate cleaning or disinfection between uses on different patients unless they become soiled. If a patient is infected or colonized with vancomycin-resistant enterocci or other multidrug-resistant microorganisms, reusable noncritical items should be cleaned with a low-level disinfectant between patient uses, or such items should be assigned to each patient (Centers for Disease Control and Prevention [CDC], 1995). Low-level disinfection can be achieved with a chemical germicide registered as a hospital disinfectant by the EPA. Semicritical items come in contact with mucus membranes or skin that is nonintact. Intact mucus membranes are generally resistant to infection but are susceptible to viruses and the tubercle bacilli. Semicritical items should be disinfected with either an intermediate or high-level disinfectant solution. Most semicritical items require a high-level disinfection with either wet pasteurization (boiling) or a chemical disinfectant approved by the Food and Drug Administration (FDA). Some semicritical items, such as tubs used for patients whose skin is not intact or thermometers placed in the patient's mouth or rectum, may require only intermediate disinfection. Intermediate level disinfection can be achieved with a chemical germicide registered as a tuberculocide by the EPA. Critical items directly enter into the bloodstream or into other normally sterile areas of the body and present a risk of infection if they are contaminated with any microorganism.

The EPA is the government agency that is responsible for overseeing the registration of sterilants, tuberculocidal disinfectants, disinfectants for human immunodeficiency virus (HIV), disinfectants for hepatitis B virus (HBV), and antimicrobial products. A list of EPA-registered products may be obtained by contacting the National Antimicrobial Information Network at (800) 447-6349 or http://www.ace.orst.edu/info/nain/index.htm. The National Antimicrobial Information

Table 8–1 Categorization of Home Care Equipment

Noncritical Items	*Semicritical Items*	*Critical Items*
Apnea monitor	Oral or rectal thermometers	Dialysate solution
Back support belt	Laryngeal mirror	IV fluids
Bandage scissors	Tub used for soaking nonintact skin	IV catheters and tubing
Bath basin	Oral suction catheter	Irrigation solution
Blood pressure cuff	Respiratory therapy equipment:	Needles
Blood glucose monitor	• Humidifier	Tracheal suction catheter
Bedpan	• Nebulizer and reservoir	Urinary catheter
Cane	• Oral airway	
Commode	• Breathing circuit of mechanical ventilators	
Crutches	• Manual ventilation bag	
Doppler unit	• Nasal cannula	
Hydrotherapy equipment		
Infusion pump		
IV pole		
Linen		
Nail clippers		
Pulse oximeter		
Scales		
Shampoo board		
Stethoscope		
Suction collection canister		
Tape measure		
Tympanic or axillary thermometer		
Ultrasonic stimulator		
Urinal		
Walker		
Wheelchair		
Work surfaces		

Source: Friedman, M. (1996) Designing an Infection Control Program to Meet JCAHO's Standards. *CARING* 15, 18–25. Used with permission.

Network is a cooperative effort between Oregon State University and the EPA.

OSHA's bloodborne pathogen regulations require that contaminated surfaces and items be decontaminated with an appropriate disinfectant. OSHA considers the following to be appropriate disinfectants:

- EPA-registered tuberculocidal disinfectants
- solutions of 5.25 percent sodium hypochlorite (household bleach) diluted between 1:10 and 1:100 with water
- EPA-registered disinfectants for HIV and HBV

An EPA-registered disinfectant for HIV and HBV can be used under limited circumstances provided that such surfaces have not become contaminated with the infective agent or with volumes or concentrations of the agent for which a higher disinfection level is recommended (OSHA, 1997).

GUIDELINES FOR CLEANING AND DISINFECTION

The choice of disinfectant used depends on the category of medical equipment or supplies used (i.e., critical, semicritical, or noncritical), the type of object to be cleaned, the length of exposure, and the methods needed to achieve the correct level of disinfection. Table 8–2 contains the methods of disinfection for the three categories of medical equipment and supplies. Types of disinfectants used in home care include alcohol, hydrogen peroxide, phenolics, iodophors, chlorine and chlorine compounds, and acetic acid.

Table 8–2 Methods of Sterilization and Disinfection

	Sterilization		*Disinfection*		
	Critical Items (will enter tissue or vascular system or blood will flow through them)		*High-level (semicritical items; will come in contact with mucus membrane or nonintact skin)*	*Intermediate Level (some semicritical items[a] and noncritical items)*	*Low-level (noncritical items; will come in contact with intact skin)*
Object	*Procedure*	*Exposure Time (hr)*	*Procedure (exposure time ≥20 min)[b,c]*	*Procedure (exposure time ≤10 min)*	*Procedure (exposure time ≤10 min)*
Smooth, hard surface[a]	A	MR	C	I	I
	B	MR	D	K	J
	C	MR	E	L	K
	D	6	F		L
	E	6	G[d]		M
	F	MR	H		
Rubber tubing and catheters[c]	A	MR	C		
	B	MR	D		
	C	MR	E		
	D	6	F		
	E	6	G[d]		
	F	MR			
Polyethylene tubing and catheters[c,e]	A	MR	C		
	B	MR	D		
	C	MR	E		
	D	6	F		
	E	6	G[d]		
	F	MR			
Lensed instruments	B	MR	C		
	C	MR	D		
	D	6	E	E	
	E	6	F	F	
	F	MR			
Thermometers (oral and rectal)[f]				I[f]	
Hinged instruments	A	MR	C		
	B	MR	D		
	C	MR	E		
	D	6	F		
	E	6			
	F				

A, Heat sterilization, including steam or hot air (see manufacturer's recommendations)
B, Ethylene oxide gas (see manufacturer's recommendations)
C, Glutaraldehyde-based formulations (2%) (caution should be exercised with all glutaraldehyde formulations when further in-use dilution is anticipated)
D, Demand-release chlorine dioxide (will corrode aluminum, copper, brass, series 400 stainless steel, and chrome with prolonged exposure)
E, Stabilized hydrogen peroxide 6% (will corrode copper, zinc, and brass)
F, Peracetic acid, concentration variable but ≤1% is sporicidal
G, Wet pasteurization at 70°C for 30 min after detergent cleaning
H, Sodium hypochlorite (1000 ppm available chlorine; will corrode metal instruments)
I, Ethyl or isopropyl alcohol (70%–90%)
J, Sodium hypochlorite (100 ppm available chlorine)
K, Phenolic germicidal detergent solution (follow product label for use-dilution)
L, Iodophor germicidal detergent solution (follow product label for use-dilution)
M, Quaternary ammonium germicidal detergent solution (follow product label for use-dilution)
MR, Manufacturer's recommendations

[a] See text for discussion of hydrotherapy.

[b] The longer the exposure to a disinfectant, the more likely it is that all microorganisms will be eliminated. Ten-min exposure is not adequate to disinfect many objects, especially those that are difficult to clean because they have narrow channels or other areas that can harbor organic material and bacteria. Twenty-min exposure is the minimum time needed to reliably kill *M. tuberculosis* and nontuberculous Mycobacteria with glutaraldehyde.

[c] Tubing must be completely filled for disinfection; care must be taken to avoid entrapment of air bubbles during immersion.

[d] Pasteurization (washer disinfector) of respiratory therapy and anesthesia equipment is a recognized alternative to high-level disinfection. Some data challenge the efficacy of some pasteurization units.

[e] Thermostability should be investigated when appropriate.

[f] Do not mix rectal and oral thermometers at any stage of handling or processing.

Source: Reprinted with permission from W.A. Rutala, Disinfection, Sterilization, and Waste Disposal in *Prevention and Control of Nosocomial Infections*, pp. 540–541, © 1997, Williams & Wilkins.

Cleaning Equipment

Removing all organic matter from the equipment to be disinfected is the most important step in the disinfection process. If the equipment is not properly cleaned first, the disinfection process will not be effective. Cleaning consists of washing an item with a detergent or a disinfectant-detergent and water, rinsing the item, and thoroughly drying it. Many items may need to be cleaned before they can be disinfected because organic material, such as total parenteral nutrition solution, enteral feeding solution, or blood, may have collected on the surface and contain high concentrations of microorganisms. Reusable equipment should not be provided to or used by another patient until it has been cleaned and reprocessed appropriately.

Disinfecting Equipment

The disinfection process usually entails cleaning the object, then soaking, spraying, or wiping down the object with the chemical disinfecting solution, and finally leaving the solution on the object for the required period of time. When medical equipment, such as a commode, is picked up at the patient's home by a delivery driver, the driver may decontaminate the equipment to make it safe for handling by spraying it down with a disinfectant and waiting the allotted time for it to dry before placing it in the delivery vehicle. The equipment may not be properly disinfected, however, because it was not first cleaned, and organic matter may inhibit the disinfection process. Therefore, when the equipment is returned to the facility, it will need to be properly cleaned and disinfected so that it is ready for patient use.

When disinfectants are used, precautions should be taken to prevent or minimize the home care staff member's exposure to either the chemical disinfectant solution or the microorganisms being removed from the equipment. Precautions should be taken by using personal protective equipment such as gloves and other items as necessary. Utility gloves are recommended when equipment is being cleaned before the disinfecting procedure because Latex or vinyl gloves can easily rip and expose the home care staff member to the chemical solution as well as potentially infectious material. When the equipment is removed from the solution after the soaking time period has been completed, clean Latex or vinyl gloves should be worn. A gown, mask, and goggles or face shield may be needed if the cleaning method may result in splashing of the solution.

How To Prepare a Bleach Disinfecting Solution

An inexpensive environmental germicide that may be used on surfaces and is effective against HIV is a 1:10 solution of 5.25 percent sodium hypochlorite (household bleach). A 1:10 bleach solution is 1 part bleach to 9 parts water, and a 1:5 solution is 1 part bleach to 4 parts water (Rutala, 1996). Exhibit 8–1 explains how to make two different bleach disinfecting solutions.

Bleach Disinfecting Solution Storage

A bleach and water solution loses its strength quickly and is weakened by organic material, evaporation, heat, and sunlight. Therefore, a 1:10 bleach solution should be mixed fresh each day to ensure that it is effective. Any leftover solution should be discarded down the sink or toilet at the end of the day. A 1:5 bleach solution may be stored for 30 days in an opaque container (or brown glass), at room temperature, and out of sunlight. Bleach must never be mixed with anything but fresh tap water. Other chemicals may react with bleach and release a toxic chlorine gas. The bleach and water solution should be stored in a cool place out of direct sunlight and out of the reach of children. Bleach is corrosive to metals, especially aluminum, and should not be used to decontaminate medical equipment with metallic parts.

Noncritical Item Disinfection Guidelines

A noncritical item is one that will not come in contact with mucus membranes or skin that is not intact. Such

Exhibit 8–1 How To Make Bleach Disinfecting Solutions

To make a 1:10 bleach disinfecting solution:
Combine 1/2 cup bleach with 1 quart water
or
1/4 cup bleach with 2 1/4 cups water
To make a 1:5 bleach disinfecting solution:
Combine 1/2 cup bleach with 2 cups water
or
1/4 cup bleach with 1 cup water

items may undergo low-level disinfection. If a noncritical item has been contaminated or is visibly contaminated with blood or other potentially infectious materials, the staff member should wear gloves and first scrub the item with detergent and water, dry it with a disposable towel, and then disinfect it. Items that cannot be cleaned and disinfected without altering their physical integrity and function should not be reused. There is a potential risk, however, of home care staff members transmitting infectious agents to other patients if their hands become contaminated by touching a contaminated noncritical item. From this derives the importance of handwashing to prevent the spread of infection.

Low-level disinfection may be accomplished by using one of the following germicides (Rutala, 1996):

- ethyl or isopropyl alcohol (70 percent to 90 percent)
- sodium hypochlorite (5.25 percent household bleach), 1:500 dilution
- phenolic germicidal detergent solution (e.g., Lysol) diluted according to the product label
- iodophor germicidal solution (e.g., povidone-iodine) diluted according to the product label
- quaternary ammonium germicidal solution diluted according to the product label

Disinfectants should be left on the product for the time specified; otherwise it will not be properly disinfected. These guidelines are recommended for patients in whom only standard precautions are utilized in the course of care. Additional cleaning measures will need to be taken for patients who are infected or colonized with multidrug resistant bacteria or those on contact precautions for other diagnosis. Refer to Chapter 7 for additional information.

Blood Pressure Cuff

Blood pressure cuffs generally only touch intact skin. According to the CDC, blood pressure cuffs placed on clean, intact skin do not have to be cleaned between patient uses (Garner & Favero, 1986). It is up to the staff member to use his or her judgment as to whether the blood pressure cuff has become contaminated. If it does become contaminated, it can be washed with a detergent or a disinfectant-detergent, rinsed, and dried. Wiping the cuff and aneroid gauge with 70 percent isopropyl alcohol or another appropriate disinfectant also may be used to clean the blood pressure cuff and aneroid gauge. If a patient's skin is not intact, the staff member should wear gloves when taking the patient's blood pressure. Other options are to leave a blood pressure cuff in the patient's home to be picked up by the home care organization for cleaning and disinfecting when the patient is discharged, providing the patient a disposable blood pressure cuff, or placing a disposable impermeable barrier between the patient's skin and the cuff to prevent the cuff from becoming soiled.

Stethoscopes

A stethoscope generally only touches intact skin. According to the CDC, a stethoscope placed on clean, intact skin does not have to be cleaned routinely between patient uses. Some home care organizations, however, choose to wipe the stethoscope with 70 percent isopropyl alcohol or another appropriate disinfectant to keep it clean after each use. Each home care organization should have written guidelines regarding how and when stethoscopes must be cleaned.

Thermometers: Axillary or Tympanic

Whenever possible, each patient should use his or her own thermometer. If a glass mercury thermometer or battery-operated digital thermometer from the nursing supply bag is utilized, a plastic protective sheath should be placed over the tip before it is used with the patient. After patient use, the plastic sheath should be discarded. Because thermometers used for taking temperatures via the axillary and tympanic routes generally are in contact with intact skin, according to the CDC they do not have to be cleaned routinely between patient uses.

Laboratory Supplies

Vacuum container sleeves and tourniquets that have become contaminated with blood should be discarded. Otherwise, for normal, routine use, a vacuum container sleeve or tourniquet that has been placed on clean, intact skin should be cleaned and disinfected with 70 percent isopropyl alcohol between patient uses.

Environmental Surfaces in the Home

Microorganisms are a normal contaminant of floors, walls, and other surfaces but are rarely associated with the transmission of infections to patients or staff members. Nevertheless, routine cleaning and removal of soil are recommended. The same routine cleaning procedures are to be performed regardless of whether the patient is on standard precautions or transmission-based precautions. Disinfecting noncritical items that a patient may come in contact with, such as stethoscopes, door knobs, faucet handles, and telephone handsets, may be indicated for certain pathogens, such as multidrug-resistant microorganisms, especially enterocci, that can survive on an inanimate object for extensive periods of time (Garner, 1996).

Linens and Laundry

Although soiled linen may be a source of a large number of pathogenic microorganisms, according to the CDC the risk of actual disease transmission is negligible (Garner & Favero, 1986). Common sense should be used for the storage and processing of soiled linen. If necessary, home care staff members having contact with contaminated linen should wear protective gloves, hold the linen away from the body, and wear an impervious apron or gown if the linen is wet.

If the fabric can tolerate contact with chlorine bleach, it should be washed on the regular wash cycle in hot water with 1 cup of chlorine bleach per full load, along with regular detergent, and dried in an automatic dryer. A chlorine bleach substitute may be used, but its effectiveness in destroying microorganisms compared with chlorine bleach has not been determined (Belkin, 1998).

If a washing machine and dryer are not available in the patient's home, contaminated linens should be soaked in a receptacle or sink in cold, soapy water in a 1:10 bleach solution for 15 minutes. The linen should be washed and the fluids discarded down the toilet or drain; the staff member should wear gloves during this washing. The linen should then be rewashed using the same procedure, but with hot soapy water. The clean linen should then be hung to dry outside in the sun or, if that is not possible, inside the home in an appropriate place. Commercial dry cleaning of fabrics soiled with blood also will eliminate the risk of pathogen transmission. Once the linen is clean, it should be stored in the home in a manner that keeps it clean. Hot water heated to at least 120°F is needed to clean, sanitize, and disinfect laundry. Very hot water (>120°F), however, can be a hazard to children.

Dishes, Glasses, Cups, and Eating Utensils

No special precautions generally are needed for dishes, glasses, cups, or eating utensils. Disposable or reusable dishes or eating utensils can be used with patients who are infected or colonized with microorganisms. The best way to wash, rinse, and disinfect dishes and eating utensils is to use a dishwasher. If a dishwasher is not available, a multicompartment sink or dishpan and a dish rack with a drain board are needed to wash, rinse, and disinfect dishes.

Noncritical Equipment

Noninvasive, reusable medical equipment, such as commode chairs, hospital beds, bedrails, bedside equipment, walkers, canes, wheelchairs, and other equipment located in the home, should be cleansed and disinfected as soon as its use is discontinued or if it becomes soiled during use. Guidelines for selecting disinfectants can be found in Table 8–2.

It has recently come to the FDA's attention that reusable (nondisposable) medical devices (e.g., ambulatory infusion pumps) rented or leased from third parties may not be properly cleaned, disinfected, and/or sterilized before delivery to the home care organization. Also, when health care facilities exchange equipment with other institutions, the equipment may be improperly cleaned, disinfected, and/or sterilized either before or after patient use. Improper handling of devices between uses can contaminate facilities and expose individuals, including health care providers and couriers, to infectious, biohazardous material. Also, the presence of residual organic material on such equipment may compromise the effectiveness of the disinfection process.

The FDA recommends that home care organizations renting or leasing reusable medical devices from a third party should review all rental and leasing contracts, agreements, and other written documents to ensure that the parties responsible for cleaning, disinfecting, and/or sterilizing the equipment are clearly identified. If the home care organization is responsible for cleaning, disinfecting, and/or sterilizing equipment for reuse, it should ensure that all appropriate personnel are aware of this responsibility and are properly trained and equipped to perform these tasks. If a third party is responsible for cleaning, disinfecting, and/or sterilizing equipment for reuse, the home care organization should review the third party's operating procedures to determine that its facilities, equipment, processes, and personnel are adequate to perform these operations. The home care organization should be sure that the third party is familiar with the manufacturer's instructions for cleaning, disinfecting, and/or sterilizing the device. The home care organization also must ensure that its own personnel are properly trained and equipped to handle, package, and label contaminated equipment for shipment back to the supplier.

In some cases, third party suppliers may also reprocess or refurbish medical devices between uses. When the contract requires third party suppliers to reprocess or refurbish medical devices, the home care organization should ensure that the supplier is familiar with the device manufacturer's specifications for the product (FDA, 1997).

Semicritical Item Cleaning and Disinfecting Guidelines

Semicritical items come in contact with mucus membranes but do not enter tissue or the vascular system. Semicritical items should be subjected to either intermediate or high-level disinfection if they are to be reused. Examples of semicritical items that may be used in home care are given in Table 8–1. The only semicritical items that may be disinfected at an intermediate level are tubs used for soaking nonintact skin and oral and rectal thermometers. All other semicritical items should be subjected to high-level disinfection.

Intermediate disinfection may be accomplished by using one of the following germicides (Rutala, 1996):

- ethyl or isopropyl alcohol (70 percent to 90 percent)
- sodium hypochlorite (5.25 percent household bleach), 1:50 dilution
- phenolic germicidal detergent solution, if necessary diluted according to the product label
- iodophor germicidal solution (e.g., povidone-iodine) diluted according to the product label

Tubs

A tub used for soaking extremities with nonintact skin (i.e., foot ulcers) should be subjected to intermediate disinfection by being cleaned with a 1:50 (Rutala, 1996) or, if necessary, a 1:10 dilution of 5.25 percent household bleach (Rutala, 1996). The tub also may be sprayed with a disinfectant product, which should be left on the surface for the time required by the manufacturer before being wiped off.

Thermometers: Oral or Rectal

Whenever possible, each patient should use his or her own thermometer. If a glass mercury thermometer or battery-operated digital thermometer from the nursing supply bag is utilized, a plastic protective sheath should be placed over the tip before it is used with the patient. After patient use, the plastic sheath should be discarded and the thermometer wiped vigorously with alcohol before being replaced in the carrying case.

Laryngeal Mirrors

Laryngeal mirrors used in speech therapy are generally left with the patient and should be wiped vigorously with 70 percent isopropyl alcohol after use.

High-Level Disinfection

All other semicritical items used in home care should be subjected to high-level disinfection, which may be accomplished by one of the following methods (Rutala, 1996):

- glutaraldehyde-based formulations (2 percent)
- stabilized hydrogen peroxide (6 percent)
- peracetic acid (variable concentration, but 1 percent or less is sporicidal)
- wet pasteurization at 70°C for 30 minutes after cleaning with a detergent
- sodium hypochlorite (5.25 percent household bleach), 1:50 dilution

Critical Item Disinfecting Guidelines

Critical items are those that will enter the tissue or vascular system or through which blood will flow; these require sterilization. Items that must be sterile generally will be purchased as sterile. Home care organizations generally do not perform sterilization procedures, but some medical equipment classified as critical items, such as urethral catheters used for intermittent catheterization and tracheal suctions catheters, may be reused. The physician's orders, the patient's health status and home environment, and the patient's or caregiver's abilities will determine whether frequently used critical items, such as respiratory catheters or urethral catheters, will be disinfected between uses or whether sterile products will be purchased and used on a one-time basis. Organizations such as the CDC, the Joint Commission on Accreditation of Healthcare Organizations, and the American Hospital Association have not taken a stance on the issue. The FDA, which regulates medical devices, only covers products on a first-time use basis and good manufacturing practices. The FDA does not regulate whether a single-use device will perform as intended after it has been cleaned and disinfected. Chapter 3 provides additional information about cleaning and disinfecting respiratory therapy equipment and intermittent urethral catheters.

STORAGE OF MEDICAL EQUIPMENT AND SUPPLIES IN THE HOME CARE ORGANIZATION'S FACILITY

Separate areas should be identified for the storage of clean and dirty equipment, cleaning and disinfecting of equipment, equipment requiring repair or maintenance, obsolete inventory, and equipment that is ready for patient use. Physically separating clean and dirty equipment does not mean that the equipment must be kept in separate rooms or locations. As long as the dirty equipment is not physically comingled with the clean equipment, then the equipment is considered properly separated. For example, in a small hospice organization, the sink in the restroom can be used to clean and disinfect small durable medical equipment after the patient no longer needs it.

Equipment that is waiting to be cleaned and disinfected can be stored according to one or more of the following methods:

- placing a sticker on the equipment to indicate that it is "dirty"
- putting the equipment on a shelf that has a "to be cleaned" label on it
- putting the equipment in a red biohazard bag
- placing the equipment in an area that has colored tape on the floor or in confined quarters with a sign on the wall to designate it as an area for equipment that is to be cleaned
- storing the equipment in any other manner selected by the home care organization that is understood by home care staff members

Once the equipment has been cleaned and disinfected, one or more of the following methods may be used to identify that it has been cleaned and is ready to be used by a patient:

- placing a tag on the equipment indicating that it has been cleaned
- putting the equipment on a shelf that has a "ready for patient use" label on it
- putting the equipment in a clear plastic bag
- placing the equipment in an area that has colored tape on the floor or in confined quarters with a sign on the wall to designate it as an area for equipment that is clean
- storing the equipment in any other manner selected by the home care organization that is understood by home care staff members

Expiration dates on medical supplies, vacuum container blood tubes, and over-the-counter medications stored in a non–pharmacy-licensed home care organization's office should be checked on a regular basis to ensure that the dates have not passed.

MEDICAL EQUIPMENT AND SUPPLIES STORAGE DURING TRANSPORT TO AND FROM THE PATIENT'S HOME

The cleanliness and/or sterility of sterile items should be maintained during storage and delivery by being kept in separate areas designated as clean or dirty/contaminated. During transport to or from the patient's home, clean equipment needs to be kept separate from dirty equipment. This is important so that the clean equipment does not become soiled or contaminated. Clean equipment can be separated from dirty equipment in the staff member's vehicle in one or more of the following ways:

- placing dirty equipment in a red or dark-colored plastic bag (rather than a clear bag, which designates that the equipment is cleaned) before placing it near clean equipment
- storing clean equipment and supplies in plastic bags or a "trunk box"
- storing clean and dirty equipment in any other manner selected by the home care organization that is understood by home care staff members

Once the dirty equipment is returned to the home care organization's facility, it should be stored in a designated area and, if required, inspected. Once the reusable items are properly cleaned, they may be returned to the area designated for clean equipment or supplies.

The delivery vehicles that are owned or leased by the home care organization, not the staff member's personal vehicles, should be cleaned and inspected on a regular basis or at a frequency determined by applicable law and regulation. If an open-back vehicle, such as a pickup truck, is used to make deliveries, equipment and supplies should not be exposed to rain, snow, or other weather conditions that may impair the supplies' integrity or contaminate the equipment and supplies being delivered.

MEDICAL EQUIPMENT AND SUPPLIES STORAGE IN THE PATIENT'S HOME

Medical supplies taken into the patient's home should be stored away from pets, small children, and confused adults. If the home is infested with pests, the supplies should be placed in a sealable plastic bag, which should be kept closed at all times to prevent the contents from becoming contaminated with pest urine or feces. Sterile supplies should also be stored in a manner that will prevent them from becoming contaminated. For example, sterile gauze pads should not be stored under a kitchen or bathroom sink, where they may become wet.

If another health care organization provides supplies to the patient, the home care staff member in the patient's home will monitor the expiration date(s) before the supplies are used. If an expiration date has passed, the staff member will contact the provider immediately, and the supplies will be rendered inactive until replaced.

CARE OF STAFF MEMBERS' CLOTHING

Most home care staff members wear either "street clothes" or a uniform when providing patient care. During the course of a day, the clothes can become heavily contaminated with pathogenic microorganisms. For that reason, the clothes should be removed when the staff member gets home and not worn again until they are washed in hot soapy water with an appropriate bleach, rinsed, and dried (Belkin, 1997).

REFERENCES

Belkin, N. (1997). Use of scrubs and related apparel in health care facilities. *American Journal of Infection Control, 25*, 401–404.

Belkin, N. (1998). Aseptics and aesthetics of chlorine bleach: Can its use in laundry be safely abandoned? *American Journal of Infection Control, 16*, 149–151.

Centers for Disease Control and Prevention. (1995). Recommendations for preventing the spread of vancomycin resistance: Recommendations of the Hospital Infection Control Practices Advisory Committee (HICPAC). *American Journal of Infection Control, 23*, 87–94.

Food and Drug Administration. Center for Devices and Radiological Health. (1997, April 17). *Public notice.* Washington, DC: Author. http://www.fda.gov/medwatch/safety/1997/device.htm

Friedman, M. (1996, July). Designing an infection control program to meet JCAHO standards. *Caring, 15*, 18–25.

Garner, J.S. (1996). Guideline for isolation precautions in hospitals. *Infection Control and Hospital Epidemiology, 17*, 53–80.

Garner, J., & Favero, M. (1986, June). CDC guideline for handwashing and hospital environmental control, 1985. *American Journal of Infection Control, 14*, 110–129.

Occupational Safety and Health Administration. (1991). Occupational exposure to bloodborne pathogens: Final rule. 29 CFR 1910.1030. *Federal Register, 56*, 64003–64282.

Occupational Safety and Health Administration (OSHA). (1997, May 15). OSHA's Environmental Protection Agency approved quaternary ammonium disinfectant products. *OSHA Standards Interpretation and Compliance Letters.* Washington, DC: Author. http://www.osha-slc.gov/OshDoc/Interp_data/I19970515.html

Rutala, W.A. (1996). APIC guideline for selection and use of disinfectants. *American Journal of Infection Control, 24*, 313–342.

Rutala, W.A. (1997). Disinfection, sterilization, and waste disposal. In R.P. Wenzel (Ed.), *Prevention and control of nosocomial infections* (3rd ed., pp. 540–541). Baltimore: Williams & Wilkins.

Spaulding, E.H. (1968). Chemical disinfection of medical and surgical materials. In C.A. Lawrence & S.S. Block (Eds.), *Disinfection, sterilization, and preservation* (pp. 517–531). Philadelphia: Lea & Febiger.

Chapter 9

Medical Waste Management

Each home care organization should have a medical waste management plan to ensure that its staff members, patients, family members, and the environment are protected from medical waste that may be generated during the course of home care. The medical waste management plan should minimally meet the recommendations of the Environmental Protection Agency (EPA), the Occupational Safety and Health Administration's (OSHA) bloodborne pathogens regulations, the Department of Transportation, and any applicable state, local, county, or municipal laws or regulations. Each state regulates the storage, transportation, and disposal of medical waste. Most states permit medical waste that is generated during the course of home care to be considered general waste and disposed of along with household waste. Other state, local, county, or municipal laws or regulations may be much stricter and would consider waste generated during a patient care procedure medical waste and require that it be disposed of by a licensed biomedical waste hauler. Therefore, it is important that each home care organization have a copy of its state or local regulations addressing medical waste disposal because the regulations may vary from state to state and from county to county. Appendix 9–A is a directory of state agencies that regulate the management of infectious waste. The rule of thumb is to follow whatever regulations are the strictest (i.e., the local, county, state, or federal laws and regulations).

EPA INFECTIOUS WASTE CATEGORIES

The EPA classifies infectious waste into seven categories (EPA, 1986):

1. *Isolation waste:* Discarded articles contaminated with body fluids from humans who are known to be infected with a highly communicable disease
2. *Cultures and stocks of infectious agents:* Live and attenuated vaccines, specimens from medical and pathology laboratories, and culture dishes and devices used to transfer, inoculate, and mix cultures from clinical, research, and industrial laboratories
3. *Human blood and blood products:* Liquid blood waste, human blood, blood products, items contaminated with blood (including dried blood), serum, plasma, and other blood products
4. *Human pathological waste:* Tissue, organs, body parts, body fluids, and specimens
5. *Contaminated sharps:* Needles, vacuum container tubes, microhematocrit tubes, injection ampules, vials, and other glassware items that may be contaminated
6. *Contaminated animal waste:* Animal body parts, carcasses, and bedding intentionally exposed to pathogens
7. *Miscellaneous contaminated waste:*
   - waste from surgery and autopsy (soiled dressings, sponges, drapes, lavage tubes, underpads, drainage sets, and surgical gloves)
   - laboratory waste (specimen containers, slides and coverslips, laboratory coats, and aprons)
   - dialysis unit waste (tubing, filters, disposable sheets, towels, gloves, aprons, and laboratory coats)
   - contaminated equipment (equipment used in patient care, medical laboratories, research, and the production and testing of certain pharmaceuticals)

Home care organizations usually generate infectious waste from categories 1, 3, 5, and 7.

SEGREGATION OF WASTE

For the purposes of identification and safe handling, waste generated by staff members should be segregated into three distinct categories: general waste, infectious or medical waste, and sharps. The EPA uses the term *infectious waste,* and OSHA uses the term *regulated waste.* For consistency, the term *medical waste* is used throughout the rest of this chapter to refer to waste that has been contaminated or visibly soiled with blood or other potentially infectious materials. When waste generated in the home is segregated, it is important that it be stored in a proper container. If the state requires that medical waste generated in the home be disposed of as medical waste and not household waste, staff need to be keenly aware of the difference between general waste and medical waste to help keep the home care organization's administrative costs low. Staff should be careful about only putting medical waste in a red bag or sharps container. Staff should also be aware of the difference between blood-saturated waste and blood-stained waste. Blood-stained waste is considered general waste and can be disposed of as household waste. For example, only blood-saturated dressings generated during a dressing change should be placed in a red bag, not all the sterile wrappers and containers. Comingling both medical waste and general waste will increase the home care organization's costs for medical waste management.

General Waste

General waste is defined as materials that have not been contaminated or visibly soiled with blood or other potentially infectious materials and can include patient products such as:

- paper towels used for drying hands
- dressing wrappers
- nonsoiled personal protective equipment used by the staff members (e.g., gown, mask, or gloves)
- old dressings that are not visibly soiled with blood or other potentially infectious materials
- diapers
- incontinence pads
- intravenous tubing

General waste should be placed in a plastic bag and the bag securely fastened. General waste is disposed of in normal consumer trash bags and stored before disposal in a trash receptacle. The general waste generated in the course of care may be discarded in the patient's regular waste receptacle. Intravenous tubing is not considered medical waste unless it has been used to administer blood or blood products in the home.

Regulated Medical Waste

Regulated medical waste may be generated by the patient, the patient's caregiver(s), and home care staff members while rendering patient care. According to OSHA, regulated waste may include the following (OSHA, 1991):

- liquid or semiliquid blood or other potentially infectious material
- contaminated items that would release blood or other potentially infectious materials in a liquid or semiliquid state if compressed
- items that are caked with blood or other potentially infectious material and are capable of releasing these materials during handling
- contaminated sharps
- pathological and microbiological wastes containing blood or other potentially infectious material

Items heavily contaminated with blood or other potentially infectious materials should be placed in a leakproof, heavy-duty plastic bag and the bag securely tied at the neck. One plastic bag is adequate if the bag is sturdy and the article can be placed in the bag without contaminating the outside of the bag; otherwise the contents should be double bagged. The bag(s) should be appropriately labeled as biohazardous or color-coded in red and securely closed before removal from the patient's home. The bags should not be overfilled (OSHA, 1991).

Liquid waste such as urine, feces, povidone-iodine, irrigating solutions, suctioned fluids, excretions, and secretions may be carefully poured down the patient's toilet, which is connected to a sanitary sewer (Centers for Disease Control and Prevention [CDC], 1998). Body fluids in amounts of less than approximately 20 mL, such as blood in a syringe withdrawn from a central venous catheter before a blood sample is obtained, may be discarded in a puncture-proof sharps container.

Surgical masks used by the patient to prevent the spread of pulmonary tuberculosis and other potentially contaminated items such as tissues used by the patient should be treated as medical waste and disposed of according to the state's regulations for the disposal of medical waste. N95 respiratory protective devices certified by the National Institute for Occupational Safety and Health (NIOSH) used by staff members as personal protective equipment may be disposed of as general waste.

All waste generated from the home administration of chemotherapy is classified as chemotherapy waste. Chemotherapy waste disposal is a hazardous materials problem, not a potential transmitter of infectious disease. All items contaminated with antineoplastic agents, such as tubing, syringes, intravenous solution bags, and gloves, should be placed in a container specifically labeled for chemotherapy waste only. Chemotherapy waste should be transported in the trunk of the vehicle and segregated from other waste in the organization's facility. A licensed hazardous materials disposal company will pick up the chemotherapy waste.

Sharps

The primary route of occupational exposure to bloodborne pathogens is accidental percutaneous (through the skin) injury. Home care staff members handle sharps devices and equipment, such as hypodermic needles, Huber needles, intravenous access devices, intravenous blood collection devices, and phlebotomy devices. Of the 800,000 needlestick injuries estimated to occur annually, as many as one third are related to the disposal process. The factors most often related to sharps injuries include the following: inadequate design or inappropriate placement of the sharps disposal container, overfilling of the sharps disposal container, and inappropriate sharps disposal practices by the user during patient care. Nursing staff and phlebotomists experience the highest number of needlestick injuries. NIOSH has developed safety performance criteria for selecting and using sharps disposal containers (Table 9–1; CDC, 1998). If the home care organization's staff members clip the patient's nails with nail clippers that are owned by the home care organization and the nail clippers are capable of penetrating the patient's skin, the clippers need to be stored in an impervious container and the container appropriately labeled for storage and transport (OSHA, 1992).

Sharps Container

All used disposable sharp instruments, needles, syringes, and hypodermic units, and other sharp items such as broken glass should be placed immediately or as soon as possible after use in a puncture-resistant, leak-proof, impervious container for disposal. The container should be labeled with a biohazard sign or color-coded, and it should remain upright. The container should be constructed with a secured lid that seals, so that the contents will not spill out if it is knocked over and injuries will not result from handling the container. The container should be readily accessible and located

Table 9–1 Criteria for Selection and Use of Sharps Containers

Criterion	*Recommendation*
Functionality	The sharps container should be durable, leak resistant, and puncture resistant under all normal environmental conditions during use.
Accessibility	The sharps container must be accessible to home care staff members who use, maintain, or dispose of sharps devices. There must be sufficient numbers of containers of sufficient volume conveniently placed with safe access to the disposal opening.
Visibility	The sharps container fill status and warning labels must be visible to the home care staff members who will use it.
Accommodation	Proper selection and use of sharps disposal containers are important. Prevention strategies through training, personal protective equipment, and engineering controls such as needleless intravenous systems and safe needle-bearing products should be considered part of a needlestick prevention plan.

Source: Reprinted from *Selecting, Evaluating, and Using Sharps Disposal Containers,* Centers for Disease Control and Prevention, National Institute for Occupational Safety and Health, January 1998.

as close as possible to the patient care or work area and other areas where sharps are commonly used in the workplace. Puncture-resistant sharps containers should be brought into the work area any time syringes and needles are used for a procedure.

Vacuum container needles should be removed by means of the device, opening, or aperture built into the lid of the sharps container. If the sharps container does not contain this feature, the entire needle and vacuum container set should be disposed of. Broken glass that may be contaminated should not be picked up directly by hand; rather, a forceps, tongs, or a brush and dustpan should be used. Care should be taken not to fill the container above the indicated safe fill line that is placed on the container by the manufacturer. Once the sharps container is full, the lid should be closed tightly and the container returned to the home care organization for disposal; the container can be disposed of as household waste if permitted by state regulations.

Recapping a Needle

Used needles and other sharps should not be recapped, bent, removed from disposable syringes, or manipulated by both hands or any technique that involves directing the point of the needle toward any part of the body unless the specific procedure requires that recapping be performed. Situations in which recapping may be required include the insertion of a needle into a vial of heparin or saline to prefill syringes used for flushing venous access devices and prefilling syringes from multidose vials. Recapping in these or other similar situations may be permissible if the one-handed "scoop" technique or a mechanical device designed for holding the needle sheath is used. Contaminated needles may be recapped only if there is no alternative method feasible through the use of resheathing instruments, self-sheathing needles and/or syringes, forceps, or other one-handed method of recapping (OSHA, 1990). To recap a needle safely using a scoop technique, place the needle and the cap horizontally on a flat surface. Using one hand, scoop the needle into the cap, tip the capped syringe upward, and tighten it to the needle hub.

Sharps Storage in the Patient's Home

When the staff member brings the sharps container into the patient's home for use during a home visit, he or she should be cautious about where the sharps container is placed. For example, the staff member should consider whether there are small children, confused adults, drug abusers, or psychiatric patients in the home. Under these circumstances, the staff member should keep the portable sharps container in his or her possession at all times. The portable sharps container should also be moved close to the patient when the staff member is setting up for a procedure in which sharps will need to be used. The sharps container should be placed within arm's reach. Once the container has been used, the lid should be closed to prevent spillage or protrusion of the contents during storage and transport. Appendix 9–B contains a brochure that may be provided to patients and families to educate them in the proper methods for disposing of sharps and other medical waste.

Sharps containers may be stored in the patient's home between staff member visits. Sharps containers should be stored in the closed position and away from pets, small children, or confused adults when they are not needed. When the sharps container is three-quarters full, it may be disposed of as general waste if permitted by the state. If it is the home care organization's policy to pick up a full sharps container from the patient's home, it should be stored in the patient's home until pickup in such a way that it will not be a risk to anyone in the home.

Sharps Storage in the Staff Member's Possession

The CDC, NIOSH, the Joint Commission on Accreditation of Healthcare Organizations, and OSHA have no official position on the manner in which sharps containers should be stored in the staff member's possession or carried in and out of the patient's home. As long as there is no immediate hazard to the home care staff member carrying the container, common sense should prevail. Factors to consider in determining the proper storage of a sharps container include the size of the container and whether the container can be completely sealed. As long as the sharps container is closed and the external surface is not visibly contaminated, it may be hand carried, placed in a separate bag, or placed inside the staff member's supply bag.

Decontaminating Sharps before Transport and Disposal

Some states that permit medical waste generated in the home to be disposed of as household waste strongly recommend that sharps first be decontaminated. If the home care organization's state requires decontamination before disposal, the staff member may decontaminate the contents of a 1-gallon size sharps container by adding $\frac{1}{2}$ teaspoon bleach and $1\frac{1}{2}$ tablespoon water to the container, closing the container tightly, and gently shaking the contents to disinfect them. Medical waste that has been decontaminated does not have to be labeled or color-coded (OSHA, 1991).

Sharps as Household Waste

Most states, but not all, permit medical waste generated in the home to be disposed of as household waste. If medical waste can be disposed of along with household waste, it should not be added to the recycle bin even though the sharps may be metal and the heavy plastic container may be suitable for recycling. Sharps should be placed in a heavy-gauge plastic or metal container that can be sealed. A container commercially manufactured specifically for sharps disposal does not have to be used. Other heavy-gauge plastic containers, including bleach bottles, laundry detergent containers, or motor oil containers, may be used. Milk containers, 2- or 3-liter plastic soda bottles, and other thin-walled plastic containers should not be used. Of course, glass containers should not be used because they can break and pose a possible threat of injury to the waste handler. If sharps are not being placed in a container designated for them, the lid of the container being used should be closed tightly and, if possible, sealed with heavy-duty tape. The home care organization's state may issue guidelines on how medical waste should be contained, taped, or labeled before disposal.

WASTE STORAGE DURING TRANSPORT TO THE HOME CARE ORGANIZATION

Some home care organizations, especially home infusion organizations, will pick up sharps containers that have been filled during the course of care. When the sharps container is taken out of the patient's home, it should be completely sealed and placed in the vehicle. In the vehicle, the container should be placed in a location that will not cause injury to passenger(s) or the driver if the driver should have to stop quickly and the sharps container were to overturn and potentially spill its contents.

During transport, the sharps container should be placed upright in the trunk of a vehicle, the back seat of a vehicle if the vehicle does not have a trunk, a cargo box in an open-bed pickup truck, or a closed container in an open cargo van. The waste should be not be exposed to rain, snow, or other weather conditions that may impair the container's integrity.

SEPARATING WASTE FROM CLEAN EQUIPMENT AND SUPPLIES

During transport from the patient's home to the home care organization, the medical waste must be kept separate from clean equipment. This is important so that the clean equipment does not become soiled or contaminated. Medical waste can be separated from clean equipment in the staff member's vehicle by storing it in a red or orange plastic bag before placing it near clean equipment. Clean equipment and supplies can be stored in clear plastic bags or trunk boxes. The medical waste and clean equipment can also be kept separate in any other manner selected by the home care organization that is understood by home care staff members.

MEDICAL WASTE STORAGE IN THE HOME CARE ORGANIZATION

If medical waste and sharps cannot be disposed of at the patient's home, the biohazard bags and sharps should be either brought back to the home care organization for storage or brought to another facility with which the home care organization has made arrangements for disposal. If the medical waste is returned to the home care organization, it should be stored in a designated area of the home care organization until it is picked up for final disposal. The medical waste and sharps containers should be placed into a secondary box or containment device provided by the biomedical waste hauler or other appropriate container that is labeled with the international biohazard symbol or color-coded. The secondary container should be of the appropriate size and material required by the state's regulations, if applicable. The storage area for the secondary container should be in a low-traffic area within the facility or in a storage area with limited access. Medical waste should be stored in the home care organization for as short a time as possible or the maximum time permitted by the state's regulations. If the secondary container is full, the contracted medical waste hauler should be contacted for a pickup. Some hospital-based home care organizations store medical waste in their office, and another hospital department will come to the organization and pick it up. Regardless of who is the responsible party for pickup, the medical waste should be picked up on a routine basis to prevent overfilling. Medical waste should not be compacted by home care staff members.

MEDICAL WASTE HAULER

The home care organization, which is considered the medical waste generator, is responsible for the medical waste until it is destroyed. Therefore, a commercial, licensed medical waste hauler should be used to transport waste for treatment and final disposal unless the organization has other capabilities (e.g., incineration) for the final disposal. For example, a hospital-based home care organization may store its medical waste in the office and have it picked up at regular intervals by a hospital staff member to be incinerated along with the hospital's medical waste. Whatever method is used, all final disposal methods should be in compliance with federal, state, and local regulations.

OSHA LABELING REQUIREMENTS

OSHA requires that a biohazard warning label be affixed to containers of medical waste; the container should be fluorescent orange or orange-red with letters or symbols in a contrasting color. A biohazard warning label is shown in Figure 9–1. The biohazard label can be either part of the container or affixed by a method that will prevent loss or removal, such as taping. If the container or bag is red, a biohazard label or sticker is not required.

If a refrigerator is used in the home care organization to store blood specimens until picked up by the laboratory courier, the refrigerator must have a biohazard label on the front. The same refrigerator that is used for storing laboratory specimens should not be used to store staff members' food and other medications.

After blood specimens are obtained in the patient's home, they should be placed in an impervious container for storage or transport. If a non-red container, such as a Rubbermaid sandwich container, is used to store blood specimens during transport, it should have a biohazard label affixed to the top. Some home care organizations teach their patients to dispose of their sharps in other impervious household containers. If it is the home care organization's policy to pick up non-red sharps containers for disposal, the container must be placed inside a red bag or labeled with a biohazard label for transport and storage. Bags of cross-matched blood, blood components, or other blood products that are labeled as to their contents and have been released for transfusion are not required to be labeled as biohazardous (OSHA, 1991).

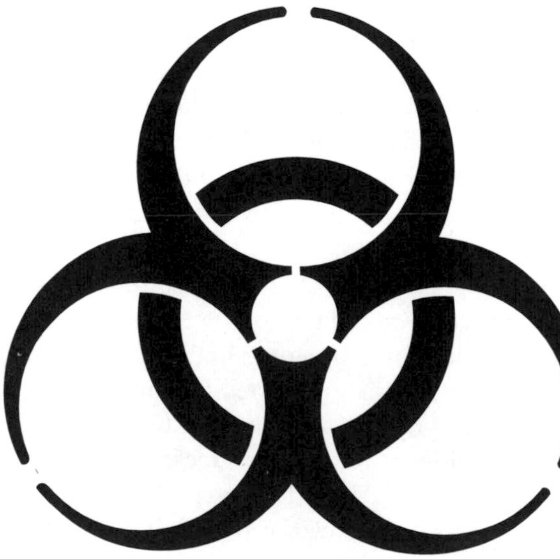

Figure 9–1 Biohazard Symbol

Source: Reprinted from *Occupational Exposure to Bloodborne Pathogens: Final Rule,* 29 CFR 1910.1030, Federal Register, Occupational Safety and Health Administration, 1991.

BLOOD SPILLS IN THE HOME

Environmental surfaces in the home may become contaminated by a blood spill, such as may occur if a full blood sample tube is dropped and broken. Gloves should be worn when spills of blood or other potentially infectious material are cleaned. Disposable towels and/or wipes should be used to wipe up the spill. Once the gross blood is removed, the surface should be cleaned and disinfected. If a blood tube is involved in the spill, the broken glass should be picked up first with tongs and placed in an impervious container for disposal, and then the blood should be wiped up with paper towels and the surface cleaned and disinfected. If the blood is not wiped up first, the diluted bleach solution or other appropriate disinfectant will not be effective because disinfectants do not work in the presence of blood. A hard, nonporous surface can be disinfected with a 1:10 dilution of 5.25 percent household bleach or another appropriate disinfectant spray or solution. The paper towels used to contain and clean the blood spill and disinfect the spill area should be bagged to prevent leakage and exposure to others. A heavy-duty plastic bag should be used for this purpose, and it should either be color-coded or have a biohazard label.

OSHA does not have any evidence to support whether decontamination of plush carpets is possible. It is OSHA's opinion that carpeted surfaces cannot be decontaminated. Under normal circumstances, carpeted surfaces are located in areas where there is minimal exposure from dermal contact; therefore, a home care provider should make a reasonable effort to clean and sanitize carpeting and plush surfaces with carpet detergent or cleaning products (OSHA, 1994). Wearing gloves, the staff member should first wipe up the blood spill with disposable towels and then clean the carpet. The carpet should then be disinfected with a solution that does not contain 5.25 percent household bleach because bleach will remove the color from the carpet fibers as well as chemically damage the tensile strength of the fiber and backing. Any other EPA-approved germicide may be used. The disinfectant should be applied according to the label instructions and allowed to remain on the carpet to air dry.

REFERENCES

Centers for Disease Control and Prevention, National Institute for Occupational Safety and Health. (1998, January). *Selecting, evaluating, and using sharps disposal containers.* Atlanta: Author. http://www.cdc.gov/niosh/sharps1.html

Environmental Protection Agency, Office of Solid Waste and Emergency Response. (1986, May). *Guide for infectious waste management* (Publication No. EPA/530-SW-014). Washington, DC: U.S. Department of Commerce.

Garner, J., & Favero, M. (1986, June). CDC guideline for handwashing and hospital environmental control, 1985. *American Journal of Infection Control, 14,* 110–129.

Occupational Safety and Health Administration. (1990, July 6). Enforcement procedures for occupational exposure to HBV and HIV. *OSHA Standards Interpretation and Compliance Letters.* http://www.osha-slc.gov/OshDoc/Interp_data/I19900706.html

Occupational Safety and Health Administration. (1991). Occupational exposure to bloodborne pathogens: Final rule. 29 CFR 1910.1030. *Federal Register, 56,* 64003–64282.

Occupational Safety and Health Administration. (1992, April, 4). Infectious materials and nail and tissue clippers as sharps. *OSHA Standards Interpretation and Compliance Letters.* http://www.osha-slc.gov/OshDoc/Interp_data/I19920404.html

Occupational Safety and Health Administration. (1994, May 6). OSHA requires the use of a tuberculocidal disinfectant to clean up blood or body fluids. *OSHA Standards Interpretation and Compliance Letters.* http://www.osha-slc.gov/OshDoc/Interp_data/I19940506.html

Appendix 9–A

State Hazardous Waste Management Agencies

State	Hazardous Waste Management Agency
Alabama	Alabama Department of Environmental Management Land Division PO Box 301463 Montgomery, Alabama 36130 (334) 271-7761
Alaska	Air and Solid Waste Management Department of Environmental Conservation 411 Willoughby Avenue Juneau, Alaska 99811 (907) 465-5350
Arizona	Arizona Department of Environmental Quality 2005 N. Central Avenue G-200 Phoenix, Arizona 85004 (602) 207-4685
Arkansas	Department of Pollution Control and Ecology Solid Waste Management Division PO Box 9583 8001 National Drive Little Rock, Arkansas 72219 (501) 682-0959
California	Department of Health Services Toxic Substances Control Division PO Box 806 Sacramento, California 95812 (916) 327-6904
Colorado	Colorado Department of Health Waste Management Division 4300 Cherry Creek S. Denver, Colorado 80222 (303) 692-3920
Connecticut	Department of Environmental Protection Bureau of Waste Management Section 79 Elm Street Hartford, Connecticut 06106 (860) 424-3022
Delaware	Department of Natural Resources and Environmental Control 98 King Highway Dover, Delaware 19901 (302) 739-3820

State	*Hazardous Waste Management Agency*
District of Columbia	Department of Environmental Programs 777 N. Capital Street, N.E. Suite 300 Washington, DC 20002 (202) 962-3200
Florida	Department of Environmental Regulation 3900 Commonwealth Boulevard Tallahassee, Florida 32399 (904) 488-0300
Georgia	Georgia Environmental Protection Division Hazardous Waste Management Program Land Protection Branch Floyd Towers East Suite 1154 205 Butler Street, S.E. Atlanta, Georgia 30334 (404) 656-2833 Toll Free: (800) 334-2373
Hawaii	Department of Health Hazardous Waste Division 1250 Punchbowl Street Honolulu, Hawaii 96813 (808) 586-4225
Idaho	Department of Health and Welfare Bureau of Hazardous Materials 1410 N. Hilton Boise, Idaho 83706 (208) 373-0502
Illinois	Environmental Protection Agency Division of Land Pollution Control 2200 Churchill Road, #24 Springfield, Illinois 62794 (217) 782-8700
Indiana	Division of Land Pollution Control 1330 W. Washington Street Indianapolis, Indiana 46204 (317) 233-6663
Iowa	Iowa Department of Natural Resources Environmental Protection Division 900 E. Grand Street Des Moines, Iowa 50319 (515) 281-8895
Kansas	Department of Health and Environment Bureau of Waste Management Forbes Field Building 740 Topeka, Kansas 66520 (913) 296-1667
Kentucky	Department of Environmental Protection Division of Waste Management 14 Reilly Road Frankfort, Kentucky 40601 (502) 564-6716

continues

Appendix 9–A continued

State	*Hazardous Waste Management Agency*
Louisiana	Department of Environmental Quality Hazardous Waste Division PO Box 82178 Baton Rouge, Louisiana 70884 (504) 765-0246
Maine	Department of Environmental Protection Bureau of Oil and Hazardous Materials Control State House Station #17 Augusta, Maine 04333 (207) 287-2812
Maryland	Department of Health and Mental Hygiene Maryland Waste Management Administration Office of Environmental Programs 2500 Broening Highway Building 40 Baltimore, Maryland 21224 (410) 631-3321
Massachusetts	Department of Environmental Quality Engineering Division of Solid and Hazardous Waste One Winter Street 7th Floor Boston, Massachusetts 02108 (617) 292-5849 (617) 292-5851
Michigan	Michigan Department of Natural Resources Hazardous Waste Division Waste Evaluation Unit PO Box 30241 Lansing, Michigan 48909 (517) 335-3383
Minnesota	Pollution Control Agency Solid and Hazardous Waste Division 520 Lafayette Road St. Paul, Minnesota 55155 (612) 296-6300
Mississippi	Department of Natural Resources Division of Solid and Hazardous Waste Management PO Box 10385 Jackson, Mississippi 39289 (601) 961-5171
Missouri	Department of Natural Resources Waste Management Program PO Box 176 Jefferson City, Missouri 65102 (573) 526-2415 (800) 361-4827
Montana	Department of Health and Environmental Sciences Solid and Hazardous Waste Bureau PO Box 200901 Helena, Montana 59620 (406) 444-5294

State	*Hazardous Waste Management Agency*
Nebraska	Department of Environmental Control Hazardous Waste Management Section 1200 North Street Suite 400 PO Box 98922 Lincoln, Nebraska 68509 (402) 471-4217
Nevada	Division of Environmental Protection Waste Management Program 333 W. Nye Lane Carson City, Nevada 89706 (702) 687-4670 ext. 3001
New Hampshire	Department of Health and Human Services Division of Public Health Services Office of Waste Management Health and Welfare Building 6 Hazen Drive Concord, New Hampshire 03301-6527 (603) 271-2925
New Jersey	Department of Environmental Protection Division of Waste Management 401 E. State Street Trenton, New Jersey 08625 (609) 984-6880
New Mexico	Environmental Improvement Division Ground Water and Hazardous Waste Bureau Hazardous Waste Section PO Box 26110 Santa Fe, New Mexico 87503 (505) 827-0169
New York	Department of Environmental Conservation Bureau of Hazardous Waste Operations 50 Wolf Road Room 212 Albany, New York 12233 (518) 457-7337
North Carolina	Department of Human Resources Solid and Hazardous Waste Management Branch PO Box 29569 Raleigh, North Carolina 27626 (919) 733-4996 ext. 254
North Dakota	Department of Health Division of Hazardous Waste Management and Special Studies PO Box 5520 Bismarck, North Dakota 58506 (701) 328-5166
Ohio	Ohio EPA Division of Solid and Hazardous Waste Management PO Box 1049 Columbus, Ohio 43216 (614) 644-2621

continues

Appendix 9–A continued

State	*Hazardous Waste Management Agency*
Oklahoma	Waste Management Service Oklahoma State Department of Health 1000 N.E. 10th Street Oklahoma City, Oklahoma 73117 (405) 745-7133
Oregon	Hazardous and Solid Waste Division 811 S.W. 6th Avenue Portland, Oregon 97204 (503) 229-6922
Pennsylvania	Bureau of Waste Management Division of Compliance Monitoring PO Box 2063 Harrisburg, Pennsylvania 17105 (717) 783-0540
Rhode Island	Department of Environmental Management Division of Air and Hazardous Materials 291 Promenade Street Providence, Rhode Island 02908 (401) 277-2797 ext. 7510
South Carolina	Department of Health and Environmental Control Bureau of Solid and Hazardous Waste Management 2600 Bull Street Columbia, South Carolina 29201 (803) 896-4173
South Dakota	Department of Water and Natural Resources Office of Air Quality and Solid Waste Foss Building 523 E. Capitol Avenue Pierre, South Dakota 57501 (605) 773-3153
Tennessee	Division of Solid Waste Management Tennessee Department of Public Health L&C Tower 5th Floor 401 Church Street Nashville, Tennessee 37243 (615) 532-0796
Texas	Texas Water Commission Hazardous and Solid Waste Division Mail Code MC-124 Austin, Texas 78711 (512) 239-6796
Utah	Department of Health Bureau of Solid and Hazardous Waste Management PO Box 144880 Salt Lake City, Utah 84114 (801) 538-6170
Vermont	Agency of Environmental Conservation 103 S. Main Street West Building Waterbury, Vermont 05671 (802) 241-3482

State	*Hazardous Waste Management Agency*
Virginia	Department of Health Division of Solid and Hazardous Waste Management PO Box 10009 Richmond, Virginia 23240 (804) 698-4327
Washington	Department of Ecology Solid and Hazardous Waste Program Wells Fargo Building Suite 700 999 3rd Avenue Seattle, Washington 98104 (206) 296-4831 (206) 296-4807
West Virginia	Division of Water Resources Solid and Hazardous Waste/Ground Water Branch 815 Quarrier Street Suite 418 Charleston, West Virginia 25301
Wisconsin	Department of Natural Resources Bureau of Solid Waste Management PO Box 7921 Madison, Wisconsin 53707 (608) 267-3548
Wyoming	Department of Environmental Quality Solid Waste Management Program Hersler Building 4th Floor 122 W. 25th Street Cheyenne, Wyoming 82002 (307) 777-7752

APPENDIX 9–B

Disposal Tips for Home Health Care

MILLIONS OF HOUSEHOLDS PRODUCE MEDICAL WASTE

Every year, Americans use over one billion sharp objects in their homes to administer health care. These "sharps" include lancets, needles, and syringes. If they are not disposed of in puncture-resistant containers, they can injure trash handlers; can increase the risk of infection if they come in contact with contaminated materials such as bandages, dressings, and surgical gloves; and can pollute the environment.

WE NEED YOUR HELP

You play an important role in safe practices associated with health care at home. Through this brochure, we are asking your help to safely dispose of sharps and other contaminated medical waste, such as bandages and soiled disposable sheets. We urge all home health care patients to read and follow the disposal tips contained in this brochure and handout.

PREVENTING INJURY AND POLLUTION

Containers with Sharps Are Not Recyclable

EPA promotes all recycling activities, and therefore encourages you to discard medical waste sharps in sturdy, nonrecyclable containers, when possible. If a recyclable container is used to dispose of medical waste sharps, make sure that you don't mix the container with other materials to be recycled. Since the sharps impair a container's recyclability, a container holding your medical waste sharps properly belongs with the regular household trash. You may even want to label the container, "NOT FOR RECYCLING." These steps go a long way toward protecting workers and others from possible injury. (Although disposing of recyclable containers removes them from the recycling stream, the expected impact is minimal.)

LOCAL PROGRAMS

Your state or community environmental programs may have other requirements or suggestions for disposing of your medical waste. You should contact them for any information you may need.

DISPOSAL TIPS FOR HOME HEALTH CARE

You can help prevent injury, illness, and pollution by following some simple steps when you dispose of the sharp objects and contaminated materials you use in administering health care in your home. You should place:

- **Needles,**
- **Syringes,**
- **Lancets, and**
- **Other sharp objects**

in a hard-plastic or metal container with a screw-on or tightly secured lid.

Source: Reprinted from *Solid Waste and Emergency Response (5305)*, United States Environmental Protection Agency, EPA530-F-027-A, November 1993.

Many containers found in the household will do, or you may purchase containers specifically designed for the disposal of medical waste sharps. Before discarding a container, be sure to reinforce the lid with heavy-duty tape. **Do not put sharp objects in any container you plan to recycle or return to a store, and do not use glass or clear plastic containers.** Finally, make sure that you keep all containers with sharp objects out of the reach of children and pets.

We also recommend that:

- **Soiled bandages,**
- **Disposable sheets, and**
- **Medical gloves**

be placed in securely fastened plastic bags before you put them in the garbage can with your other trash.

Chapter 10

Surveillance of Home Care-Acquired Infections

Wherever health care is delivered, whether in the hospital, home, long-term care facility, or hospice, there is some risk that the patient will acquire an infection related to the care rendered. It is incumbent upon the home care organization and its professional staff members to recognize this risk and to use appropriate infection control and prevention strategies to reduce the risk and prevent infection. Even with the best infection control efforts, however, the risk of infection will never be completely eliminated because it depends on the host's ability to resist infection (intrinsic factors) as well as the many circumstances that surround the delivery of care (extrinsic factors). Home care professionals have the responsibility to measure the occurrence of home care-acquired infection in their patient population to estimate risk more accurately and determine whether infection control procedures are effective. Risk assessment is accomplished through surveillance activities.

INFECTION SURVEILLANCE

Surveillance is defined as "the ongoing, systematic collection, analysis, and interpretation of health data essential to the planning, implementation, and evaluation of public health practice, closely integrated with timely dissemination of these data to those who need to know" (Centers for Disease Control and Prevention [CDC], 1988, p. 1). Surveillance is based on epidemiological principles and methods and can be applied to many types of health data (e.g., cancer incidence, mortality statistics, and risk factors for a specific disease). Infectious disease epidemiology, among the oldest applications of the science, was initially applied to the study of epidemics to determine their cause and develop interventions to control them. A classic case is the Broad Street cholera epidemic, which occurred in 1849 in London, in which many thousands of people became ill and died. The source of the infection was determined through the now famous epidemiological study conducted by John Snow, which associated drinking water from the public well with the occurrence of the disease (Snow, 1965). More recently, infectious disease epidemiology has been applied to determine the cause and risk factors for new diseases such as acquired immune deficiency syndrome and Legionnaires' disease.

Hospital epidemiology is a developing field that began in the United States in the early 1970s with newly established infection control programs (see Chapter 1). Infection control practitioners (ICPs), who are usually nurses or microbiologists, and hospital epidemiologists, who are usually physicians with training in infectious diseases or microbiology, have developed surveillance programs specifically to study nosocomial infections. Study of nosocomial infection has allowed ICPs and hospital epidemiologists to determine the expected frequency of infection (endemic rates), identify risk factors (e.g., indwelling Foley catheters), and measure the effectiveness of interventions and strategies to reduce infection (e.g., maintaining a closed urinary drainage system). These efforts are greatly enhanced through the support of the CDC and the National Nosocomial Infection Surveillance (NNIS) study. The NNIS program has developed standard definitions of nosocomial infection as well as standardized methods for data management (Emori, Culver, & Horan, 1991; Garner,

Jarvis, Emori, Horan, & Hughes, 1988). Many U.S. hospitals (more than 200 in 1996) participate in NNIS and submit their data regularly for analysis and comparison. As a result, there are published rates of infection that provide a basis for comparison with other hospitals (Jarvis et al., 1998). Although NNIS provides standardized methods and valuable data, its current focus is hospital-acquired infections.

ICPs and others involved in health care quality are now challenged to develop surveillance methods for the study of health care–acquired infections in settings outside the hospital. Standardized surveillance systems are needed in home care, ambulatory care, long-term care, subacute facilities, and other settings where patients are at risk for the development of an infection that is related to the care they are receiving. Standardized methods (e.g., definitions, data collection, and data analysis) are needed so that the occurrence of infection from nonhospital settings can be measured, compared, and reduced. Although surveillance definitions and methods used in hospitals provide an excellent model for the study of infections in other settings, in most cases they must be significantly modified to accommodate the many differences from nonhospital settings. Although hospitalized patients may represent the most severely ill in the health care system, there is increasing acuity among patients in other settings, especially home care, which puts them at risk for infection. This chapter focuses on the development of surveillance methods for the study of home care-acquired infections.

WHY STUDY HOME CARE-ACQUIRED INFECTIONS?

Ongoing surveillance and the study of endemic and epidemic nosocomial infections provide scientifically valid information to identify risk factors and reduce risk. Endemic infection is the usual or expected rate of infection in a specific population within a defined time period. For example, a certain proportion of patients with indwelling Foley catheters will develop a urinary tract infection (UTI); the frequency will never be zero percent even with the best infection control efforts. When the frequency of infection is much higher than expected, an epidemic is said to occur. These outbreaks are frequently associated with a common bacterial agent. For example, an outbreak of vancomycin-resistant enterococci (VRE) may be identified in a group of home care patients who have undergone surgery at the same hospital during the same time period.

Publication of the "normal" or "expected" endemic rates of infection can be used to compare a hospital's nosocomial infection rate with that of other hospitals and to identify an epidemic or a rate of infection that is significantly greater than expected. NNIS publishes the results of the infection data that are submitted to the CDC (Gaynes, Edwards, Jarvis, Culver, Tolson, & Martone, 1996; Martone et al., 1995; Jarvis et al., 1998). These reports provide data that other hospitals can use to compare and evaluate their own rates of infection. Even when the same definitions and methods for surveillance are employed, however, caution must be used when infection rates are directly compared. There may be a number of differences in the patient populations and the manner in which care is delivered from one organization to another that must be considered in the comparison of results. Many of these factors are discussed in Chapter 3. A home care organization providing services to Medicare patients may have more older women with long-term indwelling Foley catheters and a higher endemic rate of UTIs than an organization caring for pediatric patients with less frequent long-term urinary catheter use. A more valid comparison for a home care organization providing Medicare services is another Medicare-certified agency with a similar patient population.

Based on NNIS data and the publication of other studies, ICPs have been able to identify specific risk reduction strategies and measure their effectiveness. For example, studies of catheter-related UTIs have demonstrated that risk is reduced by maintaining a closed drainage system (Kunin & McCormack, 1966). In addition, although performed to decrease risk for UTI, routine provision of meatal care has been shown actually to increase risk (Burke, Garibaldi, Britt, Jacobson, Conti, & Alling, 1981). Based on these studies, ICPs in hospitals have developed policies and procedures and have selected products (e.g., catheters with needle ports to obtain urine samples) to minimize the need to interrupt a urinary drainage system. Routine meatal care has been eliminated, and ongoing surveillance has provided data to show a measurable reduction in the occurrence of UTIs as a result.

Reports of outbreaks have also allowed ICPs to identify potential causes of infection and eliminate them. Publication of these outbreaks and the results of the investigational methods as well as risk reduction strategies provides important references for others in the field who may experience a similar situation.

The home care industry must support the study of home care-acquired infection through the development of surveillance systems and the publication of methods and results. Only then will providers of home care have a better estimate of the endemic rates of home care-acquired infection and the contributing risk factors. Outbreaks must also be studied and published for the benefit of other patients and providers. To date, there are few valid scientific reports describing endemic rates of home care-acquired infection or outbreaks and their control in the peer-reviewed health care literature (Lorenzen & Itkin, 1992; White, 1992; White & Ragland, 1993; Danzig et al., 1995; Kellerman et al., 1996).

ASSESSMENT OF THE POPULATION

There are specific steps that should be followed in the development of a surveillance system in a home care organization (Lee, Baker, Lee, Scheckler, Steele, & Laxton, 1998; Exhibit 10–1). First, the patient population must be assessed to identify the characteristics that may affect health status as well as the intrinsic and extrinsic factors that may affect risk for developing an infection. Intrinsic risk is related to the host and immune status. For example, patients with chronic diseases, such as insulin-dependent diabetes or chronic obstructive pulmonary disease, are at increased risk for infection. Extrinsic factors are related to the care being provided and the environment. Home infusion therapy presents specific risks because it involves an invasive procedure and an indwelling medical device.

In light of limited resources, surveillance efforts should focus on patients and services that represent the greatest risk for home care-acquired infection. For example, surveillance for bloodstream infections in children receiving home infusion therapy should be a priority because of the risks related to the age of the patients as well as to the therapy provided. In contrast, pneumonia in hospice patients would be considered differently for a surveillance program. When the decision must be made about where to focus surveillance efforts, priority should be given to those infections that first, are the direct result of home care services and interventions, and second, can be reduced through specific procedures under the control of the home care staff. Infections that are not directly related to home care services (e.g., UTIs in uncatheterized older female hospice patients) should not be measured unless resources for surveillance are unlimited. Identification of infection for surveillance purposes (to reduce overall risk) must be differentiated from the identification of an infection so that the patient's physician can provide appropriate treatment. Both are important, but they have different purposes.

Although individuals in home care organizations know the general characteristics of the patient population and the types of services being provided, a more explicit assessment should be done when planning for surveillance. Exhibit 10–2 provides a list of population characteristics and types of services that may be considered when a surveillance program is being designed for a home care organization. If possible, actual data and statistics from the past 1 to 2 years that describe the home care organization's population (e.g., Medicare or pediatric patients) and the types of care that patients have received (e.g., wound care or home infusion therapy) should be used to profile the population. This planning will help ensure that the limited resources available for surveillance activities are used in the most efficient manner.

Exhibit 10–1 Steps in Developing a Surveillance Program

1. Assess the patient population.
2. Select the outcome or process for surveillance.
3. Develop or select definitions.
4. Develop data collection methods.
5. Calculate rates and analyze data.
6. Apply risk stratification methods.
7. Use data and information for risk reduction and quality improvement.

SELECTION OF OUTCOMES OR PROCESSES FOR MEASUREMENT

Selection of the specific outcomes for measurement is the next important step in planning a home care surveillance program. Surveillance activities in home care should not include identification and measurement of community-acquired infections in home care patients. Community-acquired infections include upper and lower respiratory infections (e.g., colds, flu, and pneumonia), gastrointestinal infections (e.g., nausea, vomiting, diarrhea, and viral gastroenteritis), and other com-

Exhibit 10–2 Assessment of the Population

Patients Served	*Services Provided*
Age • Newborn • Pediatric • Adult • Geriatric	Homemaker/companion services Home health aide services Skilled nursing services • Medical • Surgical
Gender	
Race	Behavioral health care
National origin	Respiratory therapy
Language spoken in the home	Home infusion therapy
Level of education	Home hemodialysis
Socioeconomic status	Ambulatory peritoneal dialysis
Living conditions and sanitation	Medical equipment and supplies
Demographics • Urban • Suburban • Rural	Neonatal/infant/pediatric care Hospice care
Frequency of disease	Physical therapy
Common diagnoses	Occupational therapy
Chronic illnesses	Speech-language pathology
	Medical social services
	Perinatal/postpartum care
	Nutritional assessment and consultation

mon illnesses that may occur as a result of exposure in the community. Although home care staff members can advise patients in how to avoid the risk of community-acquired infection (e.g., by advising older patients to avoid crowds during influenza season), they do not have control over patients or family members. In fact, community-acquired infections may frequently come from a family member living in the patient's home; this risk is difficult to avoid. In addition, community-acquired infections are generally self-limiting and not usually specifically diagnosed through cultures or other laboratory tests, so they are difficult to define for surveillance purposes.

In some home care organizations, surveillance activities measure all home care-acquired infections in all home care patients. This approach of performing total surveillance is not reasonable for several reasons. First, it may not be necessary to detect all infections for the purpose of quality improvement. Some infections may not be preventable as a result of intrinsic risk factors. Second, unless significant resources are provided to support surveillance activities and ensure the accuracy and reliability of data, the data may be inaccurate and misleading. Finally, as has been demonstrated in nosocomial surveillance, conducting surveillance of all infections and calculating a single infection rate is ill advised. An overall rate is not specific or focused enough to draw conclusions or make reasonable plans for risk reduction. A reportedly low rate may be unreliable and may not reflect actual incidence and risk in certain high-risk patients. In addition, external agencies and organizations, such as managed care organizations, may request this rate and rely on its accuracy. Requests for such data should be denied with an explanation of why they are not reasonable or valid (Bryant, 1997).

Home care organizations should measure home care-acquired infections; that is, those infections that occur as a result of the home care provided. The term *home care-acquired infection* is preferred over other recently suggested terms, such as *nosohusial* or *homocomial* (Friedman, 1996). Rather than attempt to measure all health care-acquired infections, home care organizations should assign priority to a given measurement by considering factors related to risk and preventability. These factors may include the following (Lee et al., 1998):

- frequency of infection
- negative impact, such as increases in morbidity, mortality, and/or cost
- potential for prevention by home care staff
- specific needs and risks in the patient population served
- requirements of external customers (e.g., reporting requirements of managed care organizations)
- the organization's mission and strategic goals
- relationship of the infection outcome with the process of care
- resources available for surveillance

Infections are generally categorized by body site. A list of potential types of home care acquired infections to be considered for surveillance is provided in Exhibit 10–3. Not all infections listed must or should be monitored. Each home care organization must decide which infections to measure based on the factors listed above, assessment of the home care population served, and the knowledge gained from the surveillance planning process.

Exhibit 10–3 Sites of Home Care-Acquired Infection

Urinary tract

Respiratory tract

Skin and soft tissue

Gastrointestinal system

Central nervous system

Eye, ear, nose, throat, mouth

Bloodstream

IV-related infections

- catheter-related bloodstream
- infusate-related bloodstream
- exit site
- pocket
- tunnel

Data demonstrate that a large proportion of nosocomial infections is related to medical devices (device-related infections). These devices (e.g., urinary catheters, central venous catheters [CVCs], tracheotomies, etc.) interrupt (urinary catheter) or breech (CVC) normal anatomical barriers to infection and provide a portal of entry for microorganisms that is not normally present. They may also provide a protective environment for bacteria to grow and cause infection (Goldmann & Pier, 1993). Patients with indwelling devices have a greater extrinsic risk for infection than those without devices. Device-related infections should receive priority when sites are being selected for surveillance because the home care staff are responsible for care and maintenance of the device. Home care organizations providing home infusion therapy should minimally select catheter-related bloodstream infections as part of their surveillance activities.

Although many home care organizations monitor wound infections in their surveillance activities, surgical site infections are not usually home care-acquired infections. Surgical site infections begin (are seeded) in surgery. Once the surgical wound is closed, there is little risk for external contamination of the wound if there is primary closure and no drains are left in place. The wound is generally sealed in about 12 hours. For a surgical site infection to be a home care-acquired infection, the wound would either have to be open or have some type of drain or catheter in place that is being cared for in the home. If the wound has a drain to reduce the risk of infection (e.g., a Jackson-Pratt drain after head and neck surgery), the drainage system is usually closed. A home care-acquired surgical site infection might occur if a closed drainage system is entered carelessly and contaminated. Routine surveillance of true home care-acquired surgical site infections may not be of great value because the frequency should be very low.

A home care organization may decide to identify surgical site infections in postoperative patients for other purposes. Because most surgical site infections have an incubation period of 7 to 10 days (or longer), they are not evident before hospital discharge. Although most surgical site infections become evident while the patient is receiving home care services, the infection should be considered nosocomial and not home care-acquired. A home care organization might consider identifying, recording, and reporting surgical site infections to the referring hospital's infection control department to assist in its surveillance efforts. The information can be helpful because there are many surgical procedures that are now performed on an ambulatory basis and because the length of postoperative stay for those who are admitted to the hospital has decreased significantly in the past several years. This makes surgical site infection surveillance difficult for hospital ICPs. Home care staff can greatly improve the surveillance of nosocomial surgical site infections if they report them to the infection control program of the hospital where the surgery was performed or to the ICP in the ambulatory surgery center. Other infections that are recognized during the course of home care and are suspected to be of nosocomial origin can also be reported to the hospital infection control program.

Wound infection surveillance for home care-acquired infections may more logically focus on infected decubitus ulcers and soft tissue infections that are the result of skin breakdown. Although there are many intrinsic host factors that affect the risk for decubitus ulcers and general skin integrity, there are a variety of interventions that may reduce the risk. These are logical targets for surveillance and improvement efforts.

DEVELOPING DEFINITIONS FOR HOME CARE-ACQUIRED INFECTIONS

Although home care staff can recognize infections, definitions provide specific criteria for measuring home care-acquired infections in a consistent manner. Otherwise, one staff member may interpret various clinical signs and symptoms as an infection more frequently than another staff member. Consistency among staff members in identifying and measuring infections for surveillance is referred to as interrater reliability. Ideally, the same conclusion about the presence of an infection should be reached no matter who is performing surveillance. Application of specific criteria within a definition facilitates this consistency. In addition, standard definitions are necessary if rates of infection are going to be compared with those reported by other home care organizations.

NNIS has published a full set of definitions for nosocomial infections (Garner et al., 1988). Although these definitions are widely used in hospital surveillance programs, they are not easily adapted to home care. Legitimately, the NNIS definitions rely heavily on diagnostic tests (e.g., cultures, laboratory tests, and radiological imaging) to identify and define infection. Obtaining specimens for cultures and laboratory tests is not common practice in home care. Frequently, a physician makes the diagnosis of an infection based on signs and symptoms, the patient's history and current health status, and extrinsic risk factors. Diagnosis is made for the purpose of treatment, not for surveillance. The physician will more often presume that the patient is infected and treat the infection empirically rather than underdiagnose and increase the potential for additional complications. Currently, many home care organizations use a physician's diagnosis of infection or prescription for antibiotic therapy as the sole criterion for the definition of a home care-acquired infection, but this may lead to higher than actual infection rates. A set of definitions has been developed for infections acquired in long-term care that may be helpful in the development of definitions for home care-acquired infections (McGeer et al., 1991). These definitions are less reliant on laboratory data than the NNIS definitions.

Several groups, including the Association for Professionals in Infection Control and Epidemiology and the Missouri Alliance for Home Care, have been working to develop definitions for home care-acquired infection for surveillance purposes. Other groups may also be active in this pursuit. If there are local or state groups sponsoring projects for home care infection surveillance, a home care organization should investigate these efforts and consider participating in them.

The development of definitions of infection for the purposes of surveillance should be based on several considerations. First, clinical data, including typical signs and symptoms that would occur in a normal host with the infection of interest, should be incorporated into the definition. Signs and symptoms will vary according to the site of infection and age of the patient. For example, symptoms of a UTI include frequency, burning, and pain. Signs include a fever and cloudy urine. A skin or wound infection may result in symptoms of redness, pain, and tenderness at the site. Purulent drainage may be observed as a sign of infection. Definitions of infection should take into account the fact that signs and symptoms might vary in different age groups. Neonates, infants, and children exhibit different signs and symptoms of infection than adults. For example, neonates may not develop a fever if they have a bloodstream infection, and their body temperature may be below normal. These differences must be incorporated into the definitions of infection if different age groups are served by the home care organization.

Second, some type of laboratory data should be included in the definition of a home care-acquired infection as objective evidence of infection. This is more difficult because the diagnosis of infection for the purpose of treatment in home care patients is more often empirical (based on the physician's assessment of the signs and symptoms reported) and less often based on laboratory tests. The diagnosis of a UTI is frequently based on signs and symptoms, and antibiotics are ordered without a culture. For surveillance purposes, however, it is preferable to have some confirmatory laboratory data whenever possible. Table 10–1 provides some criteria for consideration in the development of definitions for home care-acquired infections by site.

The definitions developed by the Missouri Alliance for Home Care for catheter-related UTIs and CVC infection are provided in Exhibit 10–4. According to the definition, a UTI requires the observation of a change in the character of the urine as well as at least two signs and symptoms of infection, which may include an elevated serum white blood cell count. The definition also specifies that, if a physician prescribes antibiotics for treatment of a UTI, it is counted as an infection for surveillance purposes. CVC infection also requires two or more signs and symptoms, including elevated serum white blood cell count or culture of a pathogen from the CVC.

The surveillance of infections related to home infusion therapy (see Chapter 4) is important but may be the most challenging in terms of the development of definitions. To accurately determine the incidence of infections related to intravenous (IV) therapy and identify specific risks, definitions for various types of IV-related infections must be developed. As discussed above, both clin-

Table 10–1 Criteria for Definition of Infection by Site

Site of Infection	*Clinical Data*	*Laboratory Data*
Catheter-related UTI	Change in characteristics of urine Fever Pain	Elevated serum white blood cell (WBC) count Evidence of UTI on urinalysis Evidence of WBCs on urine dipstick test Positive urine culture (>10^5 colony forming units of a single organism per milliliter of urine)
Postoperative pneumonia	Change in character of sputum Decreased breath sounds Increase in rales and rhonchi Fever Shortness of breath Pain	Elevated serum WBC Evidence of respiratory infection on sputum Gram stain Positive sputum culture Positive chest radiograph
Catheter-related bloodstream infection	Fever with chills and rigors Redness, tenderness, pain at insertion site Purulent drainage at site	Elevated serum WBC Positive blood culture Positive catheter culture (after catheter removal)
Skin and soft tissue (includes infected decubitus ulcer)	Pain, swelling, tenderness at site Inflammation and warmth Purulent drainage Fever	WBCs and organisms on Gram stain Positive culture Elevated serum WBC
Endometritis in postpartum patients	Uterine tenderness and abdominal pain Purulent vaginal drainage (lochia) Foul-smelling lochia Fever	Positive Gram stain of lochia Positive culture of lochia Elevated serum WBC

Exhibit 10–4 Missouri Alliance for Home Care Definitions of Home Care-Acquired Infections

Catheter-Related UTI	*CVC Infection**
The patient has an indwelling urethral catheter or suprapubic catheter and: 1. A change in the character of the urine • Hematuria • Increasing levels of sediment • Foul odor • Plus two or more of the following signs and symptoms: – Fever of 100.4°F or greater† – New flank pain or suprapubic pain† – Elevated serum white blood cell count† – Worsening or change in mental status† – A pathogen or pathogens cultured from the urine OR 2. A physician prescribes a course of antibiotic treatment for a suspected bladder infection	A patient with an indwelling CVC and: 1. Two or more of the following signs or symptoms: • Erythema associated with the central line • Pain associated with the central line • Purulent drainage from the exit site • Elevated serum white blood cell count† • Fever 100.4°F or greater† OR 2. A physician prescribes a course of antibiotic treatment for a suspected or confirmed CVC infection OR 3. A physician orders the removal of the CVC because of suspected or confirmed infection

*Includes central venous lines, PICC lines, implanted ports, subclavian and jugular catheters, Hickman and Broviac catheters, and Groshong catheters.

†Need to rule out other possible causes of infection, i.e., respiratory.

Courtesy of the Missouri Alliance for Home Care, Jefferson City, Missouri.

ical signs and symptoms (e.g., fever and redness at the exit site) and laboratory data (e.g., positive blood cultures) should be incorporated, with definitions. Bloodstream infection should also be distinguished by its source. Bloodstream infection may be secondary to an infection at another site (e.g., secondary to pneumonia), or it may be secondary to contaminated IV fluid. Bloodstream infection may also arise from a colonized CVC, or it may be related to an exit site infection. The specific source must be distinguished in the definition of bloodstream infection to assess the risk accurately. In addition to clinical signs and symptoms, the definition of catheter-related bloodstream infection should include positive blood culture results with cultures drawn from two separate sites. One culture specimen should be drawn through the IV catheter and a second obtained through a percutaneous blood draw. If both cultures grow the same organism (i.e., genus and species) with the same antibiotic sensitivity pattern, the infection can be considered a catheter-related bloodstream infection (Pearson, 1996).

Local IV-related infections must also be specifically defined with consideration given to the type of IV access device. Signs and symptoms of infection (e.g., redness, tenderness, and purulent drainage) may be incorporated into a definition of exit site infection related to percutaneous catheters (such as peripherally inserted central catheter lines). A tunnel infection may occur in surgically implanted catheters, such as a Hickman catheter. A tunnel infection is one that is below the skin and exit site that affects the subcutaneous tract that was created to "tunnel" the catheter below the skin and into a major vein. Subcutaneous IV access devices or ports have surgically created pockets that may become infected. They, too, should be considered in the development of definitions for IV-related infection (Pearson, 1996).

The definition of home care–acquired infection must also consider the incubation period for the infection. The incubation period is the time from the initial exposure to the pathogen to the time when the infection is evident. Most bacterial infections have an incubation period of 48 to 72 hours, but the period may be shorter or longer. The incubation time varies for viral infections; for chickenpox it is 10 to 21 days, and for influenza it is 24 to 48 hours. The incubation period must be considered to avoid counting nosocomial infections (or infections that originated at other sites of care) as home care-acquired. Therefore, if a patient discharged from a hospital with an indwelling Foley catheter exhibits signs and symptoms of a UTI within 48 hours of admission for home care, the infection should not be counted as home care-acquired because it is probably nosocomial. Specific circumstances should be considered, however. Some home care-acquired infections can occur within the first 72 hours of home care. For example, if a patient receiving home parenteral nutrition develops a fever with shaking chills and rigors the first or second day at home and immediately after a new bag of IV fluid has been hung, this should be counted as a home care-acquired bloodstream infection. Other circumstances in which it is clear that a home care intervention within the first 72 hours of care has led to an infection should be considered.

There are two specific conditions that should not be included as home care-acquired infections: colonization and inflammation. As explained in Chapter 2, colonization describes the presence of bacteria without multiplication and damage to the host tissue. A positive culture may detect colonization, but the application of the definition of infection should avoid inclusion of a case of colonization as a home care-acquired infection. Inflammation may occur without infection, such as occurs in phlebitis from a peripheral venous catheter. Again, a consistent definition of infection should be applied to avoid the identification of an inflammation as an infection.

DATA COLLECTION METHODS

Once the site definitions of infection are selected or developed, the home care organization must determine what additional information about each infected patient should be collected and analyzed. The general tendency is to collect more information than is useful, such as recording the name and dose of the antibiotic ordered to treat an infection. This approach should be avoided because data collection may be time consuming, adding to the expense of performing surveillance. To determine what specific information will be recorded, the home care organization must consider the value and future use of the specific information in elucidating more about home care-acquired infection. If the data will not be useful in describing the occurrence of home care-acquired infections and identifying risk factors, it should probably not be collected. Useful data, however, may include the specific organism that is cultured from the site of infection, which may lead to the recognition of an outbreak or specific reservoir of infection.

The data collected and recorded should include patient demographic data, data to describe the infection, and some risk data. Demographic data are information about the patient, including age, gender, and diagnosis. Other variables about the patient may be helpful but should be limited to only what is considered necessary. For example, when information is collected about bloodstream infection in children receiving home infusion therapy, in addition to the patient's identification number, the demographic data might include the child's age, gender, primary diagnosis, and primary caregiver. If the home care organization provides care in an urban setting for a diverse ethnic population, the primary language spoken in the home may be an important demographic variable. In an elderly patient population, additional information about living arrangements (e.g., lives alone, lives with daughter, lives with disabled elderly spouse) may be important.

A description of the infection should include the site of infection, date of infection onset (first day on which signs and symptoms were observed), and the results of cultures, if available. It is usually not useful to collect data on the antibiotic sensitivity report for routine surveillance. If the organism demonstrates multidrug resistance (e.g., methicillin-resistant *Staphylococcus aureus* or VRE), that information should be noted in the infection report.

The risk data collected depend on the site of infection. Some examples of risk elements are provided in Table 10–2. For example, information about IV catheter–related infections should include the type of catheter (e.g., Broviac or Hickman) and the number of lumens because these may be important risk factors. Information must be recorded in a practical, useful manner. Thus it must be categorized or coded so that it can be either entered into a database or easily counted and summarized in a table. Descriptive information that is written in sentences or phrases does not lend itself to easy analysis. Dependence on a written narrative to provide information about home care-acquired infection should be avoided. Thus an infection report form should be designed with check boxes and minimal "fill in the blank" fields. An example of an infection control report form is provided in Exhibit 10–5.

PERIOD OF SURVEILLANCE

A specified period for which data are collected and analyzed should be determined before data collection

Table 10–2 Risk Factors for Home Care-Acquired Infection by Site

Site of Infection	*Risk Factors*
Catheter-related UTI	Date of insertion Urethral versus suprapubic catheter
IV catheter-related infection	Type of catheter (Hickman, Broviac, peripherally inserted central, midline) Central or peripheral Percutaneous or implanted Number of lumens Date of insertion Type of IV therapy (total parenteral nutrition, antibiotics)
Postoperative pneumonia	Date and type of surgery
Gastrointestinal infection in patients receiving enteral nutrition	Type of enteral therapy (prepared in home or preprepared) If prepared in home, how and by whom
Peritonitis in CAPD patients	Type of catheter Date of placement

is initiated. Hospitals use surveillance periods of 1 month. Most home care organizations conduct surveillance over a 90-day time period or by quarters. Based on anecdotal experience and limited data (White, 1992), however, it appears that home care-acquired infections do not occur as frequently as hospital-acquired infections. Home care surveillance periods should be longer than 30 days so that a sufficient sample size for data analysis can be gathered, conclusions drawn, and risk reduction activities planned. Eventually, annual rates of infection by site can be calculated, but the trending of rates over short periods, such as monthly or quarterly, is much more meaningful and sensitive, provided that there is a sufficiently large sample.

DEFINING DENOMINATORS

Infections should never be reported as a number of events (e.g., 12 UTIs in May and 16 UTIs in June). Infections should be reported, analyzed, and trended as rate-based data by infection site. To develop rate-based data, it is necessary to have a numerator (number of infections) and a denominator. The denominator is the number of patients at risk for that infection (e.g., postoperative patients at risk for postoperative pneumonia during the surveillance period) or the number of days at risk (e.g., total number of catheter days for all patients with indwelling urinary catheters during the surveillance period). Days at risk provides a more accurate estimate of risk when the rate of device-related infections is calculated. The alternative measure is the number of patients with a device, no matter how long they had the device. This does not adequately or accurately represent the risk because the risk for infection increases with exposure time. The longer a device is in place, the greater the risk for infection.

A specific denominator must be developed or selected for each site of home care-acquired infection. Suggested denominators for various sites of infection are found in Table 10–3. It is important to define the denominator before surveillance begins because this will determine which patients will be monitored for the infection. Methods to identify patients with the infection of interest are discussed below.

RETROSPECTIVE VERSUS CONCURRENT DATA COLLECTION

Infections should always be identified concurrently (as they occur) rather than retrospectively (after the fact). Retrospective surveillance is usually based on chart review. Retrospective clinical record review should not be performed as the routine method of case finding mainly because it may be inaccurate. Retrospective clinical record review depends solely on what is written in the patient record and may not include important signs and symptoms; also, it is labor intensive. In addition, if the home care staff member who cared for the patient is asked to clarify information in the clinical record, recall may be incomplete or inaccurate. Finally, if a retrospective approach is taken, current problems and outbreaks of infection may be missed.

Exhibit 10–5 Infection Screening Report

Date of Report: ______________________________ Completed by: ______________________________

Patient Name: ______________________________ Identification Number: ____________ SOC date: ______

Primary Diagnosis: ______________________________ Physician Name: ______________________________

Instructions: The staff member observing the signs and symptoms should complete sections one and two and submit the report to infection control practitioner. ______________________________

Section One: Patient Signs and Symptoms ***(Check all that apply)***

Signs and Symptoms and Date Observed: ____________

□ Fever ≥ 100.5° F (oral)
□ Chills and rigors
□ Elevated serum WBC Date: ____________ Results: ____________________ or □ Copy of lab results attached
□ New antibiotic order Date: ____________ Order: ______________________________
□ New culture order—Site and date: ____________
□ Positive culture results or □ Copy of lab results attached
Date culture obtained: ____________ Site of culture: ____________________
Organism(s) isolated: ______________________________
Drug resistant organisms: □ Yes □ No Describe ____________________

Section Two: Potential Infection Site(s)

Possible catheter-associated UTI

□ Change in character of urine (Check all that apply: □ increased sediment, □ cloudiness, □ foul odor, □ hematuria)
□ New flank pain or suprapubic pain
□ Change or worsening mental status
□ WBC's in dipstick urine test

Possible bloodstream infection

□ IV catheter-related bloodstream infection
□ IV infusate-related bloodstream infection
□ Secondary to other infection site
Primary site (e.g., pneumonia, peritonitis): ____________________

Possible IV catheter-related infection (Check One: □ exit site □ tunnel □ pocket)

□ Insertion/exit site, tunnel or pocket (Check all that apply: □ redness, □ pain, □ swelling)
□ MD ordered catheter to be removed
□ Pain, tenderness at pocket site
□ Pain, tenderness along tunnel
□ Purulent drainage—Describe: ____________________
Date of catheter insertion: ____________________

Possible skin or soft tissue infection

Specific site: ______________________________
Check all that apply: □ redness □ pain or tenderness □ swelling
□ Purulent drainage—Describe: ____________________
□ Evidence of cellulitis—Describe: ____________________

Possible wound infection (Check One: □ wound □ drain site □ decubitus)

□ Redness, tenderness
□ Swelling
□ Purulent drainage—Describe: ______________________________
□ Post-operative wound Date and type of surgery: ____________________

continues

Exhibit 10–5 continued

Possible Pneumonia

□ Change in sputum (Check all that apply: □ color, □ purulence, □ thickness)
□ Increase in rales and rhonchi
□ Decrease in breath sounds
□ Pain in chest/thorax
□ Change or worsening mental status
□ Shortness of breath

Possible Postpartum Endometritis

□ Uterine tenderness
□ Abdominal pain
□ Foul-smelling lochia

Possible Peritonitis

□ Abdominal pain
□ Rebound tenderness

Possible Gastrointestinal

□ Sudden onset of nausea and vomiting
□ Diarrhea

Source: Copyright © 1999, Emily Rhinehart and Mary Friedman.

Elements from Exhibit 10–5 can be combined with elements of Exhibit 10–6 to develop a single form for screening and recording home care-acquired infections.

It may also be preferable to collect denominator data concurrently, depending on the type of data required. For example, if the denominator is the number of patients admitted for CVC care, the data may be captured from a clinical documentation system, so that counting at the end of the month may be accurate and feasible. If the denominator is the total number of days for which all patients had indwelling urinary catheters, however, a daily count (concurrent) may be necessary. Concurrent versus retrospective capture of denominator data

Table 10–3 Denominators for Infection by Site

Infection Site (Numerator)	*Denominator*	*Type of Rate*
Catheter-related UTI	Total number of catheter days for all patients with indwelling Foley catheters	Incidence density
Postoperative pneumonia	Number of patients admitted during surveillance period for postoperative care	Cumulative incidence
IV-related bloodstream infection	Total number of catheter days for all patients with venous access devices (or by device if there is a sufficient sample)	Incidence density
Skin and soft tissue infection in patients with diabetes	Number of patients with insulin-dependent diabetes mellitus admitted or cared for during surveillance period	Cumulative incidence
Gastrointestinal infection in patients receiving enteral nutrition	Number of patients receiving enteral nutrition or total number of days for which all patients received enteral nutrition	Incidence density
Endometritis in postpartum patients	Number of postpartum patients admitted during surveillance period	Cumulative incidence
Peritonitis in patients receiving continuous ambulatory peritoneal dialysis (CAPD)	Total number of days during surveillance period	Incidence density

may depend on what data are available electronically in a clinical record or billing system and what data must be compiled manually.

IDENTIFYING HOME CARE-ACQUIRED INFECTIONS

Once the specific definitions for home care-acquired infections are developed and denominators selected, case finding to identify patients with the infection of interest can begin. The home care organization must decide who will be responsible for identifying the cases and reporting or recording them for the purpose of surveillance and data analysis. In some organizations, all the professional home care staff may be responsible for identifying and recording infections. This may result in poor interrater reliability, however, if too many individuals are applying the definitions and counting infections. To improve the reliability of surveillance data, the home care organization may decide to conduct surveillance in two phases: screening all patients at risk for the specified infection, and then applying the specific definition. With this approach, all professional staff members are required to report any patient with signs and symptoms of an infection. This may include patients with fever, local signs and symptoms of infection, and a new prescription for an antibiotic. Reports should not be verbal; a screening form should be completed (a sample form is provided as Exhibit 10–6) and forwarded to the individual who has been designated as the ICP responsible for surveillance.

The designated ICP should review the screening form to determine whether the infection meets the criteria for home care-acquired infection as specified in the organization's definitions. The ICP should make this determination based on additional information obtained by reviewing the clinical record, speaking with the professional who filled out the infection control screening form, speaking with the patient's physician if necessary, reviewing laboratory data if available, and/or actually visiting the patient, if necessary, to assess for infection. Once the ICP has determined that the patient meets the definition of infection, he or she will record information about the patient, the infection, and risk factors for aggregation and further analysis. The infection reporting form (Exhibit 10–5) and the sample screening form (Exhibit 10–6) can be combined into a single surveillance form if preferred, but the two-phase approach to improve data reliability should be kept in mind.

The ICP should be a registered nurse who has had some training or additional education in infection control, including surveillance methods. In this role, the nurse not only would be responsible for surveillance but also may be responsible for developing and maintaining current infection control policies and procedures, providing staff education related to infection control, and serving as the primary resource for infection control questions (see Chapter 13).

AGGREGATION AND ANALYSIS OF INFECTION DATA

At the end of the surveillance period, all the numerator and denominator data should be aggregated. Analysis can then be performed. If surveillance data are aggregated and reported quarterly, the ICP should review them each month to ensure the completeness and accuracy of the infection reports. Denominator data should also be obtained monthly or at the end of the quarter if they have not already been collected. Data collection for a particular surveillance period usually cannot be completed until 7 to 10 days after the end of the period. This delay allows for recognition and reporting of all infections that are evidenced within the time period and for other systems to complete the tallying of denominator data. Once a complete set of numerator data and denominator data is available, however, the ICP should not delay in preparing the infection report.

An additional form or tool that may be used at this time to analyze the organization's infection surveillance data is a line listing. This form contains a summary of information for all infections identified at a specific site. A line listing can be compiled manually, or it may be generated as part of a computerized surveillance program. A line listing is frequently helpful in that all the key information about the infections can be viewed on one page. This may facilitate recognition of a specific risk factor or frequency of a specific organism. A sample line listing is provided in Exhibit 10–7.

At a minimum, the individual preparing the infection report should provide a summary of the infections that have occurred, calculate rates, and provide some analysis of the current incidence of home care-acquired infection. As discussed above, some infection rates will use the number of patients at risk as the denominator, and some will use days at risk. These two types of rates are referred to as cumulative incidence and incidence

Exhibit 10–6 Confirmed Home Care-Acquired Infection Report

Patient Name: ______________________ Identification Number: ______________________

Age: _______ Gender: M F Primary Diagnosis: ______________________

Lives alone ☐ Lives with spouse or family ☐

Primary language spoken: ☐ English ☐ Other: ______________________

Confirmed Site of Infection:	***Culture Results (if available):***

☐ Catheter-associated UTI
☐ Bloodstream infection:
  ☐ IV catheter-related bloodstream infection
  ☐ IV infusate-related bloodstream infection
  ☐ Secondary to other infection
☐ IV catheter-related infection
  ☐ Exit site infection
  ☐ IV tunnel infection
  ☐ IV pocket infection
☐ Skin or soft tissue infection
  ☐ Decubitus
  ☐ Other
☐ Surgical site infection
☐ Wound drain or G-tube site infection
  ☐ Pneumonia
  ☐ Postpartum endometritis
  ☐ Peritonitis
☐ Gastrointestinal infection
	☐ Attach a copy of culture results
	  OR complete as follows:
	Date obtained: ______________
	Site of culture:
	☐ Urine
	☐ Blood
	☐ Wound drainage or lochia
	☐ Sputum
	☐ Other
	Organism(s) isolated: ______________________
	______________________
	Multidrug-resistant ☐ Yes ☐ No
	If yes, describe: ______________________

UTI

☐ Indwelling foley Date of original insertion: ______________ Date of last insertion: ______________

☐ Indwelling suprapubic catheter Date of original insertion: ______________ Date of last insertion: ______________

IV-Related infection

☐ Central Venous Access Device Date of insertion: ______________

- ☐ Nontunneled CVC—Number of lumens: _____
- ☐ Hickman/Broviac—Number of lumens: _____
- ☐ Implanted port—Number of lumens: _______
  - ☐ Single lumen
  - ☐ Double lumen
  - ☐ Triple lumen
- ☐ PICC—Number of lumens: _____
- ☐ Other ____________________

☐ Peripheral Venous Access Device

Type: ____________________ Date of insertion: ______________

- ☐ Short line
- ☐ Midline

Pneumonia

☐ Post-operative

☐ Immobility (non–post-op) including stroke. Cause of immobility: ____________________

☐ Ventilator dependent

☐ Tracheostomy tube

☐ Enteral feeding

☐ Respiratory therapy (e.g., oxygen, nebulizer)

Type: ____________________

Surgical site infection
G-tube site infection
Type and date of surgical procedure or G-tube insertion:

____

Gastrointestinal infection
□ Enteral feeding
Feedings prepared by: ______________
Feedings provided by: ______________
Peritonitis
□ CAPD
□ Other ______________

Previous hospital or long-term care admission (date of discharge): ______________

Other risk factors:

____

____

To be completed by infection control practitioner

Screening Results
(Check One): □ Home care-acquired infection □ Nosocomial infection □ Community-acquired infection

Infection reported to, as applicable:
□ Physician (Name and date): ______________
□ Hospital ICP (Name and date): ______________
□ Pharmacist (Name and date): ______________
□ Department of Health (Name and date): ______________

Reviewed by: (Name and date) ______________

Recorded for surveillance period of: □ 1st Quarter, □ 2nd Quarter, □ 3rd Quarter, □ 4th Quarter Year ________
Additional Comments: ______________________________

____

Source:

Exhibit 10–7 Line Listing for IV Catheter-Related Bloodstream Infections

Patient ID	*Age and Gender*	*Dx*	*Date of Catheter Insertion*	*Date of Onset*	*Type of Catheter*	*Number of Lumens*	*Type of IV Therapy*	*Culture Results*
19837204	64 yo/M	Bowel obst	12/12/97	3/19/98	Broviac	1	TPN	N/A
19827684	45 yo/F	Endocarditis	1/14/98	2/2/98	PICC	1	Atb therapy	S. epidermidis
19875385	18 mo/F	Short gut	2/3/98	3/18/98	Hickman	3	TPN, meds	E. faecalis
19885490	70 yo/M	Ca bowel	1/29/98	2/28/98	Portacath	1	Chemo and meds	S. aureus
19865075	35 yo/M	AIDS	11/23/97	1/14/98	Hickman	3	Meds and Atb	C. albicans
19860974	56 yo/F	Ca—breast	2/5/98	3/22/98	PICC	1	Chemo	N/A
19892755	22 yo/M	Osteo	3/12/98	3/29/98	Peripheral	1	Atb	N/A
19843847	3 yo/F	Leukemia	1/14/98	3/15/98	Hickman	2	Chemo, Atb	E. cloacea

Exhibit 10–8 Formulas for Calculation of Infection Rates

Cumulative Incidence	*Incidence Density*
$\frac{\text{N (Number of infections)}}{\text{D (Number of patients at risk)}} \times 100 = \text{Rate}$	$\frac{\text{N (Number of infections)}}{\text{D (Number of days at risk)}} \times 1000 = \text{Rate per 1,000 days}$
N = Number of patients with postoperative pneumonia D = Number of postoperative patients	N = Number of bloodstream infections D = Number of IV catheter days
$\frac{4}{164} \times 100 = 2.4\%$ infection rate	$\frac{4}{1820} \times 1{,}000 = 2.2$ bloodstream infections per 1,000 catheter days

density. The formulas for calculating each are given in Exhibit 10–8.

The individuals in the home care organization who review infection surveillance data will usually prefer to have data provided in simple charts, graphs, and tables rather than lengthy written or verbal reports. These tables and graphs should be used to summarize data by site. Table 10–4 is an example of a summary of UTI data displayed by quarter for 1998 and 1999. In this home care organization, a risk reduction effort was focused on reducing the number of patients with Foley catheters to reduce the days of exposure. Table 10–4 shows that in the first two quarters of 1999 the home care organization was able to accomplish both goals. This apparently led to the reduction in the number of UTIs as well as the risk per 1,000 catheter days.

Other descriptive data about patients with home care–acquired infections can be placed in a table or graph. These may include data about the frequency of infection related to specific risk factors. Table 10–5 summarizes information about catheter-related bloodstream infections, including information about catheter placement (peripheral or central) and the type of therapy. The frequency of specific organisms causing home care-acquired infections can also be illustrated. Figure 10–1 is a pie chart depicting the proportion of various organisms causing IV-related bloodstream infections in 1998. The bar graph in Figure 10–2 illustrates the proportion of home care-acquired infections by site for six consecutive quarters in 1998 and 1999.

Incidence data should be tracked and trended. This lends itself to representing data on a line or run chart. Figures 10–3 and 10–4 depict time on the horizontal axis and the rate of infection on the vertical axis. This allows for easy identification of increases and decreases in the rate of infection over time.

No single table, graph, or chart may be sufficient to allow for identification of all important variables or

Table 10–4 UTI Data by Quarter

Quarter	*Number of Patients with Foley Catheters*	*Total Catheter Days**	*Mean (Range)†*	*Number of Infections*	*Incidence Density‡*
1st Q 98	108	6,912	64 (3–90)	26	3.76
2nd Q 98	112	8,064	72 (2–90)	32	3.96
3rd Q 98	102	4,896	68 (4–90)	34	6.94
4th Q 98	115	6,900	78 (2–90)	28	4.05
1st Q 99	98	6,468	66 (2–88)	22	3.40
2nd Q 99	88	4,928	56 (2–78)	18	3.65

* Obtained by adding all the catheter days from all patients with catheters.
† Mean calculated by adding all catheter days and dividing by number of patients.
Range is the fewest number of catheter days in one patient to the greatest number of catheter days in one patient.
‡ Number of UTIs/Total number of catheter days × 1000 = Incidence density

Table 10–5 Summary of Bloodstream Infections

Quarter	*Number of Patients Receiving IV Therapy*	*Number of Bloodstream Infections*	*Pediatric/ Adult Patients (%)*	*Peripheral/ Central Catheters (%)*	*Number of Infected Patients on Total Parenteral Nutrition*	*Number of Infected Patients Receiving Antibiotics*	*Number of Infected Patients Receiving Chemotherapy*
1st Q 98	230	6	66/34	36/64	2 (33%)	1 (16%)	3 (50%)
2nd Q 98	184	2	72/28	22/88	0 (0%)	0 (0%)	2 (100%)
3rd Q 98	192	4	56/44	44/56	1 (25%)	0 (0%)	3 (17%)
4th Q 98	225	8	82/18	21/89	3 (38%)	1 (12%)	4 (50%)
1st Q 99	212	3	76/24	38/62	1 (33%)	0 (0%)	2 (66%)
2nd Q 99	198	1	68/32	28/82	0 (0%)	0 (0%)	1 (100%)

causes of home care-acquired infections. The ICP may want to experiment with displaying the data in various ways, and the individuals who examine the data can determine which is most useful.

Once a full year of data is accumulated, there may be more questions about the interpretation of the data beyond simple incidence and trends over time. For example, is the increase or decrease in the incidence density of UTIs in Table 10–4 in 1999 statistically significant? Is the difference in risk of bloodstream infection related to total parenteral nutrition versus chemotherapy in Table 10–5 statistically significant? Although these questions are important, it is more important to look for trends than for statistical significance. In the UTI example, the orga-

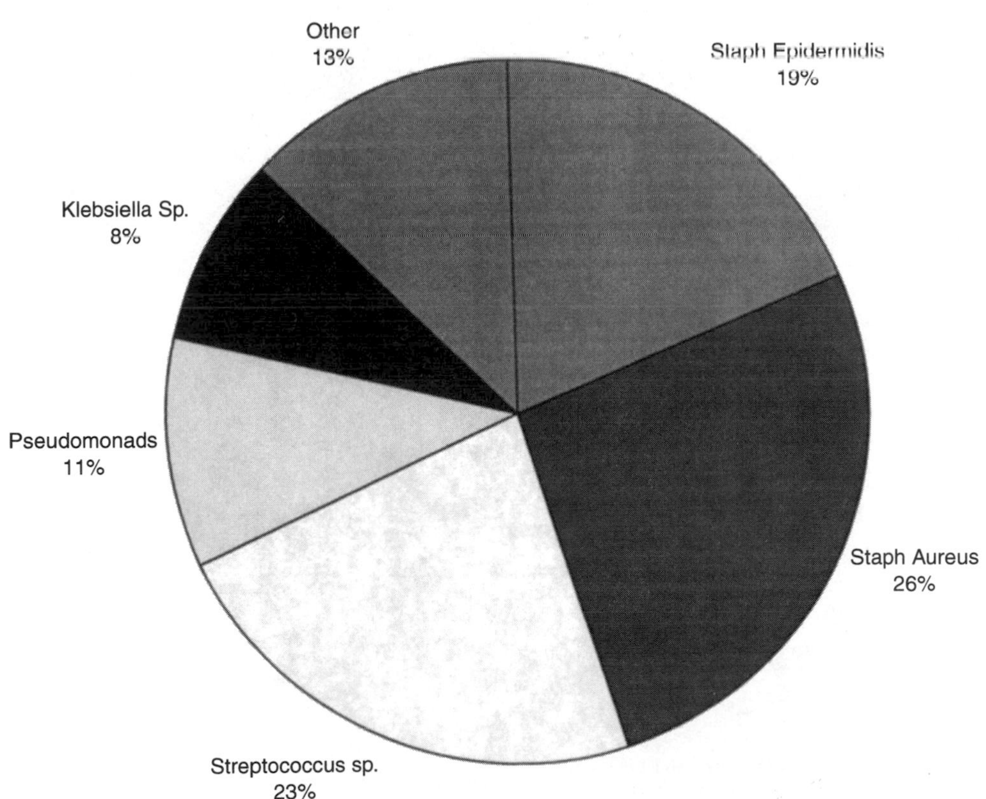

Figure 10–1 Organisms Causing IV-Related Bloodstream Infections, 1998.

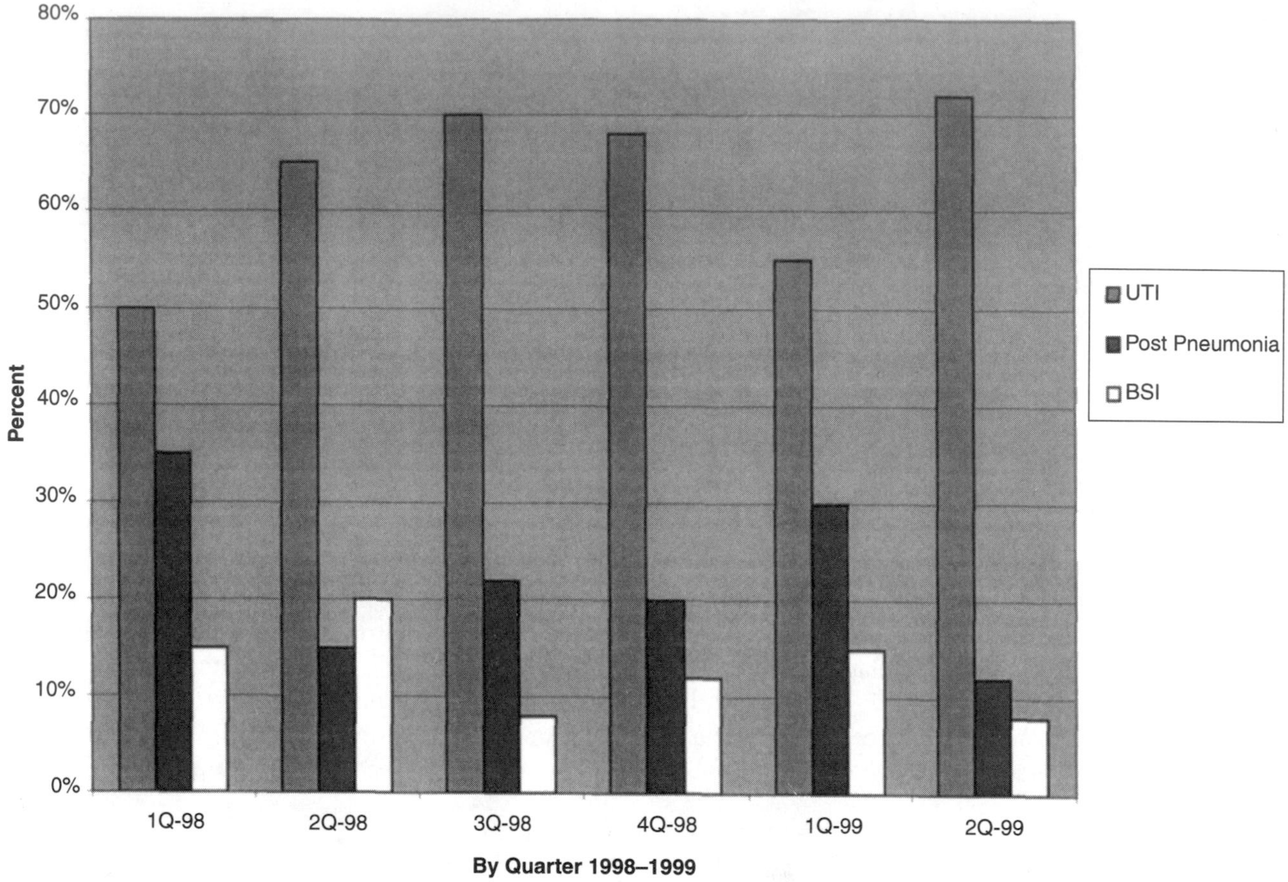

80%
70%
60%
50%
40%
30%
20%
10%
0%
Percent
UTI
Post Pneumonia
BSI
1Q-98
2Q-98
3Q-98
4Q-98
1Q-99
2Q-99
By Quarter 1998–1999

Figure 10–2 Proportions Summary of Home Care-Acquired Infection by Site, 1998–1989

12
10
8
6
4
2
0
Cumulative Incidence of Pneumonia
1Q-98
2Q-98
3Q-98
4Q-98
1Q-99
2Q-99
By Quarter 1998–1999

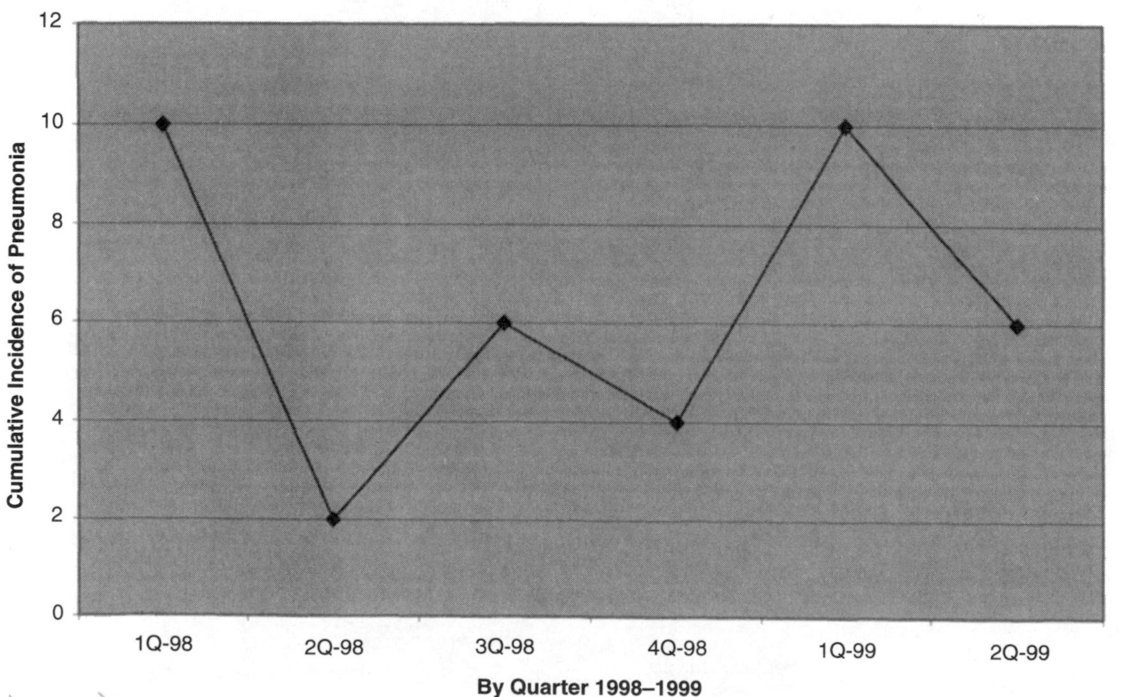

Figure 10–3 Post-operative Pneumonia (Cumulative Incidence)

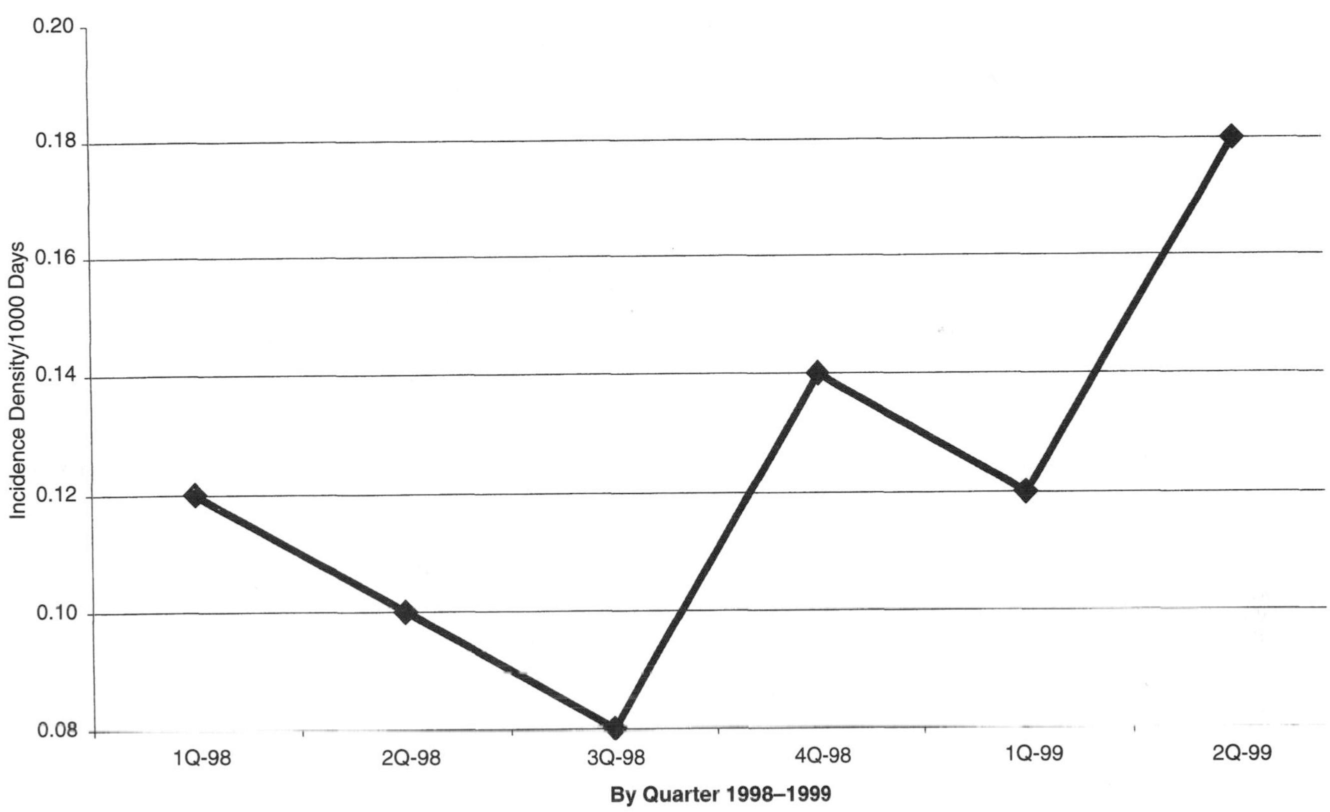

Figure 10–4 IV Catheter-Related Bloodstream Infection (Incidence Density)

nization has demonstrated a decrease in the risk associated with the use of Foley catheters, the length of time they are in place, and infection risk. This demonstrates significant quality improvement and risk reduction regardless of whether it meets statistical significance. The proportion of bloodstream infections in patients receiving chemotherapy appears to be at least two times greater than in those receiving total parenteral nutrition. This may be more related to the diagnoses among the patients and their intrinsic risk than to the infusion therapy.

Once the ICP and organization become competent in surveillance skills, further application of biostatistical methods may be sought (Checko, 1997). Initially, however, the ICP and organization should stick to the basics.

USE OF DATA FOR IMPROVEMENT OF PATIENT CARE

As discussed throughout the chapter, the purpose of infection surveillance is to reduce risk. Once confidence in the data is acquired and there is at least 1 year of data, the home care organization should select a specific area for risk reduction. Notes and minutes from surveillance planning meetings may be useful, with reference to criteria for selection of the outcome of interest. In collaboration with the quality improvement activities of the organization, a risk reduction project can be selected. Although the ICP can participate in the project, other knowledgeable clinical staff members should lead and participate as well. The ICP will provide continued support through data collection and analysis.

Risk reduction projects should use the surveillance data to identify some risk factors and provide baseline measurement. Additional resources from the literature will be necessary, however, to fully explore potential risks and their potential reduction. Most projects will focus on clinical policies and procedures that can be changed and improved to reduce risk. For example, a revised procedure for CVC dressing changes that specifies a different skin antiseptic may be tried. Various strategies to improve urinary continence can be implemented to reduce urinary catheter days and UTIs.

Whatever the approach, the plans should be well researched and then implemented. Remeasurement should not begin until the new protocol is resolved and has been fully implemented.

ONGOING MEASUREMENT

To determine whether the revised or redesigned approach to care has resulted in a reduction in risk and infection, the rate of infection should be remeasured on an ongoing basis. It is essential that the same definitions and surveillance methods be used in the postintervention period. Any change can affect the data, and actual improvement (or lack of improvement) may not be measured accurately. Focusing on a particular infection site with a revised procedure may actually result in an increase in the number of infections identified. This may result from increased interest and sensitivity in detecting the infection. Another phenomenon may be an actual decrease in infection during the initial months in which the new procedure is in place and a subsequent gradual increase over time. Surveillance should continue long enough to ensure that the organization is able to "maintain the gain" by sustaining a reduction in the infection rate over time.

VALIDATING SURVEILLANCE DATA

Accuracy of surveillance data has been a concern in nosocomial infection surveillance, and it should be a concern in home care as well. Ideally, infection rates should be as close to the actual occurrence as possible. However, efforts to improve accuracy may increase the cost of surveillance. Because home care resources are so precious, the home care organization must determine the amount of resources that can be put into surveillance to get acceptably accurate data, knowing that most systems will not be 100 percent accurate. The two main factors that can influence the accuracy of the infection rate are the case finding methods and the definitions of infection. The methods used to screen patients for home care-acquired infection should be sensitive, acknowledging that once the definition is applied it will be determined that some of the patients identified do not have a home care-acquired infection. Infection rates are more likely to be underestimated if the identification and screening methods are insufficient (requires a culture). They may be overestimated if the definition is too broad (new antibiotic order).

To perform some quality control and validation of infection data, the ICP may employ several strategies depending on how much time is allotted for surveillance and how much electronic data are available. For example, to determine whether all patients with symptoms of a UTI are being reported on screening reports, the ICP may obtain a list of all patients with indwelling Foley catheters during a specific time period (e.g., 1 month) in the past. Through clinical record review, the ICP can determine whether there were additional patients with signs and symptoms of a UTI who were not identified or reported. A broader review to identify patients who should be reported via screening would involve obtaining a list of all patients with new antibiotic orders within a selected month and comparing that list with the screening forms submitted for the same time period. Alternatively, the clinical records of all patients with CVCs can be reviewed from 1 month. Patients with evidence of bloodstream infection can be compared with those patients who are included on the line listing for that month. There may also be some coded information within an electronic patient record system that could be used to validate surveillance data.

To validate the application of the definitions of home care-acquired infection, the ICP may ask a colleague to review the patients whom he or she has determined meet the definition to determine whether there is agreement. This colleague may be the ICP from another location in a multisite organization or the ICP from the corporate office in a national organization. In a hospital-based home care organization, the hospital ICP may perform the record review.

USE OF COMPUTERS AND SOFTWARE FOR SURVEILLANCE

There are many software programs available specifically for the management and analysis of nosocomial infection data. Currently, there are no specific software programs available for home care surveillance. If a home care organization is large and sees many thousands of patients each year, computerization of surveillance data may be beneficial and necessary. Initially, however, the ICP who is developing skills for home care surveillance should rely on a sharp pencil, paper, and a hand-held calculator. Common computer applications, such as Microsoft Office (which includes Access and Excel), can be used to produce graphs, charts, and tables. Once the basics of surveillance are mastered, the ICP may wish to routinely enter the surveillance data into a database for analysis. Many database programs, including Access, are suitable for this task. The CDC offers a public software program called EpiInfo. It is available on the Internet and can perform common biostatistical functions. Additional information about EpiInfo is given in Appendix 13–B.

GETTING STARTED

Surveillance of any type requires development of definitions and methods. Skills in applying them must also be developed. Skills development requires some education and training followed by practice. A home care organization initiating a serious surveillance program should anticipate a reasonable time period to develop definitions and methods. This may be 3 to 6 months, depending on the degree of reliance on outside sources, such as the definitions from Missouri Alliance for Home Care, compared with development of internal definitions. Data collection methods will require some time for development as well. The ICP and others participating in this project will need time and resources. Once the surveillance begins, a pilot period of 1 to 3 months should be planned for training of staff, skill development, and learning. The data from this pilot period should not be used in reporting because they will probably not be reliable in the initial time period. The data will improve as the ICP's skills improve. Each organization will have to determine whether it can "trust" the initial data or whether these data should simply be considered practice data.

Development of knowledge and skills for infection surveillance will benefit other quality measurement and improvement projects. All the activities of infection surveillance should be performed in the context of the overall quality improvement program.

REFERENCES

Bryant, J. (1997). Organized systems of care. *American Journal of Infection Control, 25*, 363–364.

Burke, J., Garibaldi, R., Britt, M., Jacobson, J., Conti, M., & Alling, D. (1981). Prevention of catheter-associated urinary tract infections. Efficacy of daily meatal care regimens. *American Journal of Medicine, 70*, 655–658.

Centers for Disease Control and Prevention (CDC). (1988). *CDC surveillance update*. Atlanta: Author.

Checko, P. (1997). Use of statistics for epidemiology. In R. Olmstead (Ed.), *Infection control and applied epidemiology: Principles and practice* (pp. 4-1–4-10). St. Louis: Mosby.

Danzig, L. Short, L., Collins, K. Mahoney, M., Sepe, S., Bland, L., & Jarvis, W. (1995). Bloodstream infections associated with a needleless intravenous infusion system in patients receiving home infusion therapy. *Journal of the American Medical Association, 23*, 1862–1864.

Emori, I., Culver, D., & Horan, T. (1991). National Nosocomial Infections Surveillance System (NNIS): Description of surveillance methods. *American Journal of Infection Control, 19*, 259–267.

Friedman, M. (1996). Designing an infection control program to meet JCAHO standards. *Caring, 15*, 18–25.

Garner, J., Jarvis, W., Emori, T., Horan, T., & Hughes, J. (1988). CDC definitions for nosocomial infection. *American Journal of Infection Control, 16*, 28–40.

Gaynes, R., Edwards, J., Jarvis, W., Culver, D., Tolson, J., & Martone, W. (1996). Nosocomial infections among neonates in high-risk nurseries in the United States. National Nosocomial Surveillance System. *Pediatrics, 98*, 357–361.

Goldmann, D., & Pier, J. (1993). Pathogenesis of infections related to intravascular catheterization. *Clinical Microbiology Review, 6*, 176–192.

Jarvis, W., Gaynes, R., Horan, T., Alonso-Exhanove, J., Emori, T., Fridkin, S., Lawton, R., Richards, M., Wright, G., Culver, D., Abshire, J., Edwards, J., Henderson, J., Peavy, G. Tolson, J., & Wages, J. (1998). National Nosocomial Infection Surveillance (NNIS) system report, data summary from October 1986–April 1998, issued June 1998. *American Journal of Infection Control, 26*, 522–533.

Kellerman, S., Shay, D., Howard, J., Goes, C., Feusner, J., Rosenberg, J., Vugia, D., & Jarvis, W. (1996). Bloodstream infections in home infusion patients: The influence of race and needleless intravascular access devices. *Journal of Pediatrics, 129*, 711–717.

Kunin, C., & McCormack, R. (1966). Prevention of catheter-induced urinary tract infections by sterile closed drainage. *New England Journal of Medicine, 274*, 1155–1162.

Lee, T., Baker, O., Lee, J., Scheckler, W., Steele, L., & Laxton, C. (1998). Recommended practices for surveillance. *American Journal of Infection Control, 26*, 277–288.

Lorenzen, A., & Itkin, D. (1992). Surveillance of infection in home care. *American Journal of Infection Control, 20*, 326–329.

Martone, W., Gaynes, R., Horan, T., Danzig, L., Emori, T., Monnet, D., Stroud, L., Wright, G., Culver, D., & Banerjee, S. (1995). National Nosocomial Infections Surveillance (NNIS) semiannual report, May 1995. *American Journal of Infection Control, 23*, 377–385.

McGeer, A., Campbell, B., Emori, T., Hierholzer, W., Jackson, M., Nicolle, L., Peppler, C., Rivera, A., Schollenberger, D., & Simor, A. (1991). Definitions of infection for surveillance in long-term care facilities. *American Journal of Infection Control,* 19, 1–7.

Pearson, M. (1996). CDC guideline for prevention of intravascular device–related infection. *American Journal of Infection Control, 24*, 262–277.

Snow, J. (1965). *Snow on cholera.* Cambridge: Harvard University Press.

White, M. (1992). Infection and infection risks in home care. *Infection Control and Hospital Epidemiology, 13*, 535–539.

White, M., & Ragland, K. (1993). Surveillance of intravenous catheter–related infections among home care clients. *American Journal of Infection Control, 21*, 231–235.

CHAPTER 11

Outbreak Investigations

WHAT IS AN OUTBREAK?

The term *outbreak* is commonly used when the expected frequency of infection (endemic rate) is greatly exceeded. Public health professionals use the term *epidemic*. For the purposes of home care infection control, however, the term *outbreak* refers to an incidence of home care-acquired infection that is greater than expected or the occurrence of an unusual infection, even if it is only a few cases. The term is used to alert the home care organization's leaders that something out of the ordinary may be occurring and should be investigated. There is no specific arbitrary or statistical threshold that is used to determine whether an infectious disease, nosocomial infection, or home care-acquired infection is occurring in "epidemic proportions." It is more a matter of judgment based on experience and, if available, data. When Legionnaires' disease first appeared, it was discovered because of an outbreak of unusual pneumonia among attendees at an American Legion convention in Philadelphia. The cause of the pneumonia was eventually identified as a newly discovered bacteria, *Legionnella pneumophila* (Fraser et al., 1977). In the flu season, epidemiologists calculate how many cases of specific types of influenza A and B are expected to occur. If they occur in a large proportion of the population, it is described as an epidemic year.

WHY OUTBREAKS SHOULD BE INVESTIGATED AND REPORTED

The outbreaks of Legionnaires' disease were related to public health. In home care organizations, outbreaks occur as well. In hospitals, it is estimated that about 5 percent of all nosocomial infections are related to outbreaks. Not all outbreaks are recognized or reported, but many have been reported in the infection control and medical literature. Outbreak investigation and reporting are important for several reasons. First, the occurrence should be investigated so that a source can be identified and eliminated and so that other patients are not infected. Results of an outbreak investigation and the control measures implemented should be reported to the organization's leadership. Beyond the specific organization and its patients, it is important to report outbreak investigations and findings in the literature as a reference for other health care providers in case they should recognize a similar occurrence in their practice setting.

IDENTIFYING THE CAUSE OF AN OUTBREAK

New sources, organisms, and causes of outbreaks are reported every year, but these are usually hospital-based occurrences. At the time of this writing, only two home care–based outbreaks had been reported in the infection control literature (Danzig et al., 1995; Kellerman et al., 1996). Both reports describe the investigation of an outbreak that was recognized by home care staff when the occurrence of bloodstream infections was much greater than expected. The outbreak investigations that were performed applied epidemiological methods to collect variables about the patients involved and determine the probable cause(s) of the outbreak. In both cases, the increase in bloodstream infections was associated with the use of needleless intravenous (IV) delivery systems.

Outbreaks may be associated with a single organism, a single source, or a single cause of infection. A single organism may be a multidrug-resistant microorganism, such as methicillin-resistant *Staphylococcus aureus* (MRSA) or a vancomycin-resistant enterococcus that is recognized to colonize or infect a number of patients (Rhinehart, Shlaes, Serkey, & Keys, 1987; Rhinehart et al., 1990). A single environmental source may be identified as the reservoir of infection, such as a contaminated sink in an intensive care unit (Dandalides, Rutala, & Sarubbi, 1984) or a contaminated antiseptic solution (Sobel, Hashman, Reinherz, & Merzbach, 1982). A single source may also arise from an inanimate object that is used from one patient to another, such as an electronic thermometer (Livornese, Dias, & Samel, 1992). A person may also be a single source of infection if he or she is colonized or infected with an organism such as *S. aureus* and transmits it to patients. In the home care–based outbreaks mentioned above, the bloodstream infections were not caused by a single or unusual organism but rather were related to the improper use and management of needleless IV administration sets. These outbreaks had a common cause rather than a single source or common reservoir.

In home care, when an increase in respiratory infections is recognized, it may be associated with an outbreak in the community rather than directly related to home care services. This occurs most commonly in the winter months, when influenza and other respiratory illnesses occur at increased rates. These outbreaks should not be considered home care–acquired infections. Home care staff, however, should educate patients and families about the risk of the community-acquired infection and recommend strategies to reduce the risk. In most cases, this would involve staying out of crowded public areas, such as malls and public events, and minimizing visitors in the home. If there is an outbreak of community-acquired infection, the family should request that visitors not come into the home if they are symptomatic.

STEPS IN AN OUTBREAK INVESTIGATION

It is sometimes difficult to determine when an outbreak investigation should be undertaken. As mentioned above, there is no particular threshold or trigger that should be used. In general, if an infection control practitioner (ICP) or a home care organization has a suspicion or impression that something is out of the ordinary, either more infections than normally seen or one or two cases of an unusual infection, an investigation should be initiated. It is better to be prudent and gather the facts in an organized fashion and determine that there is no problem than to wait and eventually determine that there is a significant problem that involves many more patients than initially recognized.

Many infections in patients who are already ill, such as urinary tract infections in older women, are not preventable. By definition, infections related to an outbreak are preventable because they arise from a single source or cause. An outbreak investigation is undertaken to identify the source of the outbreak and eliminate it. That is why it is so important to conduct an outbreak investigation using the specific steps described below. If information is not gathered in an organized fashion and carefully examined, erroneous assumptions about the cause of the outbreak may be made, and the steps taken to end the outbreak will not be effective. This may lead to a further spread of the outbreak and much wasted time. It is much more preferable to approach the investigation in a planned, scientific manner rather than guess at the cause.

There are specific steps that have been prescribed for an outbreak investigation (Table 11–1; Checko, 1997). On first suspicion that an outbreak is occurring, the ICP must verify the diagnosis or identify the organism involved. For example, a home care staff member may observe that several patients receiving home infusion therapy have purulent exit site infections. Although the staff member has seen exit site infections before, he or she suspects that there are more infections in the past 2 weeks than usual. When this is reported to the ICP, the first step is to verify the diagnosis. The ICP would want to interview the staff member reporting the infections to determine the specific nature of the infections and the time frame in which they have occurred. If any cultures were performed, the results should be obtained immediately. If some patients had cultures and others did not, cultures should be obtained for those who did not.

It may take a few days to confirm that these exit site infections are occurring and that the same organism is involved. The ICP may find that there are more exit site infections than usual, but they are caused by different bacteria. To determine whether the causative organism is the same or different in each case, the ICP would review the culture results. The genus and species of the organisms may be the same (e.g., *Staphylococcus aureus*), or the cultures may show that some of the infec-

Table 11–1 Outbreak Investigation

Steps To Take	*What To Do*
1. Verify the diagnosis and identify the organism	When the potential or suspicion is reported, obtain objective, scientific data (cultures, blood tests, physician's diagnosis) to substantiate that all the potential cases have a common diagnosis, organism, or source.
2. Confirm that an outbreak exists.	Review the known cases and compare their occurrence with the expected occurrence, or determine whether a single case or small cluster of cases is so unusual that an outbreak investigation is warranted.
3. Search for additional cases.	Formulate a case definition based on the diagnosis or organism and look for additional cases among the patient population.
4. Characterize cases for common elements or exposures such as time, place, person.	Review all the cases to look for a temporal relationship and a common exposure or risk.
5. Formulate a hypothesis.	Based on information gained in step 4, formulate a possible cause of the outbreak.
6. Test the hypothesis.	Go back to each case and analyze it based on the hypothetical cause to determine whether the theory is potentially correct in all or most cases.
7. Develop control measures and implement them.	Once the potential cause is determined, develop strategies to eliminate the cause and implement them.
8. Evaluate the control measures.	Continue to watch for new cases to determine whether the control measures were effective.
9. Write a report.	Summarize the outbreak investigation findings and interventions.

tions are caused by *S. aureus* and others by *S. epidermidis* or some other organism. If the same genus and species are found, further review of the culture results is necessary. Although many bacteria have a common pattern in their sensitivity and resistance to specific antibiotics that are tested in the microbiology laboratory, the bacteria causing the outbreak infections may have a different pattern, which can differentiate the "outbreak strain." When a culture is performed, a sensitivity test for a specifically selected set of antibiotics is also done; this is referred to as sensitivity testing. Gram-positive organisms such as staphylococci and enterococci are tested against a different panel of antibiotics than Gram-negative organisms such as *Pseudomonas* and *Klebsiella* species. The results of the sensitivity testing are referred to as an antibiogram. Organisms of the same genus and species frequently have different antibiograms. This provides a means to differentiate one bacterial strain from another. For example, some strains of *S. aureus* are sensitive to gentamicin and others are resistant, just as some are sensitive to methicillin and MRSA is not. Although gentamicin is not used to treat staphylococcal infections, the resistance or sensitivity in the antibiogram can differentiate one staphylococcal strain from another.

The ICP in home care can review the antibiograms to see if there are differences or similarities in them. Some assistance in the review and analysis can be sought from the microbiologist from the laboratory. The antibiogram can be helpful in recognizing the common pattern of sensitivity and resistance (the so-called "garden variety") and discriminating it from a pattern that may be more unusual. If the antibiogram of the bacteria from the patient is different from that usually seen but the same one from all or most of the outbreak cases, that evidence is helpful in confirming an outbreak and identifying its cause. If the organisms cultured from the patients are all different, it does not necessarily mean that there is not an outbreak. It may mean that there is an increase of infection caused by different organisms.

The next step is to search for additional cases that were not identified in the initial report. Now, the ICP can develop a case definition to identify new cases. This is sometimes difficult because at this point in the investigation not much is known. The definition may be based on a combination of factors, such as the site of infection, the organisms or other laboratory data, or other clinical factors, such as the type of care (e.g., home infusion therapy) that the patients are receiving or have undergone. The case definition may initially be broad and may be changed as more information is collected (Beck-Segue, Jarvis, & Martone, 1997). The ICP must formulate a case definition, however, to continue the investigation and focus on the most likely patients who may be included as cases. To investigate an exit site infection outbreak, the ICP might formulate the following case definition: "patients receiving central venous catheter care and maintenance who have had signs and symptoms of an exit site infection within the past 30 days." Although this definition narrows the field to those patients receiving home infusion therapy, it is not so narrow that it focuses only on a specific type of catheter, type of IV therapy, or specific organism. If the definition is too narrow at this early phase of the investigation, cases may be missed.

With the case definition in hand, the ICP can identify additional cases. These patients may be identified through a record review or by interviewing staff members to ask them to recall potential cases. Review of all culture reports could also be used to identify cases. Further culturing of patients who have signs and symptoms of exit site infections may be necessary. This can be accomplished by calling the patients' physicians, explaining that a potential outbreak is occurring, and requesting an order for a culture.

Collection of data and information about the patients who are potentially involved as cases in the outbreak should be accomplished using a data collection form specifically developed for the outbreak investigation. This will assist the ICP in ensuring that all the same information is collected for each patient in an organized fashion. It will minimize the need to go back to information sources more than one time to gather data or ask questions. A sample data collection form for an investigation of exit site infections is provided in Exhibit 11–1.

Once the possible cases that meet the case definition are identified, more data on each case must be collected. The information can be put into a line listing, such as described in Chapter 10 (see Exhibit 10–7). From these data the ICP looks for particular factors re-

Exhibit 11–1 Data Collection Tool for Outbreak Investigation

Patient's name ______________________ Record # ______ Date of admission ______________

Date of onset of signs and symptoms of exit site infection ______

Type of catheter ______________________ Date placed ______________________

Setting where CVC placed ______________________ Physician who placed CVC ______________

Type of dressing ______________________ Frequency of dressing change ______________

Who performs dressing changes? Home care nurse (name) ______________________
Family member or other? (name) ______________________

Have cultures been obtained? Yes _____ No _____

Culture results:

Date of culture: ______________________

Organism(s) cultured ______________________

Provide antibiogram for each organism

lated to time, place, and person that the cases have in common. In an outbreak, one would expect that all the cases would occur in a narrow time frame. For example, six cases of *Staphylococcus aureus* exit site infection over 2 months may not constitute an outbreak (depending on the total number of patients at risk), but six cases over 2 weeks are more suspicious. A simple graph referred to as an epidemic curve can be drawn to illustrate how many cases have occurred and their relationship in time. A sample epidemic curve is shown in Figure 11–1. In home care, the place component may be related to a referral hospital where the patients were admitted or had their central venous catheter (CVC) placed. Place may also refer to a common pharmacy that was preparing the IV fluids if there was an increased occurrence of bloodstream infection related to contaminated infusate. Person refers to a common person who may have been involved in the care of the patients. In home care, a single staff member may be involved in the care of home infusion therapy patients with exit site infections caused by *S. aureus*.

Once there is enough information to characterize the infections, the ICP will draw some conclusions about what the patients have in common and subsequently will develop a hypothesis or opinion about the cause. The hypothesis should be tested by application to the cases that have been gathered to determine whether it fits. If it does fit the majority of cases, control measures to stop the outbreak should be developed based on the assumed cause. If it does not fit, further information about the cases may be necessary; there may be some important data or risk factors missing. Occasionally, observation of patient care activities may provide additional information or clues as to the cause of an outbreak. For example, if CVC exit site infections are occurring, the ICP may go on home care visits and observe dressing changes and other aspects of home infusion therapy care by several home care staff members or the patient or family members. Interviews with home care staff about how they go about providing care or education to patients and family members in performing CVC care and maintenance may also be helpful in identifying risks and potential sources of an outbreak.

Sometimes these first steps of an outbreak investigation can occur rapidly; others may occur over a few days or even a few weeks. For example, an outbreak involving contaminated IV fluids may be recognized quickly if several patients exhibit signs and symptoms (e.g., shaking chills and rigors with a sudden onset of fever temporally related to hanging a new bag of IV fluid) in the course of a day or two. Once the second or third case is reported, the ICP should have an immediate suspicion that an outbreak related to the IV fluids is occurring. Culture results may not be available, but the

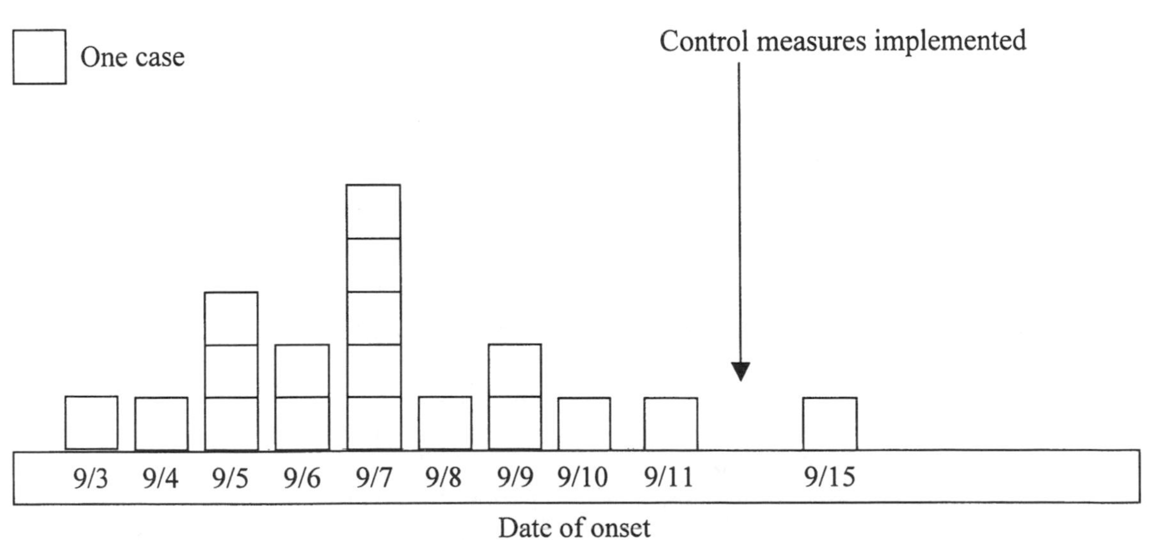

Figure 11–1 Epidemic Curve—Exit Site Infections

fact that the fluids are from the same pharmacy would be evident, and the pharmacy would be notified immediately. The pharmacy may provide home infusion therapy services to other home care organizations and have reports of similar episodes from them. In this case, the investigation would focus on the pharmacy. On the other hand, it may take a few days or weeks to identify a problem with exit site infections. Once the ICP recognizes that more infections than usual are occurring, he or she would focus on this potential problem and initiate an investigation.

CONTROL OF AN OUTBREAK

Control measures obviously depend on the assumed cause of the outbreak. If equipment is suspected, the equipment should be removed from use and inspected. Specimens from the equipment for culturing may be helpful to identify it as a source. In the contaminated fluid example, all IV fluid from the patients involved should be collected and returned to the pharmacy. Secure the suspected IV fluid and tubing (damp off at distap end) as well as any other admixtures in the home. The pharmacy staff will have a record of who mixed the IV fluid and the batch numbers or lot numbers from the manufacturer of the main fluid as well as any solution in the admixture. All the suspected fluid should be sent to a microbiology laboratory, where specific techniques for culturing the fluid will be applied.

If a person is suspected as the potential cause or source of the outbreak, the individual should be interviewed and possibly undergo a physical examination with specimens being obtained for culture. This would occur most often in an outbreak of *Staphylococcus aureus* or other organisms that can be transmitted by a human carrier. A carrier is an individual who is colonized by an organism but may not have signs or symptoms of active infection; the carrier state is therefore unrecognized until the organism causes infection in someone else. An individual who is an index case may have signs and symptoms of infection, such as a draining wound or pustule.

Once control measures are in place, the home care organization and ICP must evaluate their effectiveness by continuing surveillance and staying alert for new cases. If new cases occur, it must be determined whether they are the result of the source that has already been identified and whether the exposure occurred before or after the control measures were put in place. If it was before, the new cases are added to the data. If it was after or if they are not related to the identified source, perhaps some factor has been overlooked, and all the cases, along with the new cases, must be reexamined and new or additional control measures developed and implemented. Eventually, the control measures will be effective, the outbreak will cease, and new cases will no longer occur.

Although a formal investigation is performed in many hospital outbreaks, frequently the specific cause of the outbreak is not identified or proven, but nevertheless the outbreak terminates. It may remain unknown whether the termination is due to the specific control measures that were implemented. This common scenario may be due to several factors. First, many experts believe that, if the cause of the outbreak was not a single source but rather a combination of factors that increase risk of transmission, even though a specific cause is not identified the outbreak ends as a result of the Hawthorne effect. The Hawthorne effect refers to the phenomenon where people know that they are being observed in a critical manner and tend to perform more carefully. For example, home care staff may wash their hands more frequently if their supervisor or a Joint Commission on Accreditation of Healthcare Organizations surveyor is with them in the home. During an outbreak, health care professionals become aware of the outbreak and consciously and unconsciously improve their infection control efforts (e.g., better handwashing and compliance with transmission-based precautions). Thereby the chain of transmission is broken and the outbreak stops, but no specific source or cause is ever identified.

DOCUMENTATION OF AN OUTBREAK INVESTIGATION

A record of the steps described above should be maintained as the outbreak investigation takes place. Some documentation may occur in internal reports or memos. Most of the documentation will be recorded by the ICP as the investigation unfolds. All handwritten notes or messages should be retained for future reference. The ICP will have ongoing verbal communication about the outbreak with the home care organization's leaders. When decisions are made, more information is obtained, and specific steps are taken, some type of interim documentation (notes, memos, or brief interim reports) should be created to ensure accuracy if recall is needed. Eventually, a full report of the outbreak and investigation should be written. This report will be used to communicate the event with the group or committee in the home care organization that oversees infection control. It will also serve as a reference document if questions arise in the future. Although the document should ideally be protected from discovery if a lawsuit or claim is brought by a patient, it may also serve to demonstrate that a prudent and organized effort was initiated to investigate the outbreak and control it.

EXTERNAL ASSISTANCE

If a serious outbreak occurs involving either an unusual infectious disease or organism or a large number of patients, the home care organization should consider obtaining assistance from outside experts. In most states, the state health department is available to provide epidemiologists to assist in the investigation. The Centers for Disease Control and Prevention (CDC) has a specific division, the Epidemiologic Intelligence Service (EIS), that can also be called upon. Although some of the EIS officers are based in Atlanta, others are based within state health departments to assist in investigations. Neither the state health department nor the CDC/EIS charges for their services. In many cases, telephone consultation is sufficient to assist the home care ICP and leaders in the investigation and analysis. In other cases, the public health consultants must come on site to review clinical records and other information. Home care organizations must also be aware of whether there are any state requirements to report an outbreak of home care-acquired infections even if the organization does not need assistance from the state.

In a hospital-based home care organization, the hospital ICP and epidemiologist should be called upon initially to help determine whether an outbreak is occurring and to consult on and guide the investigation. Use of hospital-based ICPs and epidemiologists by free-standing home care organizations may depend on the relationship with a specific hospital and other resources that are available.

COMMUNICATION TO STAFF AND PATIENTS

Communication during an outbreak investigation can be tricky. On the one hand, a home care organization does not want to announce that there is a potential problem and cause undue concern among patients and families and/or draw the attention of the media. On the other hand, if there are rumors in the community that need to be corrected, some type of communication to home care staff as well as patients and families may be necessary and prudent. Home care staff should be reminded of the constant obligation to maintain confidentiality of all patient care information. They should be reminded that discussion of any potential outbreak situation outside specified parameters must be avoided. They should not discuss the situation in general or ever discuss specific patients with other patients and families. They should not discuss the situation in public places. Any discussion should be conducted within the offices of the home care organization. If telephone discussions are necessary, they should be conducted in a manner that ensures the privacy of all parties. Any information or facts that are shared outside the organization must come only from the organization's leadership. If a home care staff member is questioned by a patient or family member, he or she should be instructed to direct the questions and concerns to a specifically designated person within the organization, such as the ICP or a member of senior management. These individuals should provide information as necessary and agreed upon by the organization's leaders.

As home care expands its services to more acutely ill patients and provides more skilled, high-technology services, it can be expected that more outbreaks will occur. Although there are currently only two outbreak reports in the literature, it may be safe to assume that others have occurred and were either unrecognized or unreported. It is imperative that more home care organizations take the time to investigate outbreaks and report their findings and experiences at professional meetings and in the literature. This will benefit all providers and their patients.

REFERENCES

Beck-Segue, C., Jarvis, W., & Martone, W. (1997). Outbreak investigations. *Infection Control and Hospital Epidemiology, 18*, 138–145.

Checko, P. (1997). Outbreak investigation. In R. Olmstead (Ed.), *Infection control and applied epidemiology: Principles and practice* (pp. 4-1–4-10). St. Louis: Mosby.

Dandalides, P., Rutala, W., & Sarubbi, F. (1984). Postoperative infections following cardiac surgery: Association with an environmental reservoir in a cardiothoracic intensive care unit. *Infection Control, 5*, 378–384.

Danzig, L., Short, L., Collins, K., Mahoney, M., Sepe, S., Bland, L., & Jarvis, W. (1995). Bloodstream infections associated with a needleless intravenous infusion system in patients receiving home infusion therapy. *Journal of the American Medical Association, 273*, 1862–1864.

Fraser, D., Tsai, T., Orenstein, W., Parkin, W., Beecham, H., Sharrar, R., Harris, J., Mallison, G., Martin, S., McDade, J., Shepard, C., & Brachman, P. (1977). Legionnaires' disease: Description of an epidemic of pneumonia. *New England Journal of Medicine, 297*, 1183–1197.

Kellerman, S., Shay. D., Howard, J., Goes, C., Feusner, J., Rosenberg, J., Vugia, D., & Jarvis, W. (1996). Bloodstream infections in home infusion patients: The influence of race and needleless intravascular access devices. *Journal of Pediatrics, 129,* 711–717.

Livornese, L., Dias, S., & Samel, C. (1992). Hospital-acquired infection with vancomycin-resistant *Enterococcus faecium* transmitted by electronic thermometers. *Annals of Internal Medicine, 117*, 112–116.

Rhinehart, E., Shlaes, D., Serkey, J., & Keys, T. (1987). Nosocomial clonal dissemination of methicillin-resistant *Staphylococcus aureus*: Elucidiation by plasmid analysis. *Archives of Internal Medicine, 147*, 521–524.

Rhinehart, E., Smith, N., Wennersten, C., Gorss, E., Freeman, J., Eliopoulos, G., Moellering, R., & Goldmann, D. (1990). Rapid dissemination of beta-lactamase–producing, aminoglycoside-resistant *Enterococcus faecalis* among patients and staff on an infant–toddler surgical ward. *New England Journal of Medicine, 323*, 1814–1818.

Sobel, J., Hashman, N., Reinherz, G., & Merzbach, D. (1982). Nosocomial *Pseudomonas cepacia* infection associated with chlorhexidine contamination. *American Journal of Medicine, 73*, 183–186.

CHAPTER 12

Occupational Health

PLANNING FOR OCCUPATIONAL HEALTH

The health and well-being of the employees in a home care organization represent an important priority. Although little is known about the actual risk and incidence of occupationally acquired infectious diseases among home care staff members, there are many reports of the occurrence of these illnesses in health care providers in other settings, especially in acute care. With more and more care shifting from the hospital to home care, long-term and subacute care, and various ambulatory settings, health care staff members outside acute care may be at increased risk for occupational exposure and illness from infectious diseases. Surveillance data for human immunodeficiency virus (HIV) and hepatitis B virus (HBV) have been maintained for many years. Although there are no reports of occupational HIV infection in home care providers to date, data as of June 1997 indicate that 52 health care workers have acquired HIV through occupational exposures such as needlesticks (Centers for Disease Control and Prevention [CDC], 1997a). Immunization with HBV vaccine has reduced the risk for contracting HBV significantly since its introduction in 1982. Health care staff members in all settings, however, continue to experience needlestick injuries and other exposures to bloodborne pathogens. More data on the specific risks for occupational exposure and infection in home care are needed.

From a practical standpoint, employee absence due to illness or injury, whether occupational or nonoccupational, presents significant challenges to scheduling and providing patient care. In addition, occupationally acquired illnesses and injuries add to staff members' compensation costs. Therefore, home care organizations must take a proactive approach in identifying occupational health needs and in planning, supporting, and managing an occupational health program.

Considering that occupational health and safety programs involve many infection control issues (e.g., immunizations, follow-up of exposures, and workers' compensation claims), many home care organizations have incorporated these programs into a single management function. The occupational health program in home care should include structural elements such as policies and procedures, responsibility and authority, and organization oversight; processes for implementation, management, day-to-day application of the policies and procedures, and oversight of outsourced services; education and training of staff at all levels; and specific methods for annual assessment of the program's effectiveness.

As with other areas in the infection control program, specific knowledge and resources are necessary for maintaining and managing an occupational health program for home care. State and federal regulations, such as those promulgated by the Occupational Safety and Health Administration (OSHA), mandate certain program components. There are many additional policies and procedures for the occupational health of home care providers that should also be included in a program. Specific needs and program designs will depend on the size of the organization, scope of services, and types of patients. For example, there may be more emphasis on exposure to childhood diseases in an organization with a pediatric population than one whose focus is the care of older patients. In designing or reassessing an occupational health program for home care, the variables as listed in Exhibit 12–1 should be considered. Once these factors are examined, an appropriate and comprehensive occupational health program can be developed and implemented.

Once a program is developed and implemented, its effectiveness should be continuously monitored. This appraisal can be accomplished through ongoing indicators (e.g., number of needlesticks, frequency of exposures to contagious illnesses, and days lost as a result of occupational injuries). Although these monitors should demonstrate continuous improvement through the reduction of exposures and lost days, they may also identify areas that require increased attention and enhancement. Thus the occupational health program is linked to both the infection control program and performance improvement efforts.

The determination of who will actually provide occupational health services is very important. Although the designated manager in the home care organization (e.g., the infection control practitioner [ICP]) can administer, maintain, and improve the program through development and implementation of policies and procedures, this person should not routinely be providing occupational health services to colleagues as a health care provider. Although he or she will be called upon to evaluate specific situations (e.g., exposures) and should be available to provide interpretation of policies and direction on procedures, he or she should not be rendering direct care to employees. A registered nurse or ICP in the home care organization may perform preemployment health assessments, administer purified protein derivative (PPD) skin testing and some vaccines (e.g., HBV vaccine), and screen staff members after a potential exposure to bloodborne pathogens. The individuals involved in administrative duties, however, such as infection control and quality management, may not have the skills and experience to provide a full range of occupational health care. In addition, provision of care may create a conflict of interest and lead to confidentiality issues. For example, if an employee is exposed to blood and follow-up serologic testing is performed, the results of those tests must be kept confidential. Most states have specific laws regarding results of HIV testing. In fact, all information about employees and their health history and status must remain confidential.

Physicians with knowledge and/or experience in occupational health should be retained to provide occupational health services, such as follow-up for exposures and injuries. The initial health assessment that is performed at the time of employment should be limited and can be accomplished in the home care organization by the infection control practitioner or a designated nurse. The potential employee should be referred to a physician, however, if further assessment of a specific finding is warranted (e.g., positive PPD skin test). Many of the additional occupational health needs should be outsourced not only because they may be beyond the competencies of the individuals in the organization but also because they frequently require a physician to provide an additional assessment and/or to write orders for appropriate diagnostic tests, vaccines, or treatments. A hospital-based home care organization can use the employee health services of the hospital. A small home care organization that serves a limited geographic area may arrange for these services through a local hospital or a physician with a specialty in family practice or internal medicine. Ideally, this should be a physician with training and/or experience in occupational health. Larger agencies with multiple locations may choose to contract for services from a network provider, such as a health maintenance organization, that also provides medical management services for workers' compensation cases. The utilization of a single network may facilitate communication between the organization and the providers as well as improve the coordination of care. The network and its providers will become familiar with the home care organization's specific policies and procedures and can establish a working relationship with the infection control practitioner and others involved in workers' compensation management.

Exhibit 12–1 Considerations for the Design of an Occupational Health Program

- Type of home care organization (hospital-based or freestanding)
- Scope/type of services
- Patient population
- Size of organization
- Number of employees
- Number of locations
- Specific risks among population from which employees are drawn
- Epidemiology and risk for specific infectious diseases in the geographic area (e.g., tuberculosis)

Whatever the arrangements for provision of occupational health care, agreements and expectations should be made in writing and may include the sharing of the home care organization's policies and procedures (e.g., definition of exposure). The occupational health services should be evaluated on an annual basis for the quality of the service. Evaluation should include clinical quality (e.g., outcomes of care), functional status of employees requiring care for injuries, days lost as a result of illness, and compliance with organization procedures and nationally recognized guidelines (e.g., postexposure evaluation and treatment). Service quality should also be considered. This includes practical issues, such as accessibility for appointments (urgent and scheduled), return of phone calls, written communication and documentation, and the general willingness to work with the organization to coordinate care and minimize lost time.

RECORDKEEPING

Just as each home care staff member has a personnel file, each staff member should also have a personal health record. This record should be initiated at the time of employment and include documents such as the initial health assessment, immunizations, declinations, annual reassessments such as results of annual tuberculosis (TB) skin testing, and reports of occupational exposures or injuries, including follow-up and results of any other testing. Individual health records must be kept in a secure manner and separate from the location of the personnel file, in a separate locked cabinet, with a specific person or persons designated to have access to the files. The same standards for the confidentiality of patient information are also applied to the personal health information of home care employees.

In addition to individual health records, the home care organization must maintain a log of occupational illnesses and injuries to meet the requirements of OSHA. The OSHA 200 log must be maintained with records of all work-related injuries and illnesses, including exposures and infections. This may include back injuries, dog bites, and exposures to bloodborne pathogens, TB, and other infections (OSHA, 1993).

HEALTH ASSESSMENT AND IMMUNIZATIONS

The current recommendations for the initial health assessment of prospective employees suggest that this evaluation should be minimal. A full history and physical examination by a physician or physician extender has not proven to be cost effective or generally necessary. Instead, a general health assessment and functional status evaluation (e.g., ability to meet the physical requirements of the job) are recommended. For home care staff members who are directly involved in patient care, the initial assessment should include an infectious disease history. This evaluation should include history of infectious diseases that may be prevented by vaccines (i.e., childhood diseases and HBV), history of any condition that may increase the employee's risk for infection or increase the risk that he or she may transmit infection, selected laboratory testing (where required by organizational policies and procedures or state licensure regulations), and history of infection with TB and administration of a tuberculin skin test (PPD), if appropriate. Additional requirements that are related to state licensure should also be included. There are no recommendations to perform routine cultures of new home care employees.

VACCINE-PREVENTABLE DISEASES

The U.S. Public Health Service provides recommendations for the use of vaccines in children and adults through its Advisory Committee on Immunization Practices (ACIP). When the Food and Drug Administration brings a new vaccine to the market through its approval process, ACIP examines the data and scientific information about the specific infectious disease and the vaccine and formulates national recommendations. Subsequently, other agencies and organizations, such as the CDC and the American Academy of Pediatrics, base their recommendations for practice on those of ACIP.

Most adults born in the United States have either experienced an infection with the common childhood diseases listed in Exhibit 12–2 or received a vaccination to

Exhibit 12–2 Vaccine-Preventable Childhood Diseases

• Measles	• Tetanus
• Mumps	• Diphtheria
• Rubella	• Pertussis
• Polio	• Varicella

prevent these infections. Those born outside the United States, however, may not have been immunized or may not have had a vaccine-preventable disease. In addition, OSHA requires that all health care employers provide the HBV vaccine to at-risk employees. Other vaccines, such as for influenza, may also be offered. The initial health assessment should determine the prospective employee's immune status for these illnesses. A sample infectious disease history form for the employee health record is provided in Exhibit 12–3.

If the employee is immune by having had the infection or the vaccine, that history should be recorded in the employee's health record. This information may be important in the event that an exposure occurs. If the

Exhibit 12–3 Preemployment Health Survey/Immunization Status

Name ______________________ Work Area ______________________

Do you have contact with residents? ☐ Yes ☐ No ☐ Face-to-face ☐ Hands-on

HISTORY OF INFECTIOUS DISEASES/IMMUNIZATION (Check all boxes that apply):

Measles (Please provide physician certification of immunization or immunity.)

I was born before 1957 ☐ Yes ☐ No

I was born in or after 1957

I have had measles and offer physician certification ☐ Yes ☐ No

I have had immunization ☐ Yes ☐ No Dates ______________

(Give evidence of two live vaccinations) After first birthday? ______________

I have a positive antibody titre and offer written proof ☐ Yes ☐ No

Mumps

I was born before 1957 ☐ Yes ☐ No

I have had mumps ☐ Yes ☐ No

Rubella (Please provide physician certification of immunization or immunity.)

I have received live virus immunization after 1969 ☐ Yes ☐ No Dates ______________

I have laboratory evidence of immunity ☐ Yes ☐ No

After first birthday? ______________

Chickenpox

I have had chickenpox ☐ Yes ☐ No

To my knowledge, I have not had chickenpox ☐ Yes ☐ No

I do not know if I have had chickenpox ☐ Yes ☐ No

If negative or equivocal chickenpox history:

Did you have sibling(s) with history of chickenpox while you were living together? ☐ Yes ☐ No

Did you care for your own child with chickenpox? ☐ Yes ☐ No

I have had laboratory testing to determine immunity status ☐ Yes ☐ No

Miscellaneous	Yes	No	Last Booster Date
I have had polio vaccine series	☐	☐	______________
I have had tetanus/diphtheria vaccine series	☐	☐	______________
I have had hepatitis B vaccine series	☐	☐	______________
I have had measles-mumps-rubella (MMR) vaccine	☐	☐	______________
I am immune to the hepatitis B virus (per laboratory documentation)	☐	☐	______________

______________ ______________

Date Signature—Employee

Source: Reprinted with permission from Nancy L. Thayer, *Infection Control Program: Policy and Procedure Manual,* Baltimore, Maryland.

employee's history indicates a lack of immunity (i.e., no recall or record of having the infection or the vaccine), that also must be recorded and the employee considered susceptible until a vaccination is obtained. Home care organization policy will determine whether a simple verbal history of having a disease or vaccine is adequate to determine the employee's status. Otherwise, policy may require serologic testing for confirmation or written documentation from a physician.

The determination as to whether a home care organization will provide serologic testing and vaccination is based on several considerations: the likelihood of occupational exposure to vaccine-preventable illnesses based on the patient population served, the potential outcome of those exposures and burden for investigation and follow-up, the actual risk (proportion of employees already immune versus those who are susceptible) in the current employee population, and the cost of performing tests and providing vaccines versus the benefit to the organization, its employees, and its patients.

The question regarding who should pay for serologic testing and immunization (except for HBV) depends on the home care organization's policy. In a hospital-based home care organization, these services are frequently provided free of charge through the hospital's employee health program. This may not be reasonable in freestanding home care organizations where occupational health services are purchased, however, because it creates an additional operating expense. A more common approach is to require a potential employee to obtain proof of immunity (i.e., serologic testing and/or vaccination) from his or her personal physician. State employment laws must be considered when this policy is formulated.

Varicella

In the case of varicella, the virus that causes chickenpox and shingles, most experts agree that a verbal history of natural immunity (the employee reports that he or she had chickenpox as a child) from an adult born in the United States is reliable (97 percent to 99 percent of American adults are seropositive for chickenpox), and no serologic testing is required to confirm immunity (Kelley, Petruccelli, Stehr-Green, Erickson, & Mason, 1991). If an individual born and raised in the United States is not sure or does not know or recall whether he or she ever had chickenpox, additional questions (e.g., number and age of siblings as well as number and ages of their own children) can help determine status. For example, if the employee is a parent and reports that his or her own children had chickenpox and that he or she lived in the home and provided care for them while they were ill, it is likely that the individual is immune. Likewise, if an individual recalls siblings living in the same home and having chickenpox but cannot remember being ill himself or herself, it is likely that he or she was either immune at the time or had a mild, subclinical case that was not recognized at the time. Data indicate that, even when an individual born in the United States cannot recall or does not believe that he or she had chickenpox, a large proportion (71 percent to 93 percent) test positive (Bolyard, Tablan, Williams, Pearson, Shapiro, & Deitchman, 1998). Finally, a prospective employee can call his or her parents (if available) to ask about his or her childhood experience with chickenpox and other diseases.

An individual who was born and raised in a tropical area, such as the Caribbean, is less likely to have had chickenpox as a child. Serologic testing has demonstrated that immunity to varicella is far lower in adults who were raised in tropical and subtropical climates compared with adults raised in temperate climates, such as the United States and Europe, where the rate of immunity is more than 90 percent (Longfield, Winn, Gibson, Juchau, & Hoffman, 1990; Nassar & Touma, 1986). Consequently, an employee who has emigrated from a tropical area is more likely to be susceptible to primary varicella infection (chickenpox).

The varicella vaccine became available in the United States in 1995 and can be used in the immunization of children and adults. ACIP has recommended the immunization of health care staff members with the varicella vaccine if they are not already immune based on their history (CDC, 1997b). Although blood tests for antibodies for varicella are available, testing of employees before administration of the vaccine is not recommended because it is probably not cost effective. If a home care organization has a large number of employees who are susceptible to varicella and/or caring for high-risk children (e.g., pediatric patients with cancer or other immunosuppressive diseases), it may wish to consider providing the vaccine. Other strategies that can reduce risk can focus on avoiding the assignment of susceptible employees to high-risk children, thus reducing the risk of exposure to both.

Measles

Adults born before 1957 are likely to have natural immunity to measles because the vast majority of children caught measles and developed natural immunity before the introduction of the vaccine in 1963. Individuals born in or after 1957 may or may not have naturally acquired immunity. Measles vaccines that were used between 1957 and 1963 did not always confer immunity. That is why outbreaks of measles have occurred in persons born before 1963, when the current vaccine was made available and appropriate methods for storage and administration were determined. If any individual (including anyone born before 1957) cannot provide written documentation from a physician of having had measles (positive blood test) or of having received one dose of vaccine after the age of 1 year, serologic testing is necessary. Many states require all health care workers to be immune to measles. Once individuals who are susceptible to measles are identified, they should be immunized. Use of the trivalent vaccine for measles, mumps, and rubella (MMR) is recommended; the MMR vaccine is generally more available than a single vaccine for measles (CDC, 1997b).

Rubella

Rubella is less contagious than measles, and there may be more individuals among home care staff members who have not had rubella and are susceptible. Most women of childbearing age have been tested for rubella and may have received the rubella vaccine as part of the requirements for previous employment in health care or from a primary care or obstetric services provider to eliminate the risk of rubella during pregnancy. Even though most individuals born before 1957 are immune and many have received the vaccine, written documentation of immunity should be required. As with measles, many states require written proof of immunity to rubella for all health care staff members. Acceptable evidence of immunity may be an immunization record or results of serological testing from a physician. As with measles, individuals identified as susceptible should be immunized with the MMR vaccine. Pregnancy is a contraindication to vaccination (CDC, 1997b).

Diphtheria, Tetanus, and Pertussis

The incidence of diphtheria in the United States is extremely low, so that occupational or nonoccupational exposure is unlikely, and health care providers are not considered at any greater risk for diphtheria than the general population. Nevertheless, ACIP recommends that adults receive a tetanus and diphtheria booster every 10 years. If a potential employee has not received a booster in the past 10 years, he or she should be reminded of this recommendation. The tetanus and diphtheria vaccine is also recommended for prophylactic treatment of a traumatic wound (CDC, 1997b). The pertussis vaccine is not recommended for use in adults (CDC, 1991a). However, there is risk for exposure to pertussis among health care providers, including home care staff. The definition and treatment of exposed personnel are discussed later in this chapter.

Polio

Many adults have received polio vaccination (oral or by injection). Polio is rarely seen in the United States and is not considered a risk for home care staff. If there are circumstances that would expose home care personnel to a patient with polio (the virus is excreted through the stool), however, immunization should be provided (CDC, 1997b).

HBV TESTING AND VACCINATION

The OSHA rule on bloodborne pathogens (OSHA, 1991) requires that health care employers offer and provide HBV vaccine at no charge to all employees who are at risk for exposure. The policies and procedures related to HBV vaccination should be part of the organization's exposure control plan and should be incorporated into the occupational health program. In addition, the exposure control plan should outline the use of personal protective equipment, engineering controls, and the organization's policy and procedure for postexposure follow-up. Determination of current HBV status should be incorporated into the preemployment health assessment (see Exhibit 12–3).

A new employee who reports that he or she has received three doses of HBV vaccine during a previous employment should obtain a record of the vaccination and the results of any antibody testing that was performed. If no antibody testing was performed, the employee can be tested if there will be continued risk of exposure on the job. The year in which the vaccine series was completed and antibody test results should be recorded in the employee health record in case new recommendations for a booster dose are announced. If the employee has not had the vaccine, it must be offered within 10 days of employment in compliance with the OSHA rule. At this point, the employee may accept the vaccine or decline it. If the vaccine is declined, a declination statement should be signed by the employee to document that the vaccine was offered and declined. A sample declination statement is provided in Exhibit 12–4. Even though the employee decides not to have the vaccine at this time, the home care organization's policy must allow the employee to accept the vaccine at any subsequent time during employment.

If the employee decides to accept the vaccine, it must be provided in three doses over 6 months as prescribed. The first dose is given at a designated time. The second dose must be administered 1 month after the first dose, and the third dose must be given 6 months after the first dose (CDC, 1990a). It is important that the employee complete the series of three injections to ensure immunity. Although studies have demonstrated immunity after two doses, the best results have been obtained with three doses given at the prescribed intervals. The home care organization or the occupational health provider (or both) must implement a practical procedure to ensure that the employee gets the second and third doses.

Exhibit 12–4 Declination Form for Hepatitis B Vaccine

In order to comply with the Bloodborne Pathogens Rule of the Occupational Safety and Health Administration, we have offered you, an employee of ____________________ (name of Home Care Organization), the hepatitis B vaccination in a series of three injections. We have provided information about the benefits of the vaccine and have offered it to you at no charge. At this time, you have chosen not to receive the vaccine. Please sign below to indicate that you have declined the vaccine at this time. However, in spite of the declination at this time, we will provide the vaccine to you at any time in the future at no charge.

I, ____________________________, (print name) understand that I am eligible to receive the hepatitis B vaccine at no charge. I am declining receipt of the vaccine at this time.

____________________ ____________________
Signature Date

For example, the second and third doses may be administered by a nurse in the home care organization so that the employee does not have to make an appointment and travel to the office of the occupational health care provider.

If the series is not completed as prescribed, it may need to be reinitiated. If two doses have been administered, serological testing for antibody to HBV surface antigen (anti-HBs) should be obtained to determine if the employee has responded and developed adequate antibody (>10 μU/mL). If the employee has not developed antibody, then the series must be reinitiated (CDC, 1990a).

Serological antibody testing before initiation of the first dose of HBV vaccine is not required. Each organization can determine whether it wants to test routinely for existing immunity before giving the vaccine or whether it wants to provide this option to the employee. This decision may be based on the likelihood of identifying employees who are already immune to HBV or are chronic carriers. In most situations, testing for HBV markers before vaccine administration is not cost effective and delays the initiation of the vaccine series.

Testing for anti-HBs after the vaccine series has been completed is recommended for those who will have ongoing risk for potential exposure. This testing also helps assure the employee that the vaccine was effective and that he or she has successfully developed immunity. The antibody test should be performed 1 to 2 months after the administration of the third dose of vaccine and is considered adequate if the serum levels are 10 μU/mL or greater. If the employee has not developed adequate antibody levels after completing the three-dose series at the prescribed intervals, the CDC recommends that the vaccine series be repeated and the employee tested again. If the employee still has not developed measurable antibody, a test for HBsAg should be obtained to determine whether the individual had a previous HBV infection that may have gone unrecognized and led to chronic carriage of the virus (CDC, 1997c).

There is no current recommendation for a booster dose of HBV vaccine even though up to 60 percent of vaccine recipients who initially developed anti-HBs lose the detectable antibody 8 years after vaccination. A booster dose is not recommended based on the knowledge and experience that, even though antibody is not detectable in a blood test, an individual who initially developed antibody is still protected and will not become infected if exposed to HBV (CDC, 1997c).

TB ASSESSMENT

Initial assessment of a prospective employee must also include an evaluation of past infection with *Mycobacterium tuberculosis*. This infectious agent can cause active TB in the lungs (i.e., pulmonary TB) or other sites (e.g., renal TB). Exposure to the TB organism from an actively infected individual, however, does not always cause active infection. In most cases the exposure will cause the exposed individual's immune system to react even though he or she does not have active disease. This is still referred to as a TB infection, however, and is demonstrated by a positive TB skin test (defined below). A person with a positive skin test should be treated with prophylactic antibiotics to prevent the infection from becoming active in the future. Even after prophylaxis is complete, however, the individual's TB skin test will remain positive. A person who has had an active TB infection will also maintain a positive skin test after treatment. That is because the skin test reflects the immune system's response: unlike a culture, it is not a direct test for infection.

The assessment for TB should be included in the preemployment infectious disease history to determine the history of PPD skin test results and/or the individual's experience with an active TB infection. If an individual has had an active TB infection in the past, it can be assumed that they will have a positive PPD skin test. Further questions about treatment of the infection should be asked to make sure that adequate treatment was completed and there are no current signs or symptoms of active infection. If the employee reports a history of a positive skin test but never had an active infection, the history should be recorded in the health record, and the employee should be asked about follow-up and prophylactic treatment. A TB skin test should not be administered if the employee reports a history of active infection or a history of a previously positive PPD. Instead, a chest radiograph should be obtained by the occupational health care provider to determine current disease status and provide a baseline for future assessment (CDC, 1994).

PPD Skin Testing

For individuals who have a history of negative PPD skin tests or do not know their skin test status, a test should be administered using the Mantoux technique (0.1 mL PPD via intracutaneous administration on the dorsal surface of the forearm). Pregnant employees and those who have received the Callette-Guerin vaccination in the past should not be excluded from skin testing (CDC, 1994). An organization may elect to do PPD testing in house rather than have the occupational health care provider perform the testing. This is usually more convenient and practical. The test, however, must be administered by a nurse who has the training and skill to perform the intradermal injection. An incorrectly administered test can affect the accuracy of the results. Once the PPD is placed, the employee must return to have it read by the nurse. It is no longer acceptable to allow an employee (even a nurse or physician) to read his or her own skin test and report the results via postcard or other means. A qualified individual must read the test 48 to 72 hours after administration. From a practical standpoint, testing must be scheduled for a day that will allow the employee to return for interpretation 2 or 3 days later. Therefore, Monday and Tuesday are the best days to administer PPD skin tests.

A positive PPD test is based on the presence of induration (raised redness) at the injection site. If induration is present, it should be measured transverse to the long axis of the forearm and the measurement recorded in millimeters. Induration must not be estimated; it must be measured with a small ruler calibrated in millimeters. In general, induration of greater than 10 mm is considered positive. In some cases, however, a reaction of more than 5 mm may be interpreted as a positive result. This interpretation applies to close contacts of those with active TB, persons with positive chest radiographs and clinical symptoms of active TB, and those infected with HIV. Other factors in interpreting PPD skin tests should be considered (American Thoracic Society, 1990). A nurse performing PPD tests in a home care organization should send all individuals with newly positive reactions, also referred to as PPD converters, to an occupational health care provider, their primary care physician, or the county health department for further interpretation and follow-up.

All positive reactions must have further evaluation by a physician, who will obtain a chest radiograph to determine whether there is an active pulmonary infection. Physical assessment and additional testing may be needed to detect extrapulmonary TB.

If active infection is detected, treatment will be initiated, and work restrictions should be considered for those with pulmonary or laryngeal TB. If there is no active infection, the individual will need prophylactic treatment, usually administered as the oral antibiotic isoniazid (INH). In most cities and counties, the local health department will provide the medication and monitor the individual for side effects or adverse reactions as well as compliance. Employees with newly positive PPD skin tests do not have to be restricted from patient contact once active disease is ruled out.

Two-Step Testing

The routine use of a two-step method for PPD skin testing has been recommended for health care workers (CDC, 1994). The two-step method should be used in individuals who have not had a PPD skin test within the past 12 months. The two-step method refers to the application of a second PPD skin test 2 to 3 weeks after the initial test if the initial test is negative. This approach has been found to increase the identification of true positives through a booster effect to the immune system. The first time the PPD is placed, the immune system may not respond, but the second test "boosts" the reaction. When this occurs, the first test is interpreted as a false negative and the second test as a true positive. Some experts argue that the two-step method is necessary to identify all the true positives so that they can be provided prophylactic treatment to reduce their risk of active infection in the future. Routine use of the two-step method may not always be cost effective, however, because it requires more administrative time and the application of two PPD tests. At the time of this writing, OSHA was still considering the required use of the two-step method but had not finalized its rules. A home care organization may determine the actual benefit of the two-step method for its specific employee group by performing the two-step method with all new employees who have not had a skin test in the past year. If this method detects a significant number of true positives based on the second PPD, then it is worthwhile to continue its use (for example, if 20 percent or 25 percent of those testing negative on the first skin test are positive on the second skin test, the two-step method is detecting a significant number of true positives). If few or no positives are detected with the two-step method, consideration should be given to abandoning routine two-step testing unless circumstances change. Changes would include a substantial increase in new staff, a change in the population from which employees are hired, or a significant change in the patient population served.

Annual TB Skin Testing

Once each employee has been assessed for TB status at the time of employment, annual (or more frequent) testing should be performed. In most situations, repeating the PPD tests for all patient care employees every 12 months is adequate. In geographic areas where TB is highly prevalent and/or the organization is providing care for patients with active TB, more frequent PPD testing (e.g., every 6 months) may be required. If the organization has identified a number of employees with newly positive PPD tests (three within the past year from either occupational or nonoccupational exposures), semiannual testing should be considered (CDC, 1994).

Annual chest radiographs for those known to be PPD positive are no longer recommended because few cases of active pulmonary TB have ever been detected as a result of this expensive annual examination. Employees with a history of a positive PPD, however, should be evaluated for any clinical signs and symptoms of active TB infection annually. This assessment can be accomplished in several ways. A face-to-face assessment through an interview with the infection control practitioner or the occupational health care provider can be scheduled. A simpler way is to use a questionnaire to remind PPD-positive employees of the signs and symptoms of active TB infection and to request that they report these symptoms if they occur. Follow-up with a physician should also be recommended if symptoms are present. To document that an annual assessment of positive employees has occurred, the organization may require PPD-positive employees to answer the postcard or questionnaire and return it to the organization for placement in their health record.

INFLUENZA VACCINE

The occurrence and type of influenza are tracked around the world by the World Health Organization because the viruses that cause influenza A and B frequently change their antigenic make-up. New vaccines must be formulated for each flu season. The CDC tries to predict the potential incidence of flu in the United States for the coming season, including which viruses will be predominant, to determine the vaccine formulation for that year. Because the viruses change to some degree each year, annual immunization is recommended.

The influenza season in the United States runs from October through May. Immunization campaigns should begin during August and be completed by the end of September. Home care organizations may provide the influenza vaccine to their employees on an annual basis to reduce the incidence of influenza among home care staff members, reduce lost days due to illness, and avoid exposing patients who may be at risk. Frequently, the vaccine is provided at little or no charge from the state or local health department. Although influenza immunization must be voluntary, home care organizations should encourage all staff providing care for high-risk patients to become immunized (CDC, 1997b). This includes patients older than 65 years, those with chronic pulmonary disease, and those with other chronic illnesses, such as acquired immune deficiency syndrome (AIDS), that put them at greater risk. Some agencies provide vaccine to patients at high risk as well. Patients with chronic illnesses may not develop antibodies in response to the immunization, however, leaving them at risk for infection.

If an organization has not planned an influenza vaccination program for employees but influenza occurs in greater than predicted numbers, vaccination can still be given even though the season has begun. It takes about 10 days from the time the vaccine is administered for the recipient to develop immunity.

DEFINING AND MANAGING EXPOSURES

Home care staff may be exposed to communicable diseases to which they are susceptible either occupationally from patients and their families or nonoccupationally from their own family and friends or while in the community. In either case, some of these exposures should be reported to the home care organization and evaluated for necessary follow-up to reduce exposure of high-risk patients and other employees. Exposures to common community-acquired infections, such as upper respiratory viral infections, including colds and flu, should not require reporting to or follow-up by the home care organization. The course of the common upper respiratory infections is usually limited, and there are no recommendations for postexposure follow-up. In addition, it would be impossible to determine whether these infections were the result of occupational or nonoccupational exposure. Employees who are feeling ill (fatigue and general malaise), and especially those with a fever and severe upper respiratory symptoms of coughing, sneezing, and increased respiratory secretions, should not work. Once the initial signs and symptoms of an upper respiratory infection begin to subside and temperature returns to normal, the employee can return to work. Over-the-counter medications to reduce coughing and production of respiratory secretions may be used to decrease the risk of transmission to patients and other staff members.

There are certain infectious diseases that should be reported to the home care organization so that investigation and follow-up of an exposure by a home care staff member can be performed to reduce the risk of exposure to other home care staff and patients. A list of these infections is given in Exhibit 12–5. These are illnesses that may require specific interventions, including antimicrobial prophylaxis and/or work restrictions. The specific conditions necessary to define an exposure to any of these diseases should be included in the home care organization's policies and procedures. The written definition of an exposure is necessary not only to provide a reference when a potential exposure occurs but also to ensure that there is consistency in identifying and managing exposures.

Varicella

The varicella zoster virus causes chickenpox as a primary infection and most frequently causes illness in young children. Recurrence of varicella results in shingles and is seen more frequently in older people. Chickenpox is contagious and can be transmitted by contact and via the airborne route. Therefore, anyone who is in direct contact with an individual who is incubating chickenpox (contagion begins 48 to 72 hours before the development of the vesicular skin rash), has already developed the rash (contagion continues for about 5 days after the appearance of the rash), or has shared the air of a contagious person may have been exposed. An exposure to varicella is defined as face-to-face contact indoors for at least 10 minutes or being in the same room for longer than 10 minutes without the protection of a mask. For a home care employee who is susceptible to

Exhibit 12–5 Infectious Diseases Requiring Follow-Up for Exposures

- AIDS
- Hepatitis A
- Hepatitis B
- Hepatitis C
- Measles
- Meningococcal meningitis
- Rubella
- Pertussis
- Tuberculosis
- Varicella

chickenpox, it really does not matter whether the exposure occurs while providing care (occupational) or during nonworking hours. If the individual is susceptible, he or she may develop active infection and expose patients or other employees. Therefore, if an employee reports a chickenpox exposure, it must be determined whether he or she is susceptible. This should have been accomplished as part of the preemployment health screen and infectious disease history (CDC, 1997b).

The decision as to whether to restrict the exposed employee's work activities depends on the patients for whom the employee provides care. If the patients are adults who are probably immune to varicella, no restrictions may be necessary. In this case, the employee may be carefully monitored for early signs and symptoms of chickenpox and counseled to stay off work if a fever or prodromal symptoms, such as headache, fever, and malaise, develop. If the employee is caring for children, especially those who are at risk for varicella, work restriction or change of assignment should be seriously considered from day 7 after the first exposure through day 21 after the last exposure. This is the period in which active infection is most likely to occur. If the exposed employee is given varicella immune globulin, the incubation period is extended to 28 days after the last exposure. The specific date(s) of exposure must be obtained; in many cases the individual may have been exposed on several different days, including during the incubation period, when the infection was not yet recognized but was contagious. Work restrictions may allow for the staff member to work in the office (no patient care) if the other staff members are immune to chickenpox. Otherwise, complete work restriction may be indicated.

Susceptible employees should be encouraged to report exposure to varicella and the other infections listed in Exhibit 12–5. Financial disincentives (no sick time or paid time off) should be addressed and avoided to encourage reporting. If the employee develops chickenpox, he or she should remain off duty until all the lesions have crusted. Even though varicella is not contagious after the lesions have crusted, the organization may elect to restrict the employee from patient care if the rash remains to avoid questions or concerns from patients and their families. The individual may safely spend this time working in the office.

Although there are a few reports of health care providers developing chickenpox after direct contact with a patient with shingles, most infection control experts would only consider risk in exposures involving patients with disseminated zoster. By definition, disseminated herpes zoster is shingles that involves more than one dermatome. In disseminated zoster, the varicella zoster virus has been isolated from respiratory secretions. This may make the infection transmissible via the respiratory and/or airborne route as well as through direct contact with lesions by a susceptible host. If a susceptible home care staff member is caring for a patient with disseminated zoster and has not used a mask, the same work restrictions for a chickenpox exposure should be considered.

Measles, Rubella, Pertussis, Meningitis, and Hepatitis A

Measles is considered the most contagious infectious disease. It occurs through airborne transmission, so that exposure is similar to chickenpox: face-to-face contact for at least 10 minutes or presence in the same room for longer than 10 minutes without a mask. Measles is infrequently seen in the United States but may occur in unimmunized or improperly immunized children. Home care staff should be immune to measles by either natural immunity or vaccination. If for some reason a staff member is not immune, however, and because the virus may be shed from the respiratory tract from 5 days after the initial exposure until 21 days after the last exposure, the staff member should be restricted from working during that period. If a rash occurs, work restriction should continue for 7 days after the development of the rash (Bolyard et al., 1998).

Staff members should also be immune to rubella. An exposure to rubella, which is transmitted by respiratory droplets, may be defined as face-to-face contact without a mask for at least 10 minutes. If an exposure occurs, the infection may be contagious from day 7 after the first exposure to day 21 after the last exposure, and the person should be restricted from work. If a rash develops, the person should remain off duty for 5 days after the development of the rash (Bolyard et al., 1998).

Whooping cough or pertussis is transmitted via respiratory droplets. Face-to-face contact with a contagious individual for greater than 10 minutes may define exposure. A health care staff member who is exposed to pertussis should receive antimicrobial prophylaxis with erythromycin. If prophylaxis is provided, work restrictions may not be necessary. If the exposed individual does not receive antimicrobial prophylaxis, however, and/or develops signs and symptoms of pertussis, including a paroxysmal cough, he or she should be restricted from work until 5 days after the initiation of appropriate therapy (Bolyard et al., 1998).

Exposure to meningococcal meningitis occurs most frequently in emergency care providers, such as ambulance personnel. Nevertheless, an occupational exposure could occur in a home care staff member. Exposure to meningococcal meningitis requires interaction with the patient beyond face-to-face contact. Exposure should be defined as direct, intimate contact with respiratory secretions, such as would occur in kissing or administration of mouth-to-mouth resuscitation (thus the risk to emergency responders). If an exposure occurs, the exposed individual should be provided with prophylactic antibiotic treatment, usually rifampin. No work restriction is necessary (Bolyard et al., 1998).

Hepatitis A virus (HAV) infection is spread by the oral–fecal route. Home care staff may have some risk for exposure if they are caring for a patient with an unrecognized HAV infection or are working in a home where a family member has HAV. Although health care staff members should be adhering to standard precautions and wearing gloves when handling stool, unprotected exposures can occur while they are caring for a patient who is incontinent of stool or if they fail to perform adequate handwashing. Eating or drinking in the home of an HAV-infected person may also be considered an exposure. If there is sufficient evidence that exposure to HAV has occurred, the home care staff member should be given an intramuscular injection of immune globulin within 2 weeks of exposure. No work restrictions are necessary unless the staff member develops HAV infection. If infection occurs, the person should be restricted from patient care for 1 week after the onset of illness. HAV vaccine is not routinely recommended for health care providers (CDC, 1997b).

TB

Exposure to TB increased among all health care workers in the 1990s with the increase of TB in the general population. The incidence of TB began to decline in 1996, but exposure of home care staff continues to be a risk. Exposure to TB is defined as face-to-face contact for more than 10 minutes or remaining in the same room with an individual who has active and contagious pulmonary or laryngeal TB infection for more than 30 minutes without the use of a mask. Specific judgments must be made if the patient has an active, productive cough. In home care, such exposures may occur if the organization has not been informed that the patient or a member of the family has active TB.

Although the exposed employee should have had a baseline PPD test, another test should be administered as soon as possible after the exposure if the employee is PPD negative. Home care staff who are known to have positive PPD skin tests should not be retested. This test serves as a new baseline for the current exposure. A second PPD should be administered in 12 weeks after the exposure to determine whether infection has occurred. If the PPD is negative at 12 weeks, no further testing is necessary. If the PPD is positive, further examination by a physician and antimicrobial prophylaxis are indicated. If the employee is asymptomatic (e.g., no fevers, cough, or weight loss), work restriction is not necessary. If active disease is evident, the individual should be restricted from work until appropriate therapy has been initiated and there are three negative sputum smears for acid-fast bacilli obtained on different days (CDC, 1994).

Bloodborne Pathogens

Definitions and follow-up procedures for employees exposed to bloodborne pathogens, including HBV, hepatitis C virus (HCV), and HIV, should be incorporated in the exposure control plan and the policies and procedures for occupational health. Exposure to a bloodborne pathogen may occur through the percutaneous route (e.g., needlestick or sharps injury) or through exposure of the mucus membranes of the mouth, nose, or eyes to infected blood or body fluids. It is clear that a percutaneous exposure increases risk for infection (Cardo et al., 1997). All exposures must be reported and appropriate assessment and follow-up must be provided. Although the initial assessment to determine whether a significant exposure has occurred can be done in the organization, a physician should perform further assessment and follow-up.

A significant exposure to bloodborne pathogens occurs when a health care provider experiences a needlestick or percutaneous injury (laceration or puncture wound) with a sharp instrument or object that has been used in the care of a patient and has been contaminated with the patient's blood or potentially infected body fluids. An exposure also occurs when the mucus membranes of the health care provider's mouth, nose, or eyes are contaminated with blood or body fluid from a patient through a splash or spill. The body fluids of concern include cerebrospinal fluid, synovial fluid, pleural fluid, peritoneal fluid, pericardial fluid, amniotic fluid, semen, vaginal secretions, and any other body fluid containing visible blood. These are the fluids that have been recognized in the transmission of HBV, HCV, and HIV. It should be noted that the list does not include urine, stool, nasal secretions, sputum, sweat, tears, or vomitus unless they are visibly blood contaminated. When an employee reports an exposure, the designated individual in the organization will determine whether the circumstances meet the criteria for a significant exposure. For example, if an employee reports that he or she experienced an unprotected splash to the eyes and mouth of visibly bloody vomitus, a significant exposure has occurred. If an employee reports a needlestick from a syringe that was used to obtain a urine sample and the urine was not visibly bloody, no significant exposure has occurred. In either case, the home care organization should eventually investigate why the exposure occurred and whether the employee was complying with standard precautions. In addition, the report of the exposure should be noted in the employee's health record.

Once the significance of the exposure has been decided, the status of the source patient must be determined to provide the appropriate prophylaxis. The patient's physician should be called to determine the status for HBV, HCV, and HIV if it is not already known by the organization as part of the patient record. If the patient is known to be infected with HBV, HCV, or HIV, specific protocols for testing and prophylaxis as described below should be followed. A source patient is considered infected with HBV if he or she currently tests positive for hepatitis B surface antigen (HBsAg). A source patient should be considered infectious for HCV if he or she tests positive for antibodies to HCV. At this time, there are no serologic tests for HCV antigen, so that the antibody test must be used. HCV antibody-positive patients are considered potentially infectious for life. Similarly, a source patient who tests positive for antibody to HIV should be considered infectious. There are no serologic tests for HIV, and those infected, as demonstrated by antibody, are considered potentially infectious for life.

If the exposure occurs from an unknown source (e.g., a needlestick accident due to a contaminated needle in a sharps container for which the source patient is unknown), it should be assumed that the source is potentially infectious unless there are circumstances to indicate low risk based on the patient population. This type of exposure is less likely to occur in home care than in settings where there are many patients cared for at a single facility and where sharps and infectious waste are collected in common containers.

If exposure to HBV occurs and the exposed employee has received HBV vaccine and is a known responder, the employee should be retested for antibody to anti-HBs to confirm immunity. The report of the exposure and the results of testing should be placed in the employee's health record (CDC, 1991b).

If exposure to HBV occurs in an employee who received HBV vaccine and is a known nonresponder, either two doses of hepatitis B immune globulin (HBIG) should be administered (one at the time of exposure and the second 1 month later) or a single dose of HBIG should be administered and the employee should be revaccinated. If the employee's response to previous HBV vaccination is not known, an antibody test should be obtained. If the level of anti-HBs is adequate (greater than 10 μU/mL), no additional treatment is necessary. If it is inadequate, the exposed employee should receive a dose of HBIG and a vaccine booster. An unvaccinated employee should receive one dose of HBIG, and the vaccine series should be initiated as soon as possible. The vaccine should be administered even if the source patient tests negative for HBsAg in light of a clear risk for future exposure (CDC, 1991b).

HCV is an increasing risk for health care workers in all settings. There is currently no prophylactic treatment for HCV in the event of exposure, however. If the source patient is known to be infectious, the exposed employee should be tested for antibody to HCV immediately after exposure to provide a baseline result. Retesting should occur 6 months after the exposure to determine whether infection has occurred (CDC, 1997c). If results indicate that the employee is antibody positive, the infected employee should be counseled to seek follow-up care from his or her private physician, who should monitor the employee for development or progression of active infection. Should the disease progress, the employee's health record will confirm occupational exposure, and the employee will be eligible for workers' compensation benefits.

Provision of prophylaxis to employees exposed or potentially exposed to HIV must be immediate to achieve the best outcome. Therefore, a mechanism for reporting exposures and ensuring that the drugs recommended for postexposure prophylaxis (PEP) are available should be established in all home care organizations. When a significant exposure has occurred, the

HIV status of the source patient must be considered. In many cases, the status will be unknown unless the patient is known to have HIV or AIDS. If the patient has AIDS or is otherwise known to be HIV infected, postexposure prophylaxis should be provided to the employee within 1 to 2 hours of exposure for the best results. If the patient's HIV status is not known, potential risk based on current knowledge of the patient's history and epidemiological factors must be examined. This may be or may not be beyond the capabilities of the individual in the organization who is responsible for infection control or occupational health issues. Even if this person is capable, enlisting the involvement of the patient's own physician and the physician who will be providing postexposure prophylaxis may be prudent so that broader input in making the judgment regarding risk and need for postexposure prophylaxis is available. Frequently, the level of risk falls into three categories: no risk, questionable risk, or high risk. The level of risk should be assessed based on the patient's medical history and lifestyle. Factors to consider are provided in Table 12–1. If there is agreement that there is no known risk of HIV infection in the source patient, no testing of the patient is necessary, and the exposed employee should be informed. In such cases, no postexposure prophylaxis is recommended (CDC, 1998). Occasionally a concerned employee who has been exposed may prefer to initiate a minimal regimen of zidovudine (ZVD) for postexposure prophylaxis. More detail on postexposure prophylaxis protocols is provided below. The determination of who will pay for the drugs for postexposure prophylaxis will depend on the organization's policy and/or the state's workers' compensation laws.

If there is some concern that risk factors exist and the source patient may be infected with HIV, the source patient's physician should obtain testing within the parameters permitted by local laws. In most states, the patient must give written informed consent for testing. Some states allow testing without written consent if a health care provider has been exposed. The home care organization should be familiar with state laws and incorporate compliance into its policies for investigation of exposures. Initiation of postexposure prophylaxis should not be delayed waiting for test results. Blood samples for baseline testing of the exposed employee should be obtained as soon as possible, and postexposure prophylaxis should be initiated immediately. If there is considerable risk of HIV infection in the source patient but the HIV status is not known, the same steps as described above should be followed.

In 1990, the CDC made its initial recommendations for the use of antiviral agents as postexposure prophylaxis for health care workers occupationally exposed to HIV-infected blood or body fluids (CDC, 1990b). At that time, the CDC recommended that ZVD be provided as soon as possible and continue for 4 weeks or as long as tolerated. The CDC recommendations have changed, with updates published in 1996 and 1998 (CDC, 1996, 1998). The more recent recommendations, however, which include the consideration and use of additional antiviral agents, are based on treatment of HIV-infected patients, not on use as postexposure prophylaxis. Therefore, these recommendations remain provisional until more experience and data can be accumulated and examined.

The use of ZVD in postexposure prophylaxis for health care workers after percutaneous exposure to HIV has demonstrated a 79 percent reduction in the risk of infection. The actual risk for acquiring HIV infection if a health care worker experiences a percutaneous exposure is estimated at 0.3 percent. This risk is based on a number of factors that should also be con-

Table 12–1 Factors for Assessment of a Source Patient's Risk for HIV Infection

Lifestyle Risks	*Medical History*
Homosexuality or bisexuality	Hemophilia
Current or past history of intravenous drug use	Past blood transfusions
Current or past history of sexually transmitted diseases	Child of an HIV-infected mother
Sexual partner of a high-risk individual	Current signs and symptoms consistent with HIV infection

sidered when postexposure prophylaxis is prescribed. A case-control study has demonstrated that a deep needlestick or sharps injury from a device with visible blood contamination increased risk when the device had been placed in the source patient's vein or artery. Additional risk has been demonstrated when the source patient died of AIDS within 60 days of the exposure. This is due to the increased viral dose in the terminally ill patient with AIDS (Cardo et al., 1997).

Consequently, if an exposure of a home care staff member occurs and the source patient is known to be HIV positive or there is evidence of medium to high risk for infection, the circumstances of the exposure should be examined. If the circumstances increase the risk of infection (deep percutaneous exposure with a visibly contaminated device or similar circumstances), additional antiviral drugs should be added to the post-exposure prophylaxis regimen (CDC, 1996, 1998). The drugs that may be added to ZVD are antiviral agents that are used to treat patients with AIDS. Some of these drugs are recommended because HIV has demonstrated its ability to become resistant to ZVD. Other drugs are recommended to enhance antiviral activity. The 1998 CDC recommendations are provided in Appendix 12–A. A physician with knowledge and experience in the use of antiviral drugs should be consulted.

WORK RESTRICTIONS

There are various infections that occur among health care staff members that may pose a risk of transmission from the provider to the patient and others in the environment. A home care organization should recognize these conditions and formulate a policy for diagnosis, assessment, and work restrictions when they occur in patient care personnel. If they are occupationally acquired infections, workers' compensation benefits may be used to pay the employee who is not permitted to work. If the condition is nonoccupational, paid sick time benefits must be used, if they are provided. Table 12–2 provides a summary of recommendations for work restrictions for home care staff exposed to selected infectious diseases.

Some skin infections that occur in home care staff members may warrant a staff member's exclusion from patient care and food preparation activities. If a patient care provider has a skin infection caused by *Staphylococcus aureus*, the potential for transmission of the infective agent to the patient must be assessed. First, the specific type, location, and extent of infection should be considered. If there is a draining wound on the hands or upper extremities, there may be risk for transmission even if the wound is covered. This may depend on the extent or size of the wound and the degree of drainage. An extensive wound on the face or neck may also pose risk. A draining wound on the trunk or a lower extremity that is covered and for which the drainage is well contained, however, may not pose such a risk. In any case, the home care staff member must be attentive to conscientious handwashing if he or she is permitted to provide care or be involved in food preparation (Bolyard et al., 1998).

The other variable to consider in determining whether a provider with a staphylococcal skin infection should be providing care is the patient's risk. If the patient requires wound care or other skilled care that involves a potential portal of entry for the bacteria, he or she should not be exposed to the provider. Many home care patients have needs based on medical conditions, however, such as cerebrovascular accident, hypertension, or other conditions that do not involve a portal of entry. If the patient is immunocompetent and has intact skin, the risk may be minimal. A home care staff member known to be colonized with *S. aureus* (e.g., nasal colonization or skin carriage) should not automatically be excluded from patient care. Any exclusion should be in light of epidemiological evidence of transmission of the organism to patients.

Employees with skin and wound infections caused by *Streptococcus* species should be handled in the same manner as those with staphylococcal infections. With both organisms, if the provider is restricted, he or she may return to work when adequate treatment has been provided and/or when the wound is no longer draining. The organization may require a negative wound culture before the staff member returns to patient care.

Other skin conditions may not involve specific organisms such as *Staphylococcus aureus*, but a provider may be excluded based on appearance. For example, if a home care staff member has extensive poison ivy, it may be prudent to restrict patient care and allow the person to work in the office to avoid questions and concerns from patients and families. The same approach may be considered for staff members recovering from illnesses with viral exanthams, such as chickenpox. Although they may have passed the time of contagion, there may be concerns on the part of the patient or family if the rash remains evident.

Table 12–2 Summary of suggested work restrictions for health care personnel exposed to or infected with infectious diseases of importance in health care settings, in the absence of state and local regulations (modified from ACIP recommendations*)

Disease/problem	*Work restriction*	*Duration*	*Category*
Conjunctivitis	Restrict from patient contact and contact with the patient's environment	Until discharge ceases	II
Cytomegalovirus infections	No restriction		II
Diarrheal diseases			
Acute stage (diarrhea with other symptoms)	Restrict from patient contact, contact with the patient's environment or food handling	Until symptoms resolve	IB
Convalescent stage, *Salmonella* spp.	Restrict from care of high-risk patients	Until symptoms resolve; consult with local and state health authorities regarding need for negative stool cultures	IB
Diphtheria	Exclude from duty	Until antimicrobial therapy completed and 2 cultures obtained ≥24 hours apart are negative	IB
Enteroviral infections	Restrict from care of infants, neonates, and immunocompromised patients and their environments	Until symptoms resolve	II
Hepatitis A	Restrict from patient contact, contact with patient's environment, and food handling	Until 7 days after onset of jaundice	IB
Hepatitis B			
Personnel with acute or chronic hepatitis B surface antigemia who do not perform exposure-prone procedures	No restriction*; refer to state regulations; standard precautions should always be observed		II
Personnel with acute or chronic hepatitis B e antigenemia who perform exposure-prone procedures	Do not perform exposure-prone invasive procedures until counsel from an expert review panel has been sought; panel should review and recommend procedures the worker can perform, taking into account specific procedures as well as skill and technique of worker; refer to state regulations	Until hepatitis B e antigen is negative	II
Hepatitis C	No recommendation		Unresolved issue
Herpes simplex			
Genital	No restriction		II
Hands (herpetic whitlow)	Restrict from patient contact and contact with the patient's environment	Until lesions heal	IA
Orofacial	Evaluate for need to restrict from care of high-risk patients		II
Human immunodeficiency virus	Do not perform exposure-prone invasive procedures until counsel from an expert review panel has been sought; panel should review and recommend procedures the worker can perform, taking into account specific procedure as well as skill and technique of the worker; standard precautions should always be observed; refer to state regulations		II

*Unless epidemiologically linked to transmission of infection.

†Those susceptible to varicella and who are at increased risk of complications of varicella, such as neonates and immunocompromised persons of any age.

‡High-risk patients as defined by the ACIP for complications of influenza.

Table 12–2 continued

Disease/problem	*Work restriction*	*Duration*	*Category*
Measles			
Active	Exclude from duty	Until 7 days after the rash appears	IA
Postexposure (susceptible personnel)	Exclude from duty	From 5th day after 1st exposure through 21st day after last exposure and/or 4 days after rash appears	IB
Meningococcal infections	Exclude from duty	Until 24 hours after start of effective therapy	IA
Mumps			
Active	Exclude from duty	Until 9 days after onset of parotitis	IB
Postexposure (susceptible personnel)	Exclude from duty	From 12th day after 1st exposure through 26th day after last exposure or until 9 days after onset of parotitis	II
Pediculosis	Restrict from patient contact	Until treated and observed to be free of adult and immature lice	IB
Pertussis			
Active	Exclude from duty	From beginning of catarrhal stage through 3rd wk after onset of paroxysms or until 5 days after start of effective antimicrobial therapy	IB
Postexposure (asymptomatic personnel)	No restriction, prophylaxis recommended		II
Postexposure (symptomatic personnel)	Exclude from duty	Until 5 days after start of effective antimicrobial therapy	IB
Rubella			
Active	Exclude from duty	Until 5 days after rash appears	IA
Postexposure (susceptible personnel)	Exclude from duty	From 7th day after 1st exposure through 21st day after last exposure	IB
Scabies	Restrict from patient contact	Until cleared by medical evaluation	IB
Staphylococcus aureus infection			
Active, draining skin lesions	Restrict from contact with patients and patient's environment or food handling	Until lesions have resolved	IB
Carrier state	No restriction, unless personnel are epidemiologically linked to transmission of the organism		IB
Streptococcal infection, group A	Restrict from patient care, contact with patient's environment, or food handling	Until 24 hours after adequate treatment started	IB
Tuberculosis			IA
Active disease	Exclude from duty	Until proved noninfectious	IA
PPD converter	No restriction		

continued

Table 12–2 continued

Disease/problem	*Work restriction*	*Duration*	*Category*
Varicella			
Active	Exclude from duty	Until all lesions dry and crust	IA
Postexposure (susceptible personnel)	Exclude from duty	From 10th day after 1st exposure through 21st day (28th day if VZIG given) after last exposure	IA
Zoster			
Localized, in healthy person	Cover lesions; restrict from care of high-risk patients†	Until all lesions dry and crust	II
Generalized or localized in immunosuppressed person	Restrict from patient contact	Until all lesions dry and crust	IB
Postexposure (Susceptible personnel)	Restrict from patient contact	From 8th day aftr 1st exposure through 21st day (28th day if VZIG given) after last exposure or, if varicella occurs, until all lesions dry and crust	IA
Viral respiratory infections, acute febrille	Consider excluding from the care of high risk patients‡ or contact with their environment during community outbreak of RSV and influenza	Until acute symptoms resolved	

Source: Reprinted with permission from B. Bolyard, O. Tablan, W. Williams, M. Pearson, C. Shapiro, and S. Deitchman, CDC Guideline for Infection Control in Health Care Personnel, *American Journal of Infection Control,* Vol. 26, No. 3, pp. 299–301, © 1998, Mosby-Year Book, Inc.

Scabies may be occupationally or nonoccupationally acquired. The definition for occupational exposure should require skin-to-skin contact with an individual who has untreated scabies. This type of exposure may occur during direct care, such as bathing. If a home care employee discovers that a patient has scabies and is exposed, he or she should be observed for signs and symptoms of infestation and treated prophylactically with a scabicide preparation if they occur. Once the staff member is treated, he or she may return to patient care after he or she is assessed and found to be free of infestation. The patient's physician should be notified, and treatment for the patient should also be ordered and provided. All the patient's household contacts should also be treated to prevent reinfection of the patient. If a home care staff member is caring for a patient known to have untreated scabies, gowns and gloves should be used if the provider has not already been exposed (Bolyard et al., 1998).

Herpes simplex virus (HSV) is another skin infection that may occur in home care staff members. HSV is not usually an occupational infection. However, a home care staff member may acquire an occupational HSV infection of a finger; this is known as herpetic whitlow. This infection usually occurs when a staff member with nonintact skin around the nailbed (e.g., a hangnail) contacts oral secretions of a patient who is shedding HSV. A home care staff member with herpetic whitlow must be restricted from patient care until the lesions have healed and there is no risk of viral shedding. A physician's prescription for antiviral agents is usually necessary (Bolyard et al., 1998).

HSV infections occur more often on the mouth and face and may recur frequently. The actual risk of health care workers transmitting oral HSV to patients is not known. Most hospitals allow staff members to continue patient care activities unless their assignment includes patients with severe immunosuppression (e.g., those undergoing organ transplantation) or low-birthweight premature infants. Home care staff members with oral HSV lesions do not have to be restricted from patient care but should be reminded of the importance of careful handwashing and avoidance of touching the lesions during patient care activities. Use of antiviral agents should be encouraged to decrease viral shedding and hasten healing of the lesions. If the lesions are extensive, the home care organization may elect to exclude the staff member from patient care to avoid questions and concerns by the patient and family.

Home care staff members should be instructed to notify the organization if they are experiencing diarrhea

Table 12–3 Infectious Diseases of Concern to the Pregnant Employee

Disease	*Infection Source*	*Transmission*	*Precautions (in Addition to Standard and Hand Washing)*	*Reassignment of Pregnant Worker*
HIV/AIDS	Blood Body fluid containing blood Cerebrospinal fluid Synovial, pleural, peritoneal, pericardial, and amniotic fluid Vaginal secretion Semen	Parenteral (needlesticks) Mucus membrane Nonintact skin	None	No
Cytomegalovirus (CMV)	Urine Blood Respiratory secretions Transplant patients Day care toddlers	Close intimate contact	None (except mask, if CMV pneumonia) If children at home attend day care center, good hand washing at home	No
Hepatitis A	Feces	Fecal-oral	None	No
Hepatitis B	Blood	Parenteral Mucus membrane Nonintact skin	None Immunization with hepatitis B vaccine (safe during pregnancy)	No
Hepatitis C	Blood	As above	None	No
Herpes simplex types I and II	Lesions/vescular fluid	Direct contact with lesions Respiratory secretions Saliva	None Avoid direct contact with lesions. Double glove.	No
Herpes zoster (shingles)				
• Localized	Open, weeping lesions	Direct contact	None	The nonimmune health care worker, pregnant or not, should not have patient contact.
• Disseminated	Lesions, possibly respiratory secretions	Direct contact Droplet contact	Masks	
Rubella (German Measles)	Respiratory secretions	Droplet contact	Masks Respiratory isolation Immunization available for nonpregnant worker	The nonimmune health care worker, pregnant or not, should not care for rubella patients.
Rubeola (Measles)	Respiratory secretions	Airborne Droplet contact	Masks Airborne isolation Immunization available for nonpregnant worker	The nonimmune health care worker, pregnant or not, should not care for rubeola patients.
Toxoplasmosis	Cat feces Raw meat Unpasteurized milk	Ingestion	None	No
Tuberculosis	Airborne droplet Nuclei	Airborne	Masks NIOSH approved Airborne isolation	No
Varicella (chickenpox)	Respiratory secretions Lesion secretions	Droplet contact Airborne Contact with lesions	Masks Gowns Airborne/contact isolation	The nonimmune health care worker, pregnant or not, should not have patient contact.

* Standard Precautions are to be followed on all patients. Use gloves for contact with all moist body substances, gowns, masks, and eye shields when needed to prevent splashing.

Courtesy of Scottsdale Healthcare, Scottsdale, Arizona.

so that the situation can be assessed. If an infectious cause (e.g., viral gastroenteritis or *Salmonella* or *Shigella* infection) is suspected, the staff member should be restricted from patient care or food preparation until he or she is evaluated by a physician or the symptoms subside. Any provider who is experiencing diarrhea must pay careful attention to handwashing, especially if he or she is involved in food preparation. A home care staff member experiencing vomiting from a potentially infectious cause, such as viral gastroenteritis, should be excluded from patient care until the symptoms subside (Bolyard et al., 1998).

Occasionally a home care staff member will experience conjunctivitis that prompts concern regarding potential transmission to patients. Evaluation by an ophthalmologist should be sought if there is purulent drainage or if epidemic keratoconjunctivitis (EKC) is suspected. EKC is caused by an adenovirus, and nosocomial transmission has been associated with outbreaks in eye clinics. Therefore, EKC may be a concern if the home care staff member recently received optical care. As its name implies, EKC is very contagious. A home care staff member with bacterial conjunctivitis should be excluded from direct patient care until the infection is treated and no longer contagious or the symptoms have subsided. A home care staff member suspected to have EKC should be seen by an ophthalmologist and excluded from patient care until it is ruled out (Ford, Nelson, & Warren, 1987).

PREGNANT STAFF MEMBERS

Many home care staff members are women of childbearing age, so that concern about exposure to infectious agents while pregnant and providing patient care often arises. Pregnant staff members are at no greater risk for exposure to and infection with infectious diseases than other staff members. There are specific infections that are documented to pose some risk to a fetus, but these diseases are no more prevalent in home care patients than in the general population. All home care staff members, including women who may become pregnant, should be encouraged to obtain available vaccines, as discussed above. In addition, all staff should be instructed in the use of personal protective equipment and should employ precautions for bloodborne pathogens and other infectious agents as prescribed (Bolyard et al., 1998). Table 12–3 provides a summary of references for issues that may be of concern to pregnant home care staff.

In addition to some of the infectious diseases discussed previously, pregnant personnel may perceive increased risk if they are exposed to patients with cytomegalovirus (CMV) or parvovirus. CMV is a common virus that is a member of the herpes virus family. Many people experience asymptomatic CMV infections in childhood. The concern among home care staff members arises when they are caring for patients chronically infected with and shedding CMV. This may include pediatric patients and those who are immunosuppressed, such as solid organ transplant recipients. Perinatal CMV infection may cause hearing loss or a congenital syndrome leading to various pathologies in the newborn. Although a susceptible pregnant home care staff member is theoretically at risk for occupational infection with CMV, the risk for occupational infection is no greater than that for nonoccupational infection. In fact, it may be less because the staff member should be complying with standard precautions for the use of gowns, gloves, and masks. Pregnant providers should not be excluded from the care of patients known to be infected with CMV (Bolyard et al., 1998).

Parvovirus B19 is a rare cause of fetal loss and hydrops fetalis. Chronic infection with viral shedding may occur in patients with chronic anemia or immunosuppression. As in the case of CMV, pregnant home care staff members do not appear to be at greater risk for occupational infection than others, and transmission is rare. Droplet precautions should be employed for patients known to be shedding parvovirus B19 to protect all staff members. Pregnant staff members should not be excluded from their care (Bolyard et al., 1998).

REFERENCES

American Thoracic Society. (1990). Diagnostic standards and classification of tuberculosis. *American Review of Respiratory Diseases, 142*, 725–735.

Bolyard, B., Tablan, O., Williams, W., Pearson, M., Shapiro, C., & Deitchman, S. (1998). CDC guideline for infection control in health care personnel. *American Journal of Infection Control, 2*, 289–354.

Cardo, D., Culver, D., Ciesielski, C., Srivastava, P., Marcus, R., Abiteboul, D., Heptonstall, J., Ippolito, G., Lot, L., McKibbon, P., & Bell, D. (1997). A case-control study of HIV seroconversion in health care workers after percutaneous exposure. *New England Journal of Medicine, 337*, 1485–1490.

Centers for Disease Control and Prevention. (1990a). Protection against viral hepatitis: Recommendations of the Advisory Committee on Immunization Practices (ACIP). *Morbidity and Mortality Weekly Report, 39*(Suppl.), 1–26.

Centers for Disease Control and Prevention. (1990b). Public Health Services statement on management of occupational exposure to human immunodeficiency virus, including considerations regarding zidovudine postexposure use. *Morbidity and Mortality Weekly Report 39*(RR-4): 1–17.

Centers for Disease Control and Prevention. (1991a). Diphtheria, tetanus, pertussis: Recommendations for vaccine use and other preventative measures—Recommendations of the Advisory Committee on Immunization Practices (ACIP). *Morbidity and Mortality Weekly Report, 46*(RR-10), 1–28.

Centers for Disease Control and Prevention. (1991b). Hepatitis B virus: A comprehensive strategy for eliminating transmission in the United States through universal childhood vaccination—Recommendation of the Advisory Committee on Immunizations Practices (ACIP). *Morbidity and Mortality Weekly Report, 40*(RR-13), 1–25.

Centers for Disease Control and Prevention. (1994). Guidelines for preventing the transmission of *Mycobacterium tuberculosis* in health-care facilities. *Morbidity and Mortality Weekly Report, 43*(RR-13), 1–32.

Centers for Disease Control and Prevention. (1996). Update: Provisional Public Health Service recommendations for chemoprophylaxis after occupational exposure to HIV. *Morbidity and Mortality Weekly Report, 45*, 468–472.

Centers for Disease Control and Prevention. (1997a). *HIV/AIDS Surveillance Report.* Atlanta: Author.

Centers for Disease Control and Prevention (1997b). Immunization of healthcare workers: Recommendations of the Advisory Committee on Immunization Practices (ACIP) and the Hospital Infection Control Practices Advisory Committee (HICPAC). *Morbidity and Mortality Weekly Report, 46*(RR-18), 1–42.

Centers for Disease Control and Prevention. (1997c). Recommendations for follow-up of health-care workers after occupational exposure to hepatitis C virus. *Morbidity and Mortality Weekly Report, 46*, 603–606.

Centers for Disease Control and Prevention. (1998). Public Health Service guidelines for the management of health-care worker exposures to HIV and recommendations for postexposure prophylaxis. *Morbidity and Mortality Weekly Report, 47*(RR-07), 1–6.

Ford, E., Nelson, K., & Warren, D. (1987). Epidemiology of epidemic keratoconjunctivitis. *Epidemiology Reviews, 9*, 244–261.

Kelley, P., Petruccelli, B., Stehr-Green, P., Erickson, R., & Mason, C. (1991). The susceptibility of young adult Americans to vaccine-preventable infections. A national serosurvey of U.S. Army recruits. *Journal of the American Medical Association, 226*, 2724–2729.

Longfield, J., Winn, R., Gibson, R., Juchau, S., & Hoffman, P. (1990). Varicella outbreaks in Army recruits from Puerto Rico. Varicella susceptibility in a population from the tropics. *Archives of Internal Medicine, 150*, 970–973.

Nassar, N., & Touma, H. (1986). Brief report: Susceptibility of Filipino nurses to the varicella-zoster virus. *Infection Control, 7*, 71–72.

Occupational Health and Safety Administration. (1991). Occupational exposure to bloodborne pathogens: Final rule. CFR part 1910.1030. *Federal Register, 56*, 64004–64182.

Occupational Health and Safety Administration, U.S. Department of Labor. (1993). *Criteria for recording on OSHA form 200.* Washington, DC: Author.

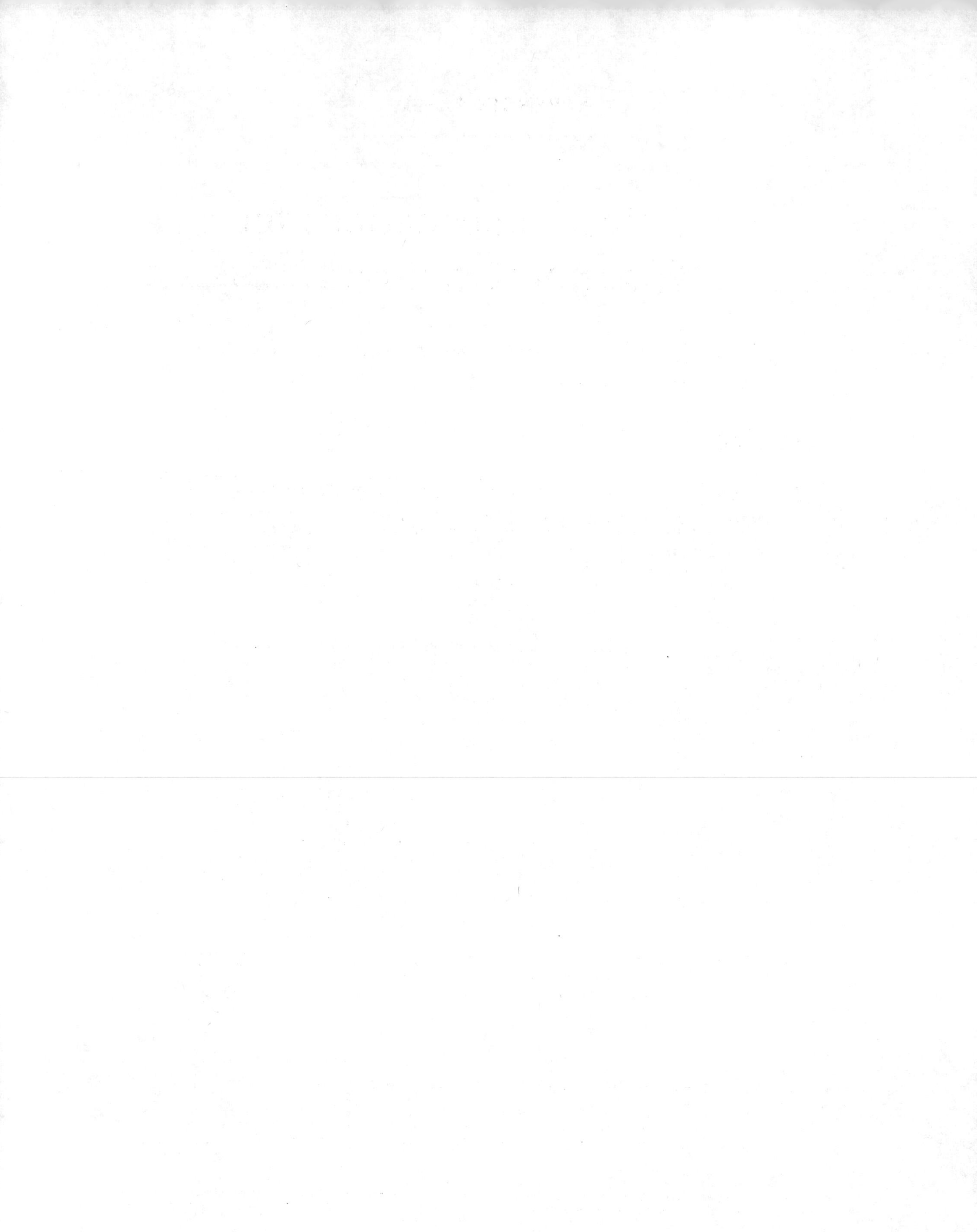

Appendix 12–A

CDC Recommendations for HIV Postexposure Prophylaxis

The following algorithm is intended to guide initial decisions about PEP and should be used in conjunction with other guidance provided in this document.

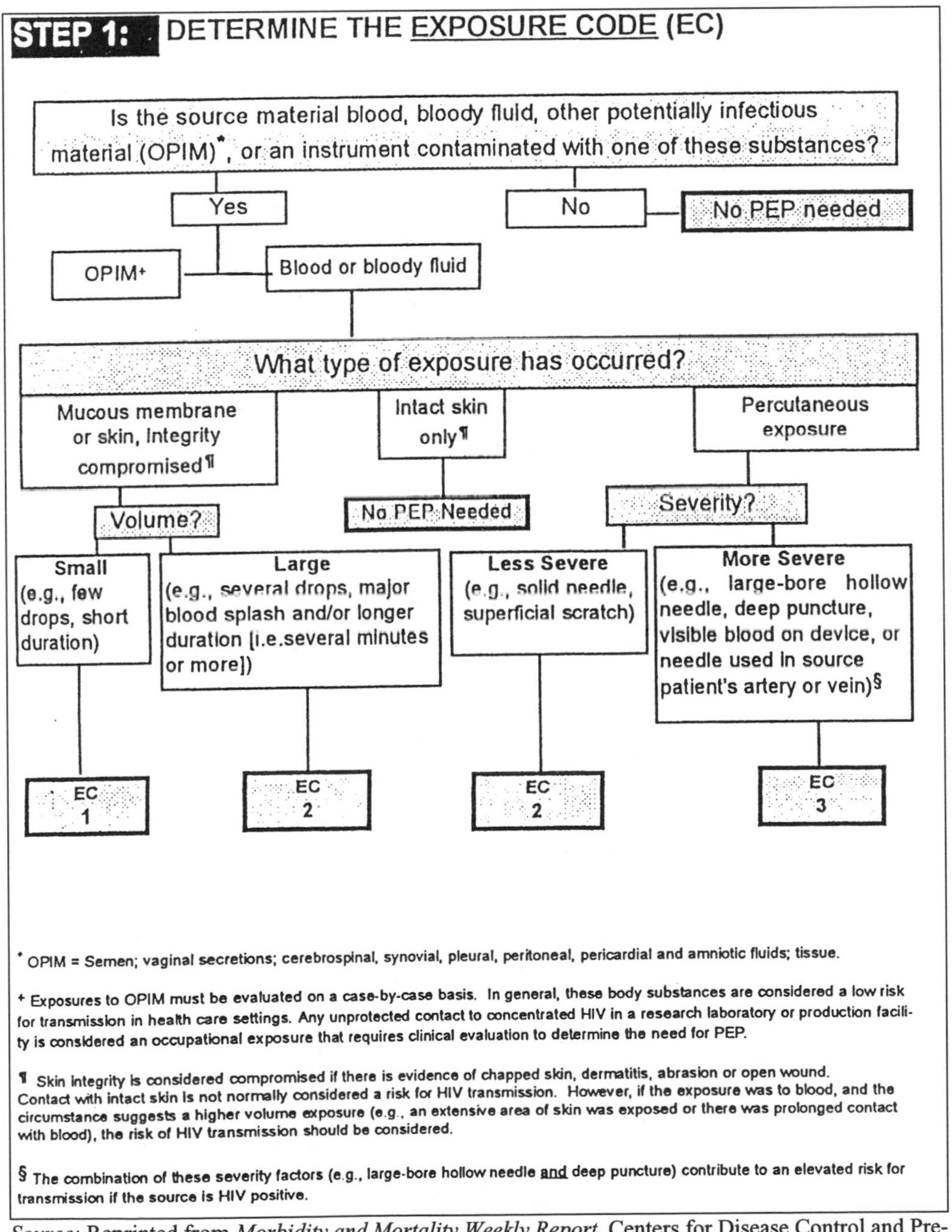

* OPIM = Semen; vaginal secretions; cerebrospinal, synovial, pleural, peritoneal, pericardial and amniotic fluids; tissue.

+ Exposures to OPIM must be evaluated on a case-by-case basis. In general, these body substances are considered a low risk for transmission in health care settings. Any unprotected contact to concentrated HIV in a research laboratory or production facility is considered an occupational exposure that requires clinical evaluation to determine the need for PEP.

¶ Skin integrity is considered compromised if there is evidence of chapped skin, dermatitis, abrasion or open wound. Contact with intact skin is not normally considered a risk for HIV transmission. However, if the exposure was to blood, and the circumstance suggests a higher volume exposure (e.g., an extensive area of skin was exposed or there was prolonged contact with blood), the risk of HIV transmission should be considered.

§ The combination of these severity factors (e.g., large-bore hollow needle <u>and</u> deep puncture) contribute to an elevated risk for transmission if the source is HIV positive.

Source: Reprinted from *Morbidity and Mortality Weekly Report,* Centers for Disease Control and Prevention, National Institute for Occupational Safety and Health, 1998.

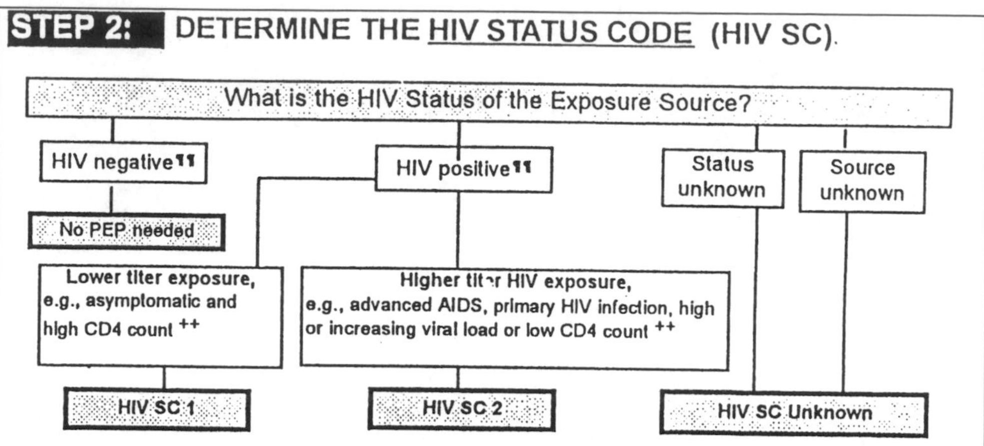

¶¶ A source is considered to be negative for HIV infection if there is laboratory documentation of a negative HIV antibody, HIV PCR or HIV p24 antigen test result from a specimen collected at or near the time of exposure and there is no clinical evidence of an acute or recent retroviral-like illness. **A source is considered to be infected with HIV (HIV Positive)** if there has been a positive laboratory result for HIV antibody, HIV PCR or HIV p24 antigen or physician-diagnosed AIDS.

++Examples are used as surrogates to estimate the HIV titer in an exposure source for purposes of considering PEP regimens and do not reflect all clinical situations that may be observed. Although a high HIV titer (status code 2) in an exposure source has been associated with an increased risk of transmission, the possibility of transmission from a source with a low HIV titer also must be considered.

STEP 3: DETERMINE THE PEP RECOMMENDATION

EC	HIV SC	PEP recommendation
1	1	**PEP may not be warranted.** Exposure type does not pose a known risk for HIV transmission. Whether the risk of drug toxicity outweighs the benefit of PEP should be decided between the exposed HCW and treating clinician.
1	2	**Consider basic regimen.** Exposure type poses a negligible risk for HIV transmission;a high HIV titer in the source may justify consideration of PEP. Whether the risk of drug toxicity outweighs the benefit of PEP should be decided between the HCW and treating clinician.
2	1	**Recommend basic regimen.** Majority of HIV exposures are in this category; no increased risk of HIV transmission has been observed but use of PEP is appropriate.
2	2	**Recommend expanded regimen.** Exposure type represents an increased HIV transmission risk.
3	1 or 2	**Recommend expanded regimen.** Exposure type represents an increased HIV transmission risk.
	Unknown	If the source or, in the case of an unknown source, the setting where the exposure occurred, suggests a possible risk for HIV exposure and the EC = 2 or 3, consider PEP basic regimen.

RECOMMENDED PEP REGIMENS

Basic regimen = 4 weeks of ZDV 600mg/day in two or three divided doses, <u>and</u> 3TC, 150 mg, BID

Expanded regimen = Basic regimen plus <u>either</u> indinavir 800 mg qh8 <u>or</u> nelfinavir 750mg, TID

CHAPTER 13

Organizing for Infection Control in Home Care

A program as comprehensive as the infection control function must be carefully managed and integrated into the overall organizational structure. There are several support functions that should be implemented to reduce the risk for infection through the continuous measurement and improvement processes. In addition to infection control, these support functions include risk management, clinical quality improvement, service/operational quality improvement, patient/family satisfaction, and occupational health and safety. All these functions may be incorporated under the umbrella of quality management or performance improvement because they share a common purpose and goal: to improve quality and reduce risk. Within a home care organization, these quality management functions may be most effective and efficient if they are connected in some way. Their connection can be based on the management structure, a committee structure, or both. The approach selected will depend on the size and complexity of the home care organization.

ORGANIZATIONAL STRUCTURE

There are no regulatory or accrediting body (e.g., Joint Commission on Accreditation of Healthcare Organizations) requirements for an infection control committee (Joint Commission, 1998). In a small home care organization with a single or few locations, the quality management/performance improvement committee structure may incorporate all the functions listed above, including infection control. This would allow the members of the committee or management team to share and review related information. For example, workers' compensation issues from the occupational health and safety function may include infection control problems. Infection control data may have an overall impact on clinical care and patient/family satisfaction. Review, discussion, and management of these issues within one committee would appear to be most efficient. The effectiveness of the approach may depend on the authority given to such a committee and the implementation and management of its decisions and recommendations.

In a larger home care organization with multiple sites doing business in several states, infection control may be integrated into other quality management/performance improvement functions at the local level, but there may be significant benefit to having a separate infection control function and committee at the corporate level (Figure 13–1). This allows for a more focused examination of infection control issues across clinical sites and more concentrated analysis of infection risk data. If the home care organization has many sites and regions, internal benchmarking of home care infection data may be possible. Internal comparisons of rates may be performed, provided that they are done appropriately to control for different risk factors and to identify locations with the best results to serve as models and mentors for other locations. Locations with higher than expected infection rates may be identified as well and may benefit from risk reduction activities developed at other locations.

Eventually, the organization leaders, including the governing body, must receive the infection control data for their information and/or action. This is a requirement of the Joint Commission and is based on sound

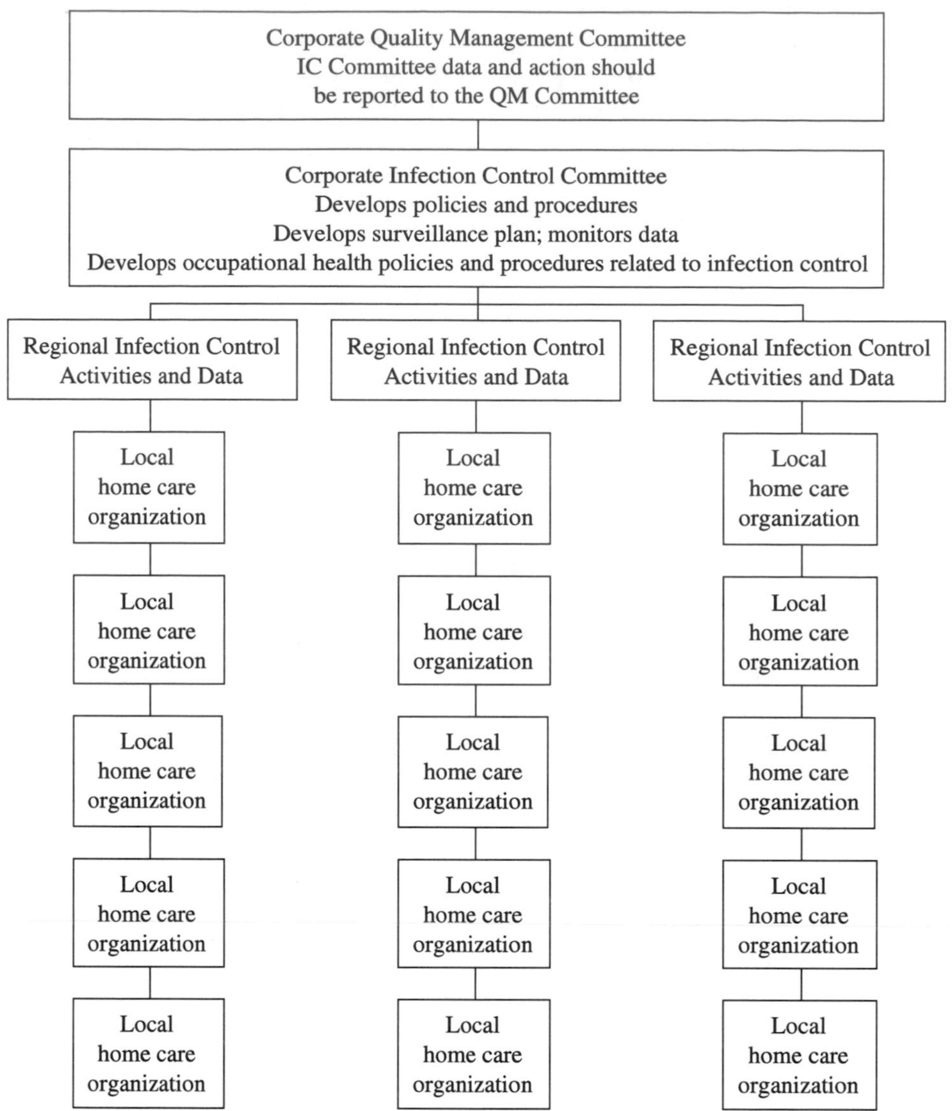

Figure 13–1 Organizational Model for Infection Control in a Corporate Setting

management principles (Joint Commission, 1998). Infection data will provide information to manage and improve home care services and may indicate specific quality issues that require attention and resources. These data may also provide information about increasing costs of care if the development of a home care-acquired infection increases patients' need (e.g., more frequent or prolonged wound care, more visits to provide intravenous antibiotics, etc.). In the Medicare prospective payment system, this may significantly affect a Medicare-certified home care agency's expenses. Infection data may also be useful in recognizing potential legal risk. Individual patients and families may bring claims of negligence if the patient develops a home care-acquired infection. Although there is not much current experience or claims data in this area, some experts are anticipating an increase in home care professional liability claims with the changes in reimbursement that will occur over the next several years (Rhinehart & Weller, 1998). A well-organized infection control program that can demonstrate proactive efforts to prevent home care-acquired infection may serve the home care organization well in defending against claims of negligence.

As mentioned in Chapter 12, infection control issues can also affect workers' compensation costs. The home care organization's leaders should review data that track home care staff needlesticks and other occupational exposures, injuries, and illnesses. Again, there can be significant financial implications if risks are not minimized to prevent the occurrence of occupational illnesses. Occupationally acquired bloodborne illnesses can be costly to any health care organization. Early detection and reduction of risk may be critical not only for the safety of staff, but also for the reduction of costs.

DAILY MANAGEMENT OF INFECTION CONTROL

Infection control is a specific health care discipline with a growing body of scientific knowledge. Designation of a single individual as the infection control practitioner in a home care organization to serve as an infection control resource and to manage routine infection control issues seems sensible and practical. A registered nurse with significant experience and knowledge in clinical care and, ideally, with a special interest in infection control is a model candidate for this role. This individual may eventually demonstrate his or her competence by becoming certified in infection control through the Certification Board of Infection Control and Epidemiology, Inc. to demonstrate their competence. This role may be assumed as part of a staff nurse's position and might provide an opportunity for advancement. More commonly, it is made part of a management position that also is responsible for related quality management functions and/or occupation health, safety, and workers' compensation. The incorporation of the infection control function into another job will depend on the individual who is available and interested in the role as well as the organization of other clinical and support functions. As mentioned above, the size and complexity of the home care organization will dictate the amount of resources allocated to this function. In a multilocation organization, a corporate infection control practitioner may support individuals in the field who manage local infection control issues as part of another role. This model may promote efficient use of internal resources by designating one individual to maintain knowledge of current infection control issues and share that information and knowledge with others. Specific responsibilities for an infection control practitioner in home care are listed in Exhibit 13–1.

Exhibit 13–1 Infection Control Practitioner Responsibilities

- Develop and maintain policies and procedures for infection control
- Review patient care policies and procedures for infection control content
- Develop and maintain policies and procedures for occupational health related to infection control
- Identify and maintain infection control resources (books, articles, etc.)
- Serve as an organizational resource for infection control practice
- Perform surveillance of home care-acquired infections
- Aggregate, report, and analyze surveillance data
- Facilitate infection control education (orientation and continuing)
- Assist in identifying risk reduction projects for infection control

PREPARATION AND RESOURCES FOR INFECTION CONTROL

If a single individual is designated to manage the infection control function on a daily basis at either a corporate or local level, that individual should be provided specific training and resources. Basic training for infection control can be obtained through many sources; a list of basic training courses is provided in Appendix 13–A. Although these courses are designed for acute care settings, they provide the principles and content needed for infection control activities to be performed in any setting, including home care. Membership in the Association for Professionals in Infection Control and Epidemiology, Inc. (APIC) will also benefit the individual designated to manage infection control. Attendance at local APIC chapter meetings will provide a network for support and information. APIC has a special membership section for home care. Information about contacting APIC is provided in Appendix 13–A. Reference texts and periodicals are also necessary resources for infection control. Again, most resources focus on infection control in the hospital setting. Various resources, including textbooks, periodicals, and software, are provided in Appendix 13–B.

Although information and data related to infection control in home care are currently scant, there is no doubt that resources will expand as this segment of health care grows. With a greater volume of patients receiving home care who are more acutely ill and have increasing needs for skilled nursing care and rehabilitation, the discipline of infection control in home care will grow.

INFECTION CONTROL PLANNING

Just as a home care organization plans for the services it will provide, it should devote a degree of planning to infection control to ensure a comprehensive and appropriate approach. There is no requirement by the Joint Commission for a written infection control plan (Joint Commission, 1999), but during an accreditation survey an organization must demonstrate that the approach to infection control is thoughtful and comprehensive.

The infection control program should include policies and procedures for patient care activities (Exhibit 13–2), a plan for occupational health and safety (Exhibit 13–3), and a plan for surveillance of home care-acquired infections (see Chapter 10). Hospital-based home care organizations should be cautious about adopting the hospital's infection control policies and procedures "as is." Many require specific adaptation before they can be used in the home care setting. This includes patient care policies and procedures (e.g., use of precautions) as well as definitions and methods for surveillance.

All the infection control activities must be coordinated within the organization. Staff members must be aware of their responsibility for infection control, and the leaders must be kept informed of infection control activities and data on an ongoing basis. How this goal is accomplished within an organization may vary. The Joint Commission has no prescribed or required approach, but during an accreditation survey the surveyor would expect to see some evidence of communication and coordination. Inservice outlines and records of attendance can assist in demonstrating communication and education to staff members. Minutes and other written documents of communication are not required but can assist in demonstrating the participation of the management and leadership within the organization.

In addition to supporting and facilitating the coordination of infection control, the organization's leadership is expected by the Joint Commission to identify specific infection risks in patients and staff and to organize and support risk reduction activities. Patient risk can be identified through surveillance activities. For example, if there is an opportunity to reduce the risk of catheter-related bloodstream infection in patients receiving home infusion therapy, documentation of these risk reduction efforts and the role of leadership is important. Refer to Chapter 10 for additional information about conducting surveillance activities in home care.

In employee health and safety, an organization may track needlesticks and sharps exposures and determine that efforts to reduce these occurrences are appropriate. The selection of risk reduction projects, specific strategies and efforts, and the follow-up data should be documented and made available for an accreditation survey.

Exhibit 13–2 Patient Care Practices, Policies, and Procedures

Handwashing
Use of personal protective equipment
Handling and transport of medical waste and laboratory specimens
Cleaning, disinfection, or sterilization of medical equipment and supplies
Exposure control plan for bloodborne pathogens
Airborne respiratory protection plan (tuberculosis control)
Isolation precautions
Follow-up procedures after occupational exposures
Work restrictions for staff with potentially infectious diseases
Surveillance and reporting of home care-acquired infections and occupational incidents

Source: Friedman, M. (1996) Designing an Infection Control Program to Meet JCAHO's Standards. *CARING* 15, 18–25. Used with permission.

Exhibit 13–3 Occupational Health Policies and Procedures

- Initial assessment and health history
- Immunity and/or vaccines required
- Annual testing (e.g., TB skin testing)
- Identification of occupational exposures and follow-up
- Exclusions from patient care activities
- Surveillance of occupational health risks

TRAINING AND EDUCATION OF STAFF

Home care staff members must be introduced to these responsibilities during orientation and subsequently receive continuing education. Content for orientation to infection control must include the use of standard precautions and the overall exposure control plan as well as the other organizational policies and procedures for infection control. Exhibit 13–4 provides a sample outline for orientation to infection control. The orientation content will depend on the role of the home care staff member and will differ for paraprofessional staff (e.g., home health aides, homemakers, sitters, and companions) and professional staff.

Ongoing education related to infection control must include an annual inservice on the exposure control plan as required by the Occupational Safety and Health Administration. A sample outline is given in Exhibit 13–5. Additional topics to support the staff in their infection control efforts should also be included. Some criteria for consideration as educational topics are listed in Exhibit 13–6.

Providing inservice education to home care staff is logistically challenging. Innovative approaches such as conference calls, audio and videotapes that can be taken home, and computer-based approaches can be considered. If there is a particular publication related to

Exhibit 13–4 Infection Control Orientation Content

Role of infection control in home care
- Patient care
- Occupational health

Patient care practices
- Handwashing
- Use of proper technique
- Standard precautions
- Transmission-based precautions

Handling inanimate objects
- Cleaning and disinfection
- Waste handling
- Laboratory specimens

Role in surveillance
- Identification of any home care-acquired infections
- Risk-reduction efforts

Occupational health
- Employee safety
- Reporting exposures

Tuberculosis control plan
- Skin testing
- Use of protective equipment
- Reporting of exposures
- Follow-up of exposures

Exhibit 13–5 Sample Outline: Annual Education for Bloodborne Pathogens

Exposure control plan
- Brief review and how to obtain a copy

Tasks that may lead to exposure

Definition of an exposure

Use of engineering controls, personal protective equipment
- Types and provision of personal protective equipment
- Selection of personal protective equipment
- Use, decontamination, and disposal of personal protective equipment
- Limitations of personal protective equipment

Hepatitis B vaccine
- Benefits, efficacy, safety
- Method of administration
- Availability and testing

Handling emergencies with risk of exposure

Exposure incidents
- Reporting and evaluation
- Medical follow-up and testing
- Postexposure prophylaxis

Questions and answers*

*A knowledgeable individual must be available to answer questions, even when a video is used.

Source: Adapted from OSHA Model Exposure Control Plan.

Exhibit 13–6 Criteria for Selecting Infection Control Continuing Education Topics

- Newly implemented policies and procedures with infection control implications
- Newly offered patient services with infection control implications
- Newly introduced patient care equipment
- Report of surveillance findings
- Report of risk reduction activities
- Newly implemented occupational health policies and procedures
- Report of community-based infection risks (e.g., tuberculosis data, human immunodeficiency virus data)
- Report of newly implemented infection prevention strategies
- Review of clinical topics (e.g., multidrug-resistant microorganisms, wound care)
- Case discussion (review of a specific patient with a home care-acquired infection)

infection control in home care that can be shared among the staff, this should also be incorporated into infection control education.

ACCREDITATION SURVEY

If a home care organization has thoughtfully considered the infection control strategies, policies, and procedures that need to be in place to provide patient care and to address occupational health issues, its preparation for an accreditation survey should be minimal. Staff members who provide direct patient care should be aware of the policies and procedures and be able to demonstrate compliance during the survey. For example, if the procedure for wound care requires that gloves be changed after the removal of the wound dressing, home care staff members must follow the organization's procedure if observed providing wound care. Handwashing should also be accomplished according to policy and procedures. Staff should be knowledgeable about their role and responsibility in surveillance and reporting of potential infections in patients. They should also know which specific exposures or illnesses that they may experience (occupational and nonoccupational) should be reported to the home care organization as well as how to report them. A Joint Commission surveyor may ask them about this. Their response should be consistent with the organization's policies. Knowledge and compliance with the organization's policies and procedures extends to contracted personnel as well.

BEYOND PLANNING

As the application of infection control principles and practices in home care continues to develop and evolve, each home care organization should continuously examine its own approaches and strategies, track and trend its own experience, and identify new information and data that should be considered. Review of current policies and procedures and response to external data and recommendations are important to maintain an infection control program that provides optimal benefit to patients and staff.

Quality improvement, performance measurement, and infection surveillance should not simply include collecting data and reporting them. Results of surveillance and other performance measures must be examined, analyzed, tracked, and trended, and evidence must be available that there has been some conclusion as to how the risks related to adverse outcomes and complications can be reduced.

REFERENCES

Friedman, M. (1996, July). Designing an infection control program to meet JCAHO Standards. *Caring, 15,* 18–25.

Joint Commission on Accreditation of Healthcare Organizations. (1998). *Comprehensive accreditation manual for home care.* Oakbrook Terrace, IL: Author.

Rhinehart, E., & Weller, P. (1998, October). Admission and termination policies: Minimizing risk and liability. *Caring, 17,* 32–35.

APPENDIX 13–A

Infection Control Training Programs

Association for Professionals in Infection Control and Epidemiology, Inc.
APIC Basic Training Course
1275 K Street NW, Suite 1000
Washington, DC 20005-4006
Tel: (202) 789-1890
Fax: (202) 789-1899
http://www.apic.org

Society for Healthcare Epidemiology of America (SHEA)
Epidemiology Course
SHEA Meetings Department
875 Kings Highway
Suite 200
Woodbury, NJ 08096-3172
Tel: (609) 845-1720
Fax: (609) 853-0411

Certification Board of Infection Control and Epidemiology, Inc.
4700 W. Lake Avenue
Glenview, IL 60025-1485
Tel: (847) 375-4732
Fax: (847) 375-4777
http://www.cbic.org

Infection Control Theory and Practice
Winthrop University Hospital
Mineola, NY
Barbara Yannelli, RN, Director
Tel: (516) 663-2724
Fax: (516) 663-2753

Basic Infection Control Course
Hartford Hospital
Hartford, CT
Brian Cooper, MD, Director
Tel: (860) 545-2056
Fax: (860) 545-2878

Program for New Infection Control Professionals
California APIC Coordinating Council
Harriett Pitt, MS, RN, CIC, Director
Tel: (562) 933-0389
Fax: (562) 981-1411

Extension Training Program for Infection Control Practitioners
University of Iowa College of Medicine
Elyse Miller, Director
Tel: (319) 356-2981

APPENDIX 13–B

Journals and Books for Infection Control

American Journal of Infection Control (official publication)
Infection Control and Applied Epidemiology, R. Olmstead, Ed.
Association for Professionals in Infection Control and Epidemiology, Inc.
1275 K Street NW, Suite 1000
Washington, DC 20005-4006
Tel: (202) 789-1890
Fax: (202) 789-1899

Infection Control and Hospital Epidemiology (official publication)
Society for Healthcare Epidemiology of America
Slack, Inc.
6900 Grove Road
Thorofare, NJ 08086-5991
Tel: (609) 848-1000
Fax: (609) 853-5991

The Red Book: Report of the Committee on Infectious Diseases
American Academy of Pediatrics, Committee on Infectious Diseases
141 N. River Rd.
Elk Grove, IL 60009-0927
Tel: (708) 228-5005
Fax: (708) 228-5097

Control of Communicable Diseases in Man, A.S. Benenson, Ed.
American Public Health Association
1015 15th St., NW
Washington, DC 20005
Tel: (202) 789-5600
Fax: (202) 789-5681

Hospital Infections (4th ed.), J. Bennett and P. Brachman
Hospital Epidemiology and Infection Control, C. Glen Mayhall, Ed.
Prevention and Control of Nosocomial Infections (3rd ed.), Richard P. Wenzel, Ed.
Lippincott Williams & Wilkins
227 East Washington Square
Philadelphia, PA 19106
Tel: 1-800-638-3030

Saunders Infection Control Reference Service, E. Abrutyn, D. Goldmann, W. Scheckler, Eds.
W.B. Saunders Company
The Curtis Center
Independence Square West
Philadelphia, PA 19106
Tel: 1-800-545-2522

Software:
EpiInfo
USD, Inc.
2075 A West Park Place
Stone Mountain, GA 30081
Tel: (404) 469-4098

APPENDIX A

Model Exposure Control Plan for Home Care: A Guide for Hospice/Home Agencies on the Bloodborne Pathogens Standards

U.S. Department of Labor
Robert B. Reich, Secretary
Occupational Safety and Health Administration
Joseph A. Dear, Assistant Secretary
Office of Occupational Nursing 1994

INTRODUCTION

The Model Exposure Control Plan for Home Care is intended to serve as an employer guide to the OSHA standard, "Occupational Exposure to Bloodborne Pathogens." Home health agencies have unique issues in protecting their workers from exposure. A central component of your effort will be the development of an exposure control plan (ECP).

Acquired immunodeficiency syndrome (AIDS) and hepatitis B are diseases that warrant serious concerns for workers occupationally exposed to blood and certain other body fluids that have been shown to transmit bloodborne pathogens. It is estimated that more than 5.6 million workers in health care and public safety occupations are potentially exposed. In recognition of these potential hazards, the Occupational Safety and Health Administration (OSHA) promulgated a standard to help protect workers from these health hazards: Title 29 *Code of Federal Regulations* 1910.1030, "Occupational Exposure to Bloodborne Pathogens," published December 6, 1991.

The major intent of this standard is to prevent the transmission of bloodborne diseases due to occupational exposure. The standard is expected to reduce and prevent employee exposure to the hepatitis B virus (HBV), the human immunodeficiency virus (HIV—the virus that causes AIDS), and other bloodborne pathogens. OSHA estimates the standard could prevent approximately 200 deaths and 9,000 infections per year from HBV alone. The standard requires that employers follow universal precautions, which means that all blood and other potentially infectious materials (OPIM) must be treated as though they are infected with HIV and HBV. Each employer must determine whether the standard applies by performing an occupational exposure determination. If occupational exposure, as defined by the standard, is present, the standard mandates a number of requirements. One of the major requirements is the development of an exposure control plan (ECP), which details the company's method of implementing engineering controls, work practices, personal protective equipment, housekeeping, HB vaccinations, and training. The standard also mandates practices and procedures for post-exposure follow-up and recordkeeping.

Employers who have additional questions concerning this standard may contact the nearest OSHA Area Office. Employers who desire a free on-site consultation visit may contact the appropriate State Consultation Project. A directory is listed in Appendix A–3.

The information contained in this publication is not considered a substitute for the Occupational Safety and Health Act of 1970 or any provisions of OSHA standards. It provides general guidance on a particular standards-related topic but should not be considered as the legal authority for compliance with OSHA requirements. The reader should consult the OSHA standard in its entirety for specific compliance requirements.

Unless otherwise noted, in this Model Exposure Control Plan, the term "employer" refers to an agency that sends health care workers into patients' private homes.

Acknowledgement

This document was developed by Alice Lind, Nurse Intern in the Office of Occupational Health Nursing, Di-

Source: Reprinted from *Mordibity and Mortality Weekly*, Centers for Disease Control and Prevention, National Institute of Occupational Safety and Health, 1998.

rectorate of Technical Support with guidance from the Office of Health Compliance Assistance, Directorate of Compliance Programs. The format is based upon the "Employer Guide and Model Exposure Control Plan" developed by the New York State Department of Labor.

USING THIS DOCUMENT

Generally, home health agencies are required to comply with the bloodborne pathogens standard. However, OSHA will not hold home health employers responsible for complying with certain site-specific provisions of the standard. These include activities that take place in clients' homes and are therefore difficult to monitor. This relaxation of the standard's requirements is due to a decision of the United States Circuit Court of Appeals for the Seventh Circuit, which generally upheld the standard but, among other things, vacated it with respect to conditions at sites not controlled by home health agencies [*American Dental Association* v. *Martin,* 984 F. 2d 823, 829-31 (7th Cir. 1993), *cert. denied* 62 U.S.L.W. 3233 (U.S. Oct. 4, 1993) (No. 93-7)].

The Exposure Control Plan should include the following elements:

- Determination of employee exposure
- Methods of exposure control, including:
  - Universal precautions
  - Engineering and work practice controls
  - Personal protective equipment
  - Housekeeping
- Hepatitis B vaccine
- Post-exposure evaluation and follow-up
- Communication of hazards to employees
- Recordkeeping
- Procedures for evaluating circumstances surrounding an exposure incident

Before proceeding with this document, read the bloodborne pathogens standard, in Appendix A–2. After you have familiarized yourself with the standard, follow the model control plan in the order in which it is presented, adding information specific to your worksite wherever indicated. You will note that in several places within the model plan, it will be necessary for you to exercise judgment as to how you will proceed. Where new terms are used, the "Definitions" section of the standard will be helpful.

The Model Exposure Control Plan for Home Care also contains, in Appendix A–1, forms that may be used to comply with recordkeeping requirements of the standard. A resource list is provided in Appendix A–4 to assist employers with the training provisions of the standard.

Contents

POLICY

The (Company Name) is committed to providing a safe and healthful work environment for our entire staff. In pursuit of this endeavor, the following exposure control plan (ECP) is provided to eliminate or minimize occupational exposure to bloodborne pathogens in accordance with OSHA standard 29 CFR 1910.1030, "Occupational Exposure to Bloodborne Pathogens."

The ECP is a key document to assist our firm in implementing and ensuring compliance with the standard, thereby protecting our employees. This ECP includes:

- Determination of employee exposure
- Implementation of various methods of exposure control, including:
  - Universal precautions
  - Engineering and work practice controls
  - Personal protective equipment
  - Housekeeping
- Hepatitis B vaccination
- Post-exposure evaluation and follow-up
- Communication of hazards to employees
- Recordkeeping
- Procedures for evaluating circumstances surrounding an exposure incident

The methods of implementation of these elements of the standard are discussed in the subsequent pages of this ECP.

PROGRAM ADMINISTRATION

- ____________ is (are) responsible for the implementation of the ECP. ____________will maintain, review, and update the ECP at least annually, and whenever necessary to include new or modified tasks and procedures. Contact location/phone number: ________________________
- Those employees who are determined to have occupational exposure to blood or other potentially infectious materials (OPIM) must comply with the procedures and work practices outlined in this ECP.
- __________________ will maintain and provide all necessary personal protective equipment (PPE), engineering controls (e.g., sharps containers), labels, and labelled or red bags as required by the standard. _____________ will ensure that adequate supplies of the aforementioned equipment are available in the appropriate sizes. Contact location/phone number: _____________________
- ________________will be responsible for ensuring that all medical actions required are performed and that appropriate medical records are maintained. Contact location/phone number:______________
- __________________ will be responsible for training, documentation of training, and making the written ECP available to employees, OSHA, and NIOSH representatives. Contact location/phone number: ______________

Notes to Employer

The names or job titles of the program administrators should be used to ensure that authority and responsibility have been designated. In a small business, the responsibilities for the program may be held by one individual. In this case, these duties can be combined.

"Other potentially infectious materials" (OPIM) means (1) The following human body fluids: semen, vaginal secretions, cerebrospinal fluid, synovial fluid, pleural fluid, pericardial fluid, peritoneal fluid, amniotic fluid, saliva in dental procedures, any body fluid that is visibly contaminated with blood, and all body fluids in situations where it is difficult or impossible to differentiate between body fluids; (2) Any unfixed tissue or organ (other than intact skin) from a human (living or dead); and (3) HIV-containing cell or tissue cultures, organ cultures, and HIV- or HBV-containing culture medium or other solutions; and blood, organs, or other tissues from experimental animals infected with HIV or HBV.

EMPLOYEE EXPOSURE DETERMINATION

I. Employee Exposure Determination

A. As part of the exposure determination section of our ECP, the following is a list of all job classifications at our establishment in which all employees have occupational exposure:

JOB TITLE	*DEPARTMENT/LOCATION*

B. The following is a list of job classifications in which some employees at our establishment have occupational exposure. Included is a list of tasks and procedures, or groups of closely related tasks and procedures, in which occupational exposure may occur for these individuals:

JOB TITLE	*DEPARTMENT/LOCATION*	*TASK PROCEDURE*

All exposure determinations were made without regard to the use of PPE.

Notes to Employer

You are not necessarily required to complete both sections A and B; you may complete only the section(s) that apply. Registered and licensed practical/vocational nurses, home health aides, and personal care providers generally fall into category A. Examples of category B would include secretarial or housekeeping staff who handle laboratory specimens or contaminated waste (e.g., sharps containers) only when they are brought into the agency office from a client's home, or office staff who are expected to clean contaminated durable medical equipment. See paragraph (c)(2) of the standard for Exposure Determination.

"Good Samaritan" acts are unanticipated events that occur when employees who do not have occupational exposure are exposed to blood or OPIM (e.g., assisting a client's child with a nosebleed). These are not included in the scope of the bloodborne pathogens standard. OSHA, however, encourages employers to offer post-exposure evaluation and follow-up in such cases.

METHODS OF IMPLEMENTATION AND CONTROL

II. Methods of Implementation and Control

A. Universal Precautions

All employees will utilize universal precautions. Universal precautions is an infection control method which requires employees to assume that all human blood and specified human body fluids (OPIM) are infectious for HIV, HBV, HCV, and other bloodborne pathogens, and must be handled accordingly.

B. Exposure Control Plan

1. Employees covered by the bloodborne pathogens standard will receive an explanation of this ECP during their initial training session. It will also be reviewed in their annual refresher training. All employees will have an opportunity to review this plan at any time during their work shifts by contacting ______________________. A copy of the plan will be made available free of charge and within 15 days of the request.

2. ______________________will be responsible for reviewing and updating the ECP annually or more frequently if necessary to reflect any new or modified tasks and procedures which affect occupational exposure and to reflect new or revised employee positions with occupational exposure.

C. Engineering Controls and Work Practices

1. Engineering controls and work practice controls will be used to prevent or minimize exposure to bloodborne pathogens. The specific engineering controls and work practice controls which we will use, and where they will be used, are listed below:
    - ______________________________________
    - ______________________________________
    - ______________________________________
    - ______________________________________

2. Sharps containers in the office will be inspected and maintained or replaced by _____________ every _________________ or whenever necessary to prevent overfilling.

3. New technology for safer needles and sharps will be evaluated and implemented whenever possible to further prevent needle-sticks and cuts. Our engineering controls will be evaluated by: ___________________.

Notes to Employer

State the person responsible for examining the effectiveness of the engineering controls used and a defined schedule for this review.

Examples of engineering controls include sharps containers, self-sheathing needles, and mechanical needle recapping devices. Needleless systems or recessed needle systems should replace exposed hypodermic needles in intravenous lines. The FDA Safety Alert (April 16, 1992) states that "devices with the following characteristics have the potential to reduce the risk of needlestick injuries:

- A fixed safety feature to provide a barrier between the hands and the needle after use; the safety feature should allow or require the worker's hands to remain behind the needle at all times.
- The safety feature as an integral part of the device, and not an accessory.
- The safety feature in effect before disassembly and remaining in effect after disposal, to protect users and trash handlers, and for environmental safety.
- The safety feature as simple as possible, and requiring little or no training to use effectively."

The Exposure Control Plan must address the disposal of sharps and sharps containers.

Due to the court of appeals decision, home health employers will not be held responsible by OSHA for ensuring that employees use proper work practice controls off of the employer's premises. However, employees must receive training in the work practice controls found in paragraph (d)(2) of the standard which include, but are not limited to, the following:

- Washing hands immediately or as soon as feasible after glove removal
- Using interim hand washing measures at sites which lack hand-washing facilities, such as antiseptic hand cleansers or towelettes

- Washing body parts as soon as possible after skin contact with blood or OPIM
- Prohibiting the recapping, bending, or breaking of contaminated needles
- Performing all procedures involving blood or OPIM in such a manner as to minimize splashing, splattering, and generation of droplets
- Placing specimens of blood or OPIM in a container which prevents leakage and is appropriately labeled for transport
- Examining equipment which may become contaminated with blood or OPIM in the client's home, and decontaminating such equipment as necessary; bagging and/or labeling such items for safe removal if not completely decontaminated (The purpose of decontamination of equipment in the home is to prevent exposure of the worker during transport or use of the equipment, as well as to prevent the exposure of other workers when the equipment is returned to the office.)
- Placing contaminated sharps in appropriate containers immediately after use
- Prohibiting eating, drinking, or smoking where there is a likelihood of exposure

---

D. Personal Protective Equipment (PPE)

1. PPE will be provided at no cost to employees. Training will be provided by ______________ in the use of the appropriate PPE for the tasks or procedures employees will perform.
2. The types of PPE available to employees are as follows:

   ____

   ____

3. Refer to written procedures (e.g., the agency's policy and procedure manual) for instructions on the use of PPE for specific tasks which may expose workers to blood or OPIM.
4. PPE is located ______________________ and may be obtained through _____________. (Specify how employees are to obtain PPE, and who is responsible for ensuring that it is available.)
5. All employees using PPE must observe the following precautions:
   - Wash hands immediately or as soon as feasible after removal of gloves or other PPE.
   - Remove PPE after it becomes contaminated, and before leaving the work area.
   - Used PPE may be disposed of in the client's home or returned to the office in appropriate containers for storage, laundering, decontamination, or disposal.
   - Wear appropriate gloves when it can be reasonably anticipated that there may be hand contact with blood or OPIM, and when handling or touching contaminated items or surfaces; replace gloves if torn, punctured, contaminated, or if their ability to function as a barrier is compromised.
   - Utility gloves may be decontaminated for reuse if their integrity is not compromised; discard utility gloves if they show signs of cracking, peeling, tearing, puncturing, or deterioration.
   - Never wash or decontaminate disposable gloves for reuse.
   - Wear appropriate face and eye protection when splashes, sprays, spatters, or droplets of blood or OPIM pose a hazard to the eye, nose, or mouth.
   - Remove immediately or as soon as feasible any garment contaminated by blood or OPIM, in such a way as to avoid contact with the outer surface.
6. The procedure for handling contaminated PPE is as follows: (may refer to specific agency procedure by title or number and last date of review)

   ____

   ____

   (For example, how and where to decontaminate face shields, eye protection, resuscitation equipment)

Notes to Employer

It is imperative that employees be provided with appropriate protection when occupational exposure is anticipated. PPE is considered "appropriate" only if it does not permit blood or OPIM to pass through or reach the employee's clothes, skin, eyes, mouth, or other mucous membranes. The type and characteristics of PPE will depend upon the task and degree of exposure anticipated. For example:

- Gloves are used when employees have contact with blood, OPIM, non-intact skin, and mucous membranes, e.g., dressing changes, bathing client with broken skin, or phlebotomy. Hypoallergenic gloves, glove liners, powderless gloves, or other similar alternatives must be provided for employees who are allergic to the gloves that are normally provided.
- Masks and eye protection are used when blood or OPIM may be splashed or sprayed, e.g., suctioning, oral care, tracheostomy care.
- Protective clothing is worn to protect against contamination of the employee's personal clothing with blood or OPIM, e.g., central venous line insertion.

Employees covered by the standard who make visits to clients in their homes must be provided with appropriate PPE. For employees who have occupational exposure, gloves, gowns or aprons, and disinfectant towelettes or antiseptic hand cleanser for hand washing in the absence of running water must be provided. Employees who perform invasive procedures must additionally be provided with face masks and eye protection. Employees using disposable sharps will be provided with portable sharps disposal containers. Employees who are expected to perform CPR as a function of their job must be provided with resuscitation bags or mouthpieces.

Due to the court of appeals decision, home health employers will not be held responsible for violating those provisions of paragraph (d) (3) in the bloodborne pathogens standard which require that the employer ensure that the PPE is actually used, or that employees wear PPE.

E. Housekeeping

1. The procedure for handling sharps containers is: (may refer to specific agency procedure by title or number and last date of review)

   ____

   ____

   ____

2. The procedure for handling other regulated waste is: (may refer to specific agency procedure by title or number and last date of review)

   ____

   ____

   ____

3. Contaminated sharps shall be discarded immediately or as soon as possible in containers that are closable, puncture-resistant, leakproof on sides and bottoms, and labeled or color-coded appropriately.
4. Sharps containers shall be easily accessible and as close as feasible to the immediate area where sharps are used, i.e., the nurse should bring the container into the client's home if sharps will be used during the visit.
5. Bins and pails (e.g., wash or emesis basins) must be cleaned and decontaminated as soon as feasible after visible contamination.
6. Broken glassware which may be contaminated must be picked up using mechanical means, such as a brush and dust pan.

Notes to Employer

Due to the court of appeals decision, employers will not be held responsible by OSHA for site-specific violations of the bloodborne pathogens standard regarding housekeeping requirements and the handling and disposal of regulated waste which occur outside the employer's premises. However, employees must be trained in the proper procedures.

Many questions have arisen about the proper handling and disposal of regulated waste in the home care setting. To assess whether the material in question meets the definition of regulated waste, see paragraph (b) of the standard (page 210 of this document). Regulated waste is defined very specifically for the purposes of this standard, and the employer should become familiar with the definition.

The procedures for the handling and disposal of regulated waste are set forth in paragraph (d) (4) (iii) of the bloodborne pathogens standard. Agency procedures must incorporate the following: Regulated waste shall be placed in containers which are closable, constructed to contain all contents and prevent leakage, appropriately labeled or color-coded (see Labels), and closed prior to removal to prevent spillage or protrusion of contents during handling. These criteria also apply to the secondary container, which must be used if the primary container is contaminated or if leakage is possible.

The disposal of regulated waste must be "in accordance with applicable regulations of the United States, States and Territories, and political subdivisions of States and Territories" [29 CFR 1910.1030 (d) (4) (iii) (C)]. Each home health agency should direct queries to the county and state agencies (e.g., public health department, transportation department, and/or environmental protection agency) for approval of procedures on disposal and transportation of regulated waste.

Procedures allowed under paragraph (d)(4) (iii) of the bloodborne pathogens standard include:

- Sharps containers may be left in the client's home between visits, and removed by employees before they overfill. Employees may need to carry an empty sharps container on all visits to prevent overfilling of the container.
- The container may be placed in a second container or bag for transportation in an employee's or company vehicle, if this is allowed by local regulation.
- Small, magnetized containers may replace the need for large plastic sharps containers.
- The home health agency may designate one employee to remove containers and return them to the office. Alternatively, the container may be removed by a company which is specifically licensed to transport and/or dispose of regulated waste.
- In some areas, sharps disposal is handled for the client by the pharmacy which supplies their syringes. In others, hospitals have agreements with home health agencies and/or their clients to accept properly contained regulated waste.
- Containers must be appropriately labeled or color-coded; see section G.
- The specific procedure should be spelled out or referred to in the ECP.

F. Laundry

1. The following contaminated articles will be laundered by this company:

   ______________________________ ______________________________

2. Laundering will be performed by ________________ at (time and/or location).
3. The following laundering requirements must be met:
   - handle contaminated laundry as little as possible, with minimal agitation
   - place wet contaminated laundry in leak-proof, labeled or color-coded containers before transporting
   - use *(red bags or bags marked with biohazard symbol)* if the facility where items are laundered does not use universal precautions
   - wear appropriate PPE when handling and/or sorting contaminated laundry

- normal laundry cycles should be used according to the washer and detergent manufacturer's recommendations, as per CDC "Guidelines for Prevention of Transmission of HIV and HBV," MMWR 6/23/89 *38*, No. S-6.

Notes to Employer

Contaminated laundry is defined as laundry which has been soiled with blood or other potentially infectious material, or may contain sharps. OSHA prohibits home laundering of PPE by the employee. Disposable PPE can be used to eliminate or greatly reduce the need for laundering.

Procedures for handling contaminated laundry allowed under paragraph (d) (4) (iv) of the standard and subsequent interpretations are as follows:

- Contaminated laundry and/or PPE may be laundered in the client's home.
- Alternatively, it may be removed for laundering to the agency office or a commercial laundromat, provided that the worker is not exposed to blood or OPIM in the process.
- Appropriate bagging to prevent contamination of the vehicle used for transportation is needed.
- Laundering of contaminated clothing or linen in the worker's home or on unpaid time are not allowed under the provisions of the standard.

Due to the court of appeals decision, home health employers will not be held responsible by OSHA for violations of the laundry provisions occurring outside the employer's premises.

G. Labels

1. The following labeling method(s) will be used:

EQUIPMENT TO BE LABELED	*LABEL TYPE* (size, color, etc.)
____________________	____________________
(e.g., specimens, contaminated laundry, etc.)	____________________

2. ______________ will ensure warning labels are affixed or red bags are used as required if regulated waste or contaminated equipment is brought into the office. Employees are to notify ____________ if they discover regulated waste containers, refrigerators containing blood or OPIM, contaminated equipment, etc. without proper labels.

Notes to Employer

Red bags or red containers may be substituted for warning labels. Labels or red bags must be used for contaminated laundry, containers of regulated waste, refrigerators containing blood or other potentially infectious material, and other containers used to store, transport, or ship blood or OPIM. Exemptions are listed under paragraph g(1)(i)(E, F, and G).

The BIOHAZARD symbol is the required legend for labels in this section. See the bloodborne pathogens standard, section g, "Communication of Hazards to Employees" (page 217 of this document), for the legend and specific language about labeling requirements.

Due to the court of appeals decision, home health employers will not be held responsible for violations of labeling and color-coding requirements occurring outside the employer's premises.

HEPATITIS B VACCINATION

III. Hepatitis B Vaccination

A. ______________________ will provide training to employees on hepatitis B vaccinations, addressing the safety, benefits, efficacy, methods of administration, and availability. The hepatitis B vaccination series will be made available at no cost after training and within 10 days of initial assignment to employees who have occupational exposure to blood or OPIM *unless:* 1) documentation exists that the employee has previously received the series, 2) antibody testing reveals that the employee is immune, or 3) medical evaluation shows that vaccination is contraindicated.

B. All employees are strongly encouraged to receive the hepatitis B vaccination series. However, if an employee chooses to decline vaccination, the employee must sign a declination form. Employees who decline may request and obtain the vaccination at a later date at no cost. Documentation of refusal of the vaccination will be kept in _______________ with the employee's other medical records.

C. Vaccination will be provided by ________(name and title)________ at ________(location)________.

D. For hepatitis B vaccinations, the health care professional's written opinion will be limited to whether the employee requires the hepatitis vaccine, and whether the vaccine was administered. (See page 198 for sample form.)

Notes to Employer

The exact language for the declination statement can be found in Exhibit 1 of the bloodborne pathogens standard. (See page 220 of this document.) Employees must sign a statement when declining the vaccination.

Participation in pre-screening must not be a prerequisite for receiving the vaccine.
Employees must not be required to waive liability in order to receive the vaccine.
Hepatitis B vaccine is to be provided even if an employee declines but later requests it.
Vaccine is to be given in accordance with U.S. Public Health Service recommendations.
Booster doses must be made available to employees if recommended in the future by USPHS.

A copy of the health care professional's written opinion, stating whether hepatitis B vaccine is indicated and/or has been received, must be provided to the employee within 15 working days. (Page 198, or alternate form, should be returned to the employee after the first dose of the vaccine, and updated after the third dose.)

If the schedule of vaccinations has been interrupted, the entire course does *not* need to be restarted. According to current U.S. Public Health Service recommendations, vaccine doses administered at longer intervals (than the recommended schedule) provide equally satisfactory protection, but optimal protection is not conferred until after the third dose. If the vaccine series is interrupted after the first dose, the second and third doses should be given separated by an interval of 3–5 months. Persons who are late for the third dose should be given this dose when convenient. Post-vaccination testing is not considered necessary in either situation. These recommendations may be updated by the USPHS; call 404-332-4555 for current information. Reasonable effort should be made to vaccinate the employee on schedule, unless the employee declines vaccination.

POST-EXPOSURE EVALUATION AND FOLLOW-UP

IV. Post-Exposure Evaluation and Follow-up

A. Should an exposure incident occur, contact ______________________ immediately at the following number: ______________________.

B. An immediately available confidential medical evaluation and follow-up will be conducted by (health care professional)____________. The following elements will be performed:

- Document the routes of exposure and how the exposure occurred.
- Identify and document the source individual (unless the employer can establish that identification is infeasible or prohibited by state or local law).
- Obtain consent and make arrangements to have the source individual tested as soon as possible to determine HIV and HBV infectivity; document that the source individual's test results were conveyed to the employee's health care provider.
- If the source individual is already known to be HIV and/or HBV positive, new testing need not be performed.
- Ensure that the exposed employee is provided with the source individual's test results and with information about applicable disclosure laws and regulations concerning the identity and infectious status of the source individual (e.g., laws protecting confidentiality).
- After obtaining consent, collect exposed employee's blood as soon as feasible after exposure incident, and test blood for HBV and HIV serological status.
- If the employee does not give consent for HIV serological testing during collection of blood for baseline testing, preserve the baseline blood sample for at least 90 days; if the exposed employee elects to have the baseline sample tested during this waiting period, perform testing as soon as feasible.

Notes to Employer

An exposure incident is defined in the standard as "a specific eye, mouth, other mucous membrane, non-intact skin, or parenteral contact with blood or other potentially infectious materials that results from the performance of an employee's duties." Employees may document each exposure on a form such as that provided on page 203 of this document, EPINet Universal Blood and Body Fluid Exposure Report, and on the OSHA No. 200 log, if appropriate.

If consent is not obtained from the source individual, the employer must show that the required consent could not be obtained. Where consent is not required by law, the source individual's blood, if available, shall be tested and the results documented. This must be done whether or not the employee elects baseline testing and follow-up.

Following an exposure incident, prompt evaluation and prophylaxis is imperative. Timeliness is, therefore, an important factor in effective treatment. The American Nurses' Association Position Statement on "Post-Exposure Programs in the Event of Occupational Exposure to HIV/HBV" (September, 1991; cited with permission) includes the following Guidelines for Immediate Treatment:

1. Wound Care/First Aid
   A. Clean wound with soap and water.
   B. Flush mucous membranes with water or normal saline solution.
   C. Other wound care as indicated.
2. Notification of Responsible Parties
   A. Notify supervisor or on-call staff member at the 24-hour hotline number after wound care has been provided.

Procedures for reporting an exposure should be in place which apply to any and all working hours. Following immediate wound care and supervisor notification, the post-exposure evaluation must be provided as in IV. B., above.

C. Health Care Professional's Follow-Up
   1. ____________ will ensure that health care professionals responsible for employee's hepatitis B vaccination and post-exposure evaluation and follow-up be given a copy of OSHA's bloodborne pathogens standard.

2. _____________ will ensure that the health care professional evaluating an employee after an exposure incident receives the following:
   - a description of the employee's job duties relevant to the exposure incident
   - route(s) of exposure
   - circumstances of exposure
   - if possible, results of the source individual's blood test
   - relevant employee medical records, including vaccination status
3. _____________ will provide the employee with a copy of the evaluating health care professional's written opinion within 15 days after completion of the evaluation. (See page 199 for sample form.)
4. The written opinion for post-exposure evaluation and follow-up will be limited to whether or not the employee has been informed of the results of the health evaluation and of any health conditions which may require further evaluation and treatment.
5. All other diagnoses must remain confidential and are not to be included in the written report to our firm.

Notes to Employer

See pages 199 and 200 for sample forms for post-exposure: Health Care Professional's Written Opinion for Post-Exposure Evaluation, and Bloodborne Pathogen Exposure Evaluation Form.

If the employer is also the health care professional, the employer must ensure that the results of the employee's post-exposure evaluation remain confidential and are not disclosed to his/her co-workers, managers, and supervisors, except to the extent absolutely necessary to comply with the standard or other legal requirements.

Post-exposure counseling is mandatory under the standard. The American Nurses' Association recommendations for exposed health care worker counseling are provided as an example. (From the Position Statement on Post-Exposure Programs, September, 1991.)

- Counseling should be provided by skilled personnel through previously established agency protocol.
- Counseling should include the following: meaning of test results; discussion of personal life factors such as safer sex practices, conception/contraception, and informing sexual partners; discussion regarding avoidance of blood, semen, and tissue donation.
- Counseling should include a validation of the health care workers' concerns and fears, and the implications of disclosure to other persons in their support system.
- The health care worker should be encouraged to monitor for signs/symptoms of acute sero-conversion illness (fevers, myalgias, rash, etc.) and to report these symptoms to designated personnel immediately.
- Information regarding workers' compensation, disability, and other benefits should be provided.

PROCEDURES FOR EVALUATING THE CIRCUMSTANCES SURROUNDING AN EXPOSURE INCIDENT

V. Procedures for Evaluating the Circumstances Surrounding an Exposure Incident

A. _____________ will review the circumstances of all exposure incidents to determine:
   - why the exposure incident occurred;
   - if procedures were being followed; and

- if procedures, protocols, and/or training need to be revised.

B. If it is determined that revisions need to be made, ______________ will ensure that appropriate changes are made to this ECP. (Changes may include an evaluation of needleless systems, adding employees to the exposure determination list, etc.)

C. Documentation of this evaluation should accompany the exposure report.

EMPLOYEE TRAINING

VI. Employee Training

A. All employees who have occupational exposure to bloodborne pathogens will receive training conducted by ______(name & title)______.

B. All employees who have occupational exposure to bloodborne pathogens will receive training on the epidemiology, symptoms, and transmission of bloodborne pathogen diseases. In addition, the training program will cover, at a minimum, the following elements:

- a copy and explanation of the standard
- an explanation of our ECP and how to obtain a copy
- an explanation of methods to recognize tasks and other activities that may involve exposure to blood and OPIM, including what constitutes an exposure incident
- an explanation of the use and limitations of engineering controls, work practices, and PPE
- an explanation of the types, uses, location, removal, handling, decontamination, and disposal of PPE
- an explanation of the basis for PPE selection
- information on the hepatitis B vaccine, including information on its efficacy, safety, method of administration, the benefits of being vaccinated, and that the vaccine will be offered free of charge
- information on the appropriate actions to take and persons to contact in an emergency involving blood or OPIM
- an explanation of the procedure to follow if an exposure incident occurs, including the method of reporting the incident and the medical follow-up that will be made available
- information on the post-exposure evaluation and follow-up that the employer is required to provide for the employee following an exposure incident
- an explanation of the signs and labels and/or color coding required by the standard and used at this facility
- an opportunity for interactive questions and answers with the person conducting the training session

---

Note to Employer

The training materials, such as overheads, workbooks, and handouts may be included in the ECP. Self-study modules, videos, and interactive computer programs may all be used as part of the training program. However, a person knowledgeable in the subject matter and who can accurately answer employee questions must be accessible for interaction during the training session.

C. Training Records

1. Training records will be completed for each employee upon completion of training. These documents will be kept with the employee's records at ________________. (See page 202 for sample form.)
2. Training records will be maintained by ____________________.

3. The training records shall include:
   - the dates of the training sessions
   - the contents or a summary of the training sessions
   - the names and qualifications of persons conducting the training
   - the names and job titles of all persons attending the training sessions
4. Training records will be maintained for a minimum of three (3) years from the date on which the training occurred.
5. Employee training records will be provided upon request to the employee or the employee's authorized representative within 15 working days.

Note to Employer

Training shall be provided:

- at initial assignment to tasks where occupational exposure may take place
- when new exposure is created by a change in tasks or procedures
- at least annually after initial training
- at no cost to the employee, during working hours
- with material appropriate to educational level, literacy, and language of employees
- by a person knowledgeable in the subject matter being presented, as it relates to home care

---

RECORDKEEPING

VII. Medical Records

A. Medical records are maintained for each employee with occupational exposure in accordance with 29 CFR 1910.20, "Access to Employee Exposure and Medical Records."

B. ______________(name & title)______________ is responsible for maintenance of the required medical records. They are kept at ______________________________.

C. In addition to the requirements of 29 CFR 1910.20, the medical record will include:
- the name and social security number of employee
- a copy of the employee's hepatitis B vaccinations and any medical records relative to the employee's ability to receive vaccination
- a copy of all results of examinations, medical testing, and follow-up procedures as required by the bloodborne pathogens standard
- a copy of all health care professional's written opinion(s) as required by the bloodborne pathogens standard

D. All employee medical records will be kept confidential and will not be disclosed or reported without the employee's express written consent to any person within or outside the workplace except as required by the standard or other legal provisions.

E. Employee medical records shall be maintained for at least the duration of employment plus 30 years in accordance with 29 CFR 1910.20.

F. Employee medical records shall be provided upon request of the employee or to anyone having written consent of the employee within 15 working days.

Notes to Employer

The medical records discussed in section VII are similar to "patient records" and enjoy the protection of strict confidentiality. Only the health care professional's written opinions are to be released to the employer.

The medical records of employees who have worked for less than one year for the employer need not be retained beyond the term of the employment if they are provided to the employee upon the termination of employment.

Appendix A–1

Sample Forms

The following pages contain sample forms that may aid your company in compliance with the bloodborne pathogens standard. None of these forms are specifically required by the standard, but it is hoped that your company can benefit from the information.

Sample Forms:

HEALTH CARE PROFESSIONAL'S WRITTEN OPINION FOR HEPATITIS B VACCINATION

Employee Name ______________________________

Date of Office Visit ______________________________

Health Care Facility Address ______________________________

____

Health Care Facility Telephone ______________________________

As required under the bloodborne pathogen standard:

Hepatitis B vaccination is ________ is not ________ recommended for the employee named above.

The employee named above is scheduled to receive the hepatitis B vaccination on the following dates:

First of three ______________________________

Second of three ______________________________

Third of three ______________________________

______________________________ ______________________________

(Signature of Health Care Provider) (Printed or typed name of health care provider)

This form is to be returned to the employer, and a copy provided to the employee, within 15 days.

Employer Name: ______________________________

Title: ______________________________

Address: ______________________________

____

____

HEALTH CARE PROFESSIONAL'S WRITTEN OPINION FOR POST-EXPOSURE EVALUATION

Employee Name ____

Date of Incident ____

Date of Office Visit ____

Health Care Facility Address ____

____

Health Care Facility Telephone ____

As required under the bloodborne pathogen standard:

________ The employee named above has been informed of the results of the post-exposure health evaluation.

________ The employee named above has been told about any health conditions resulting from exposure to blood or other potentially infectious materials which require further evaluation or treatment.

________ Hepatitis B vaccination is _______ is not _______ indicated.

____

(Printed or typed name of health care provider)

____ ____

(Signature of Health Care Provider) (Date)

This form is to be returned to the employer and a copy provided to the employee within 15 days. Please label the outside of the envelope "Confidential."

Employer Name: ____

Title: ____

Address: ____

____

BLOODBORNE PATHOGEN EXPOSURE EVALUATION FORM

(Send with employee at the time a health evaluation is needed. Form to be completed and kept by health care provider only. *Information on this form is confidential.* Do not send this form to employer.)

Employee Name ______________________ Today's Date ______________

Social Security # ______________________ Date of Birth ______________

Home Phone # ____

Job Title ____

Date of exposure ____

(See Exposure Report for circumstances under which exposure incident occurred)

Source of exposure: ____

(Circle response and complete explanation as appropriate)

Yes No Blood of source individual has been tested with consent of individual as applicable. If no, please explain and/or indicate if HIV and/or HBV is already known.

____

____

Yes No Results of source individual's testing conveyed to employee.
(Explain) ____

Yes No Employee informed of applicable laws and regulations concerning disclosure of the identity and infectious status of the source.
(Explain) ____

Yes No Exposed employee's blood collected and tested with obtained consent.
(Explain) ____

Yes No If employee declines HIV testing, blood stored for 90 days from exposed incident.
(Explain) ____

Yes No Post-exposure prophylaxis initiated if medically indicated.
(Explain) ____

Yes No Hepatitis B vaccination is indicated. Elaborate on treatment given: ______________

____

Status of employee vaccination:

One of three: Date __________ Type __________ Lot # __________ Site __________

Administered by: ______________________________

Two of three: Date __________ Type __________ Lot # __________ Site __________

Administered by: ______________________________

Three of three: Date __________ Type __________ Lot # __________ Site __________

Administered by: ______________________________

Yes No Employee informed of results of evaluation.

(Explain) ______________________________

Yes No Employee has been informed of any health conditions resulting from exposure to blood or other potentially infectious materials which require further evaluation or treatment.

(Explain) ______________________________

Assessment/Observations/Plan:

____

____

Action: __________ Confidential post-exposure evaluation entered into employee's individual health record.

__________ Copy of health care professional's written opinion for post-exposure evaluation completed and sent to employer.

__________ Copy of health care professional's written opinion for post-exposure evaluation given to employee.

Note: All other findings shall remain confidential and shall not be included.

EMPLOYEE EDUCATION AND TRAINING RECORD

Employee Name	Job Title

Subject	Date	Trainer Initials
The Standard		
Epidemiology & Symptoms of Bloodborne Diseases		
Modes of Transmission		
Exposure Control Plan		
Recognizing Potential Exposure		
Use & Limitations of Exposure Control Methods		
Personal Protective Equipment (Types, Uses, Disposal, etc.)		
Selection of PPE		
HBV Vaccination Program		
Emergencies Involving Blood or OPIM		
Exposure Follow-up Procedures		
Post-exposure Evaluation & Follow-up		
Signs and Labels		
Opportunity To Ask Questions		
Additional Education: Subjects		

Trainer Name	Initials	Trainer Qualifications

EPINET UNIFORM BLOOD AND BODY FLUID EXPOSURE REPORT

The form found in this appendix was developed by Janine Jagger, Director of the Health Care Worker Safety Project, at the University of Virginia Health Sciences Center. It has been adapted for the first time for use in home health care for incorporation in this Model Exposure Control Plan. Dr. Jagger describes the tool below:

The EPINet (Exposure Prevention Information Network) system consists of:

1. data collection forms to be filled out by employees reporting sharps object injuries or blood and body fluid exposures, and
2. software already programmed for entering data from the report forms, and for accessing and analyzing the data.

"The data entry and analysis program, Epi Info, is a public domain computer program—it can be copied freely—for MS-DOS (IBM) compatible computers developed by the Centers for Disease Control. It is ideal for use with EPINet because it was designed for surveillance programs like this one, and it is easy to use, flexible, and available at nominal cost. The data collection forms, Epi Info, and the EPINet program diskette provide you with a complete surveillance, prevention and evaluation system that can be up and running in the time that it takes you to install the diskettes and photocopy the report forms."

Epi-Info and EPINet can be ordered through USD, Inc. at 404-469-4098. Even agencies who do not utilize computers for tracking employee health and illness may find this tool useful for reporting exposures. You may copy the forms found in this appendix, or request original forms from the Health Care Worker Safety Project, at 804-982-0702.

Please note the box at the bottom right corner of pages 205 and 208, "Is this incident OSHA reportable?" The exposure incident must be recorded on the OSHA No. 200 form, "Log and Summary of Occupational Injuries and Illnesses," if the employee receives medical treatment, or if the incident results in lost workdays, restriction of work or motion, transfer to another job, illness, or death. Each reportable injury or illness must be logged on this form within six working days from the time the employer learns of it. In addition, the OSHA No. 101 form, "Supplementary Record of Occupational Injuries and Illnesses," or an equivalent which contains all the required information, must be completed.

EXPOSURE
PREVENTION
INFORMATION
NETWORK

Uniform Needlestick and Sharp Object Injury Report

Name: ______________________ **Hospital ID:** [ ][ ][ ][ ]

1. ID: [ ][ ][ ][ ] **2. Date of injury:** [ ][ ] month [ ][ ] day [ ][ ] year

3. Job Category: *(check one)*

1	M.D. *(attending/staff)*	10	clinical laboratory worker
2	M.D. *(intern/resident/fellow)*	11	technologist *(non-lab)*
3	medical student	12	dentist
4	nurse RN/LPN	13	dental hygienist
5	nursing student	14	housekeeper/laundry worker
6	respiratory therapist	15	home health aide
7	surgery attendant	16	chore worker/personal care provider
8	other attendant	99	other, describe ______________
9	phlebotomist/venipuncture/I.V. team		

4. Where did the injury occur? *(check one)*

1	patient room *(in hospital)*	9	dialysis facility
2	outside patient room *(hallway, nurses' station, etc.)*	10	procedure room *(X-ray, EMG, etc.)*
3	emergency department	11	clinical laboratories
4	intensive/critical care unit	12	autopsy/pathology
5	operating room	13	service/utility area *(laundry, central supply, loading dock, etc.)*
6	outpatient clinic/office *(incl. home health office)*	14	patient's home *(home health care)*
7	blood bank	15	transport vehicle *(car, ambulance, helicopter, etc.)*
8	venipuncture	99	other, describe ______________

5. Was the source patient known?

[1] yes [2] no [3] unknown [4] not applicable

6. Was the injured worker the original user of the sharp item?

[1] yes [2] no [3] unknown [4] not applicable

7. Was the sharp item: *(check one)*

1	contaminated *(known exposure to patient or contaminated equipment)*
2	uncontaminated *(no known exposure to pt. or contaminated equipment)*
3	unknown

8. For what purpose was the sharp item originally used: *(check one)*

1	unknown/not applicable
2	injection, intramuscular/subcutaneous, or other injection through the skin *(syringe)*
3	heparin or saline flush *(syringe)*
4	other injection into (or aspiration from) I.V. injection site or I.V. port *(syringe)*
5	to connect I.V. line *(intermittent I.V./piggyback/I.V. infusion/other I.V. line connection)*
6	to start I.V. or set up heparin lock *(I.V. catheter or Butterfly™-type needle)*
7	to draw a venous blood sample → if used to draw blood, was it a: [1] direct stick [2] draw from a line
8	to draw an arterial blood sample *(ABG)* → (see item 7)
9	to obtain a body fluid or tissue sample *(urine/CSF/amniotic fluid/other fluid, biopsy)*
10	fingerstick/heel stick
11	suturing
12	cutting *(surgery)*
13	electrocautery
14	to contain a specimen or pharmaceutical *(glass items)*
99	other, describe ______________

9. Did the injury occur: *(check one)*

1	before use of item *(item broke or slipped, assembling device, etc.)*
2	during use of item *(item slipped, patient jarred item, etc.)*
3	between steps of a multistep procedure *(between incremental injections, passing instruments, etc.)*
4	disassembling device or equipment
5	in preparation for reuse of reusable instrument *(sorting, disinfecting, sterilizing, etc.)*
6	while recapping a used needle
7	withdrawing a needle from rubber or other resistant material *(rubber stopper, I.V. port, etc.)*
8	other after use, before disposal *(in transit to trash, cleaning up, left on bed, table, floor, or other inappropriate place, etc.)*
9	from item left on or near disposal container
10	while putting the item into the disposal container
11	after disposal, stuck by item protruding from opening of disposal container
12	item pierced side of disposal container
13	after disposal, item protruded from **trash bag** or **inappropriate** waste container
99	other, describe

10. What device or item caused the injury?

(refer to the list of items and enter the item code number here): [|]

If the item is coded as "other" (29, 59, 79), then please describe the item:

____

11. If the item causing the injury was a needle, was it a "safety design" with a shielded, recessed, or retractable needle?

[1] yes [2] no/not applicable

12. Mark the location of the injury:

Front: 33 39 34 40 32 45 31 46 35 41 30 47 36 42 37 43 38 44

Back: 51 57 52 58 50 63 49 64 53 59 48 65 54 60 55 61 56 62

Right: 1 2 3 4 5 6 7 8 9 10 11 12 13 14

Left: 15 16 17 18 19 20 21 22 23 24 25 26 27 28

13. Was the injury: *(check one)*

1	superficial *(little or no bleeding)*
2	moderate *(skin punctured, some bleeding)*
3	severe *(deep stick/cut, or profuse bleeding)*

14. Describe the circumstances leading to this injury:

____

____

____

____

Costs: for office use only *(round to nearest dollar)*

				laboratory charges for employee and source *(Hb, HIV, other tests)*
				treatment, prophylaxis *(H-BIG, Hb vaccine, tetanus, AZT, other treatments)*
				service charges *(Emergency Department, Employee Health other services)*
				other costs *(Worker's Compensation, surgery, other)*
				total

Is this incident OSHA reportable?

- *Medical treatment (H-BIG, Hepatitis vaccine, gamma globulin, AZT, etc; Not first aid, not tetanus)*
- *Restricted/lost work time: transferred*
- *Illness/death*

[1] yes [2] no

If yes, enter:

days away from work			
days restricted work activity			

EXPOSURE PREVENTION INFORMATION NETWORK

Items Causing Needlestick and Sharp Object Injuries

NEEDLE

(for suture needle see "surgical instruments")

Item Codes

(1) disposable syringe *(includes standard syringes, insulin, tuberculin syringes)*
(2) prefilled cartridge syringe *(includes Tubex™*/Carpuject™*-type syringes)*
(3) blood gas syringe *(ABG)*
(4) syringe, other type or not sure what kind
(5) needle on I.V. line *(includes piggybacks and I.V. line connections)*
(6) winged steel needle I.V. set *(includes Butterfly™*-type devices)*
(7) I.V. catheter *(stylet)*
(8) vacuum tube blood collection holder/needle *(includes VACUTAINER™**-type devices)
(9) spinal or epidural needle
(10) unattached hypodermic needle

(28) needle, not sure what kind
(29) other needle *(please describe device on the report form)*

SURGICAL INSTRUMENT OR OTHER SHARP ITEM

(For glass items see below)

(30) lancet *(finger or heel sticks)*
(31) suture needle
(32) scalpel blade
(33) razor
(34) pipette *(plastic)*
(35) scissors
(36) bovie electrocautery device
(37) bone cutter
(38) bone chip
(39) towel clip
(40) microtome blade
(41) trocar
(42) vacuum tube *(plastic)*
(43) specimen/test tube *(plastic)*
(44) fingernails/teeth

(58) sharp item, not sure what kind
(59) other item *(please describe item on the report form)*

GLASS

(60) medication ampule
(61) medication vial *(small volume with rubber stopper)*
(62) medication/I.V. bottle *(large volume)*
(63) pipette *(glass)*
(64) vacuum tube *(glass)*
(65) specimen/test tube *(glass)*
(66) capillary tube
(78) glass item, not sure what kind
(79) other glass item *(please describe item on the report form)*

* Tubex™ is a trademark of Wyeth Ayerst; Carpuject™ is a trademark of Sanofi Winthrop; Butterfly™ is a trademark of Abbott Laboratories; VACUTAINER™ is a trademark of Becton Dickinson. Identification of these product categories does not imply involvement of these specific brands.

EXPOSURE
PREVENTION
INFORMATION
NETWORK

Uniform Blood and Body Fluid Exposure Report

Name: ______________________ **Hospital ID:** [ ][ ][ ][ ]

1. ID: [ ][ ][ ][ ] **2. Date of injury:** [ ][ ] month [ ][ ] day [ ][ ] year

3. Job Category: *(check one)*

1	M.D. *(attending/staff)*	10	clinical laboratory worker
2	M.D. *(intern/resident/fellow)*	11	technologist *(non-lab)*
3	medical student	12	dentist
4	nurse RN/LPN	13	dental hygienist
5	nursing student	14	housekeeper/laundry worker
6	respiratory therapist	15	home health aide
7	surgery attendant	16	chore worker/personal care provider
8	other attendant	99	other, describe ______
9	phlebotomist/venipuncture/I.V. team.		

4. Where did the exposure occur? *(check one)*

1	patient room	9	dialysis facility
2	outside patient room *(hallway, nurses' station, etc.)*	10	procedure room *(X-ray, EMG, etc.)*
3	emergency department	11	clinical laboratories
4	intensive/critical care unit	12	autopsy/pathology
5	operating room	13	service/utility area *(laundry, central supply, loading dock, etc.)*
6	outpatient clinic/office	14	patient's home *(home health care)*
7	blood bank	15	transport vehicle *(car, ambulance, helicopter, etc.)*
8	venipuncture	99	other, describe ______

5. Was the source patient known? *(check one)*

[1] yes [2] no [3] unknown [4] not applicable

6. Which body fluids were involved in the exposure? *(check all that apply)*

- [ ] blood or blood product
- [ ] vomit/gastric contents
- [ ] CSF
- [ ] peritoneal fluid
- [ ] pleural fluid
- [ ] amniotic fluid
- [ ] urine
- [ ] saliva
- [ ] sputum
- [ ] feces
- [ ] other, describe ______

7. Was the exposed part: *(check all that apply)*

- [ ] intact skin
- [ ] non-intact skin
- [ ] eye(s)
- [ ] nose
- [ ] mouth
- [ ] other, describe ______

8. Did the blood or body fluid: *(check all that apply)*

- [ ] touch unprotected skin
- [ ] touch skin through gap between protective garments
- [ ] soak through protective garment
- [ ] soak through clothing

9. Which items were worn at the time of the exposure? *(check all that apply)*

- [ ] single pair latex/vinyl gloves
- [ ] double pair latex/vinyl gloves
- [ ] goggles
- [ ] eyeglasses
- [ ] faceshield
- [ ] surgical mask
- [ ] surgical mask with attached eyeshield
- [ ] surgical gown
- [ ] plastic apron
- [ ] lab coat, cloth
- [ ] lab coat, other, ______
- [ ] other, describe ______

over

10. Was the exposure the result of: *(check one)*

1	direct patient exposure	6	other body fluid container spilled/leaked
2	specimen container leaked/spilled	7	touched contaminated equipment
3	specimen container broke	8	touched contaminated drapes/sheets/gowns, etc.
4	IV tubing/bag/pump leaked	9	unknown
5	trach/NG tubing broke/sprayed, etc. specify tubing: ______	99	other, describe ______

11. For how long was the blood or body fluid in contact with your skin or mucous membranes? *(check one)*

1	less than 5 minutes
2	5–14 minutes
3	15 minutes to 1 hour
4	more than 1 hour

12. Estimate the quantity of blood/body fluid that came in contact with your skin or mucous membranes: *(check one)*

1	small amount *(up to 5 cc. or up to a teaspoon)*
2	moderate amount *(up to 50 cc. or up to a quarter cup)*
3	large amount *(more than 50 cc)*

13. Mark the size and location of the exposure:

14. Describe the circumstances leading to this exposure:

______

______

______

______

______

______

Costs: for office use only *(round to nearest dollar)*

				laboratory charges for employee and source *(Hb, HIV, other tests)*
				treatment, prophylaxis *(H-BIG, Hb vaccine, tetanus, AZT, other treatments)*
				service charges *(Emergency Department, Employee Health other services)*
				other costs *(Worker's Compensation, surgery, other)*
				total

Is this incident OSHA reportable?

- *Medical treatment (H-BIG, Hepatitis vaccine, gamma globulin, AZT, etc; Not first aid, not tetanus)*
- *Restricted/lost work time: transferred*
- *Illness/death*

1	yes
2	no

If yes, enter:

days away from work			
days restricted work activity			

APPENDIX A–2

Text of the Standard

29 CFR 1910.1030, Occupational Exposure to Bloodborne Pathogens

TEXT OF THE DEPARTMENT OF LABOR (OCCUPATIONAL SAFETY AND HEALTH ADMINISTRATION) STANDARD 1910.1030, OCCUPATIONAL EXPOSURE TO BLOODBORNE PATHOGENS

Authority. Secs. 6 and 8, Occupational Safety and Health Act, 29 U.S.C. 655, 657, Secretary of Labor's Orders Nos. 12-71 (36 FR 8754), 8-76 (41 FR 25059), or 9-83 (48 FR 35736), as applicable; and 29 CFR Part 1911.

(a) Scope and Application.

This section applies to all occupational exposure to blood or other potentially infectious materials as defined by paragraph (b) of this section.

(b) Definitions.

For purposes of this section, the following shall apply:

"Assistant Secretary" means the Assistant Secretary of Labor for Occupational Safety and Health, or designated representative.

"Blood" means human blood, human blood components, and products made from human blood.

"Bloodborne pathogens" means pathogenic microorganisms that are present in human blood and can cause disease in humans. These pathogens include, but are not limited to, hepatitis B virus (HBV) and human immunodeficiency virus (HIV).

"Clinical laboratory" means a workplace where diagnostic or other screening procedures are performed on blood or other potentially infectious materials.

"Contaminated" means the presence or the reasonably anticipated presence of blood or other potentially infectious materials on an item or surface.

"Contaminated laundry" means laundry which has been soiled with blood or other potentially infectious materials or may contain sharps.

"Contaminated sharps" means any contaminated object that can penetrate the skin including, but not limited to, needles, scalpels, broken glass, broken capillary tubes, and exposed ends of dental wires.

"Decontamination" means the use of physical or chemical means to remove, inactivate, or destroy bloodborne pathogens on a surface or item to the point where they are no longer capable of transmitting infectious particles and the surface or item is rendered safe for handling, use, or disposal.

"Director" means the Director of the National Institute for Occupational Safety and Health, U.S. Department of Health and Human Services, or designated representative.

"Engineering controls" means controls (e.g., sharps disposal containers, self-sheathing needles) that isolate or remove the bloodborne pathogens hazard from the workplace.

"Exposure incident" means a specific eye, mouth, other mucous membrane, non-intact skin, or parenteral contact with blood or other potentially infectious materials that results from the performance of an employee's duties.

"Handwashing facilities" means a facility providing an adequate supply of running potable water, soap and single use towels or hot air drying machines.

"Licensed healthcare professional" is a person whose legally permitted scope of practice allows him or her to independently perform the activities required by paragraph (f) Hepatitis B Vaccination and Post-exposure Evaluation and Follow-up.

"HBV" means hepatitis B virus.

"HIV" means human immunodeficiency virus.

"Occupational exposure" means reasonably anticipated skin, eye, mucous membrane, or parenteral contact with blood or other potentially infectious materials that may result from the performance of an employee's duties.

"Other potentially infectious materials" means (1) The following human body fluids: semen, vaginal secretions, cerebrospinal fluid, synovial fluid, pleural fluid, pericardial fluid, peritoneal fluid, amniotic fluid, saliva in dental procedures, any body fluid that is visibly contaminated with blood, and all body fluids in situations where it is difficult or impossible to differentiate between body fluids; (2) Any unfixed tissue or organ (other than intact skin) from a human (living or dead); and (3) HIV-containing cell or tissue cultures, organ cultures, and HIV- or HBV-containing culture medium or other solutions; and blood, organs, or other tissues from experimental animals infected with HIV or HBV.

"Parenteral" means piercing mucous membranes or the skin barrier through such events as needlesticks, human bites, cuts, and abrasions.

"Personal protective equipment" is specialized clothing or equipment worn by an employee for protection against a hazard. General work clothes (e.g., uniforms, pants, shirts or blouses) not intended to function as protection against a hazard are not considered to be personal protective equipment.

"Production facility" means a facility engaged in industrial-scale, large-volume or high concentration production of HIV or HBV.

"Regulated waste" means liquid or semi-liquid blood or other potentially infectious materials; contaminated items that would release blood or other potentially infectious materials in a liquid or semi-liquid state if compressed; items that are caked with dried blood or other potentially infectious materials and are capable of releasing these materials during handling; contaminated sharps; and pathological and microbiological wastes containing blood or other potentially infectious materials.

"Research laboratory" means a laboratory producing or using research-laboratory-scale amounts of HIV or HBV. Research laboratories may produce high concentrations of HIV or HBV but not in the volume found in production facilities.

"Source individual" means any individual, living or dead, whose blood or other potentially infectious materials may be a source of occupational exposure to the employee. Examples include, but are not limited to, hospital and clinic patients; clients in institutions for the developmentally disabled; trauma victims; clients of drug and alcohol treatment facilities; residents of hospices and nursing homes; human remains; and individuals who donate or sell blood or blood components.

"Sterilize" means the use of a physical or chemical procedure to destroy all microbial life including highly resistant bacterial endospores.

"Universal precautions" is an approach to infection control. According to the concept of universal precautions, all human blood and certain human body fluids are treated as if known to be infectious for HIV, HBV, and other bloodborne pathogens.

"Work practice controls" means controls that reduce the likelihood of exposure by altering the manner in which a task is performed (e.g., prohibiting recapping of needles by a two-handed technique).

(c) Exposure Control.

(1) Exposure Control Plan.

(i) Each employer having an employee(s) with occupational exposure as defined by paragraph (b) of this section shall establish a written exposure control plan designed to eliminate or minimize employee exposure.

(ii) The exposure control plan shall contain at least the following elements:

(A) The exposure determination required by paragraph (c)(2).

(B) The schedule and method of implementation for paragraphs (d) Methods of Compliance, (e) HIV and HBV Research Laboratories and Production Facilities, (f) Hepatitis B Vaccination and Post-Exposure Evaluation and Follow-up, (g) Communication of Hazards to Employees, and (h) Recordkeeping, of this standard, and

(C) The procedure for the evaluation of circumstances surrounding exposure incidents as required by paragraph (f)(3)(i) of this standard.

(iii) Each employer shall ensure that a copy of the exposure control plan is accessible to employees in accordance with 29 CFR 1910.20(e).

(iv) The exposure control plan shall be reviewed and updated at least annually and whenever necessary to reflect new or modified tasks and procedures which affect occupational exposure and to reflect new or revised employee positions with occupational exposure.

(v) The exposure control plan shall be made available to the Assistant Secretary and the Director upon request for examination and copying.

(2) Exposure Determination.

(i) Each employer who has an employee(s) with occupational exposure as defined by paragraph (b) of this section shall prepare an exposure determination. This exposure determination shall contain the following:

(A) A list of all job classifications in which all employees in those job classifications have occupational exposure;

(B) A list of job classifications in which some employees have occupational exposure, and

(C) A list of all tasks and procedures or groups of closely related tasks and procedures in which occupational exposure occurs and that are performed by employees in job classifications listed in accordance with the provisions of paragraph (c)(2)(i)(B) of this standard.

(ii) This exposure determination shall be made without regard to the use of personal protective equipment.

(d) Methods of Compliance.

(1) General. Universal precautions shall be observed to prevent contact with blood or other potentially infectious materials. Under circumstances in which differentiation between body fluid types is difficult or impossible, all body fluids shall be considered potentially infectious materials.

(2) Engineering and Work Practice Controls.

(i) Engineering and work practice controls shall be used to eliminate or minimize employee exposure. Where occupational exposure remains after institution of these controls, personal protective equipment shall also be used.

(ii) Engineering controls shall be examined and maintained or replaced on a regular schedule to ensure their effectiveness.

(iii) Employers shall provide handwashing facilities which are readily accessible to employees.

(iv) When provision of handwashing facilities is not feasible, the employer shall provide either an appropriate antiseptic hand cleanser in conjunction with clean cloth/paper towels or antiseptic towelettes. When antiseptic hand cleansers or towelettes are used, hands shall be washed with soap and running water as soon as feasible.

(v) Employers shall ensure that employees wash their hands immediately or as soon as feasible after removal of gloves or other personal protective equipment.

(vi) Employers shall ensure that employees wash hands and any other skin with soap and water, or flush mucous membranes with water immediately or as soon as feasible following contact of such body areas with blood or other potentially infectious materials.

(vii) Contaminated needles and other contaminated sharps shall not be bent, recapped, or removed except as noted in paragraphs (d)(2)(vii)(A) and (d)(2)(vii)(B) below. Shearing or breaking of contaminated needles is prohibited.

(A) Contaminated needles and other contaminated sharps shall not be bent, recapped or removed unless the employer can demonstrate that no alternative is feasible or that such action is required by a specific medical or dental procedure.

(B) Such bending, recapping or needle removal must be accomplished through the use of a mechanical device or a one-handed technique.

(viii) Immediately or as soon as possible after use, contaminated reusable sharps shall be placed in appropriate containers until properly reprocessed. These containers shall be:

(A) puncture resistant;

(B) labeled or color-coded in accordance with this standard;

(C) leakproof on the sides and bottom; and

(D) in accordance with the requirements set forth in paragraph (d)(4)(ii)(E) for reusable sharps.

(ix) Eating, drinking, smoking, applying cosmetics or lip balm, and handling contact lenses are prohibited in work areas where there is a reasonable likelihood of occupational exposure.

(x) Food and drink shall not be kept in refrigerators, freezers, shelves, cabinets or on countertops or benchtops where blood or other potentially infectious materials are present.

(xi) All procedures involving blood or other potentially infectious materials shall be performed in such a manner as to minimize splashing, spraying, spattering, and generation of droplets of these substances.

(xii) Mouth pipetting/suctioning of blood or other potentially infectious materials is prohibited.

(xiii) Specimens of blood or other potentially infectious materials shall be placed in a container which prevents leakage during collection, handling, processing, storage, transport, or shipping.

(A) The container for storage, transport, or shipping shall be labeled or color-coded according to paragraph (g)(1)(i) and closed prior to being stored, transported, or shipped. When a facility utilizes universal precautions in the handling of all specimens, the labeling/color-coding of specimens is not necessary provided containers are recognizable as containing specimens. This exemption only applies while such specimens/containers remain within the facility. Labeling or color-coding in accordance with paragraph (g)(1)(i) is required when such specimens/containers leave the facility.

(B) If outside contamination of the primary container occurs, the primary container shall be placed within a second container which prevents leakage during handling, processing, storage, transport, or shipping and is labeled or color-coded according to the requirements of this standard.

(C) If the specimen could puncture the primary container, the primary container shall be placed within a secondary container which is puncture-resistant in addition to the above characteristics.

(xiv) Equipment which may become contaminated with blood or other potentially infectious materials shall be examined prior to servicing or shipping and shall be decontaminated as necessary, unless the employer can demonstrate that decontamination of such equipment or portions of such equipment is not feasible.

(A) A readily observable label in accordance with paragraph (g)(1)(i)(H) shall be attached to the equipment stating which portions remain contaminated.

(B) The employer shall ensure that this information is conveyed to all affected employees, the servicing representative, and/or the manufacturer, as appropriate, prior to handling, servicing, or shipping so that appropriate precautions will be taken.

(3) Personal Protective Equipment.

(i) Provision. When there is occupational exposure, the employer shall provide, at no cost to the employee, appropriate personal protective equipment such as, but not limited to, gloves, gowns, laboratory coats, face shields or masks and eye protection, and mouthpieces, resuscitation bags, pocket masks, or other ventilation devices. Personal protective equipment will be considered "appropriate" only if it does not permit blood or other potentially infectious materials to pass through to or reach the employee's work clothes, street clothes, undergarments, skin, eyes, mouth, or other mucous membranes under normal conditions of use and for the duration of time which the protective equipment will be used.

(ii) Use. The employer shall ensure that the employee uses appropriate personal protective equipment unless the employer shows that the employee temporarily and briefly declined to use personal protective equipment when, under rare and extraordinary circumstances, it was the employee's professional judgment that in the specific instance its use would have prevented the delivery of healthcare or public safety services or would have posed an increased hazard to the safety of the worker or co-worker. When the employee makes this judgement, the circumstances shall be investigated and documented in order to determine whether changes can be instituted to prevent such occurrences in the future.

(iii) Accessibility. The employer shall ensure that appropriate personal protective equipment in the appropriate sizes is readily accessible at the worksite or is issued to employees. Hypoallergenic gloves, glove liners, powderless gloves, or other similar alternatives shall be readily accessible to those employees who are allergic to the gloves normally provided.

(iv) Cleaning, Laundering, and Disposal. The employer shall clean, launder, and dispose of personal protective equipment required by paragraphs (d) and (e) of this standard, at no cost to the employee.

(v) Repair and Replacement. The employer shall repair or replace personal protective equipment as needed to maintain its effectiveness, at no cost to the employee.

(vi) If a garment(s) is penetrated by blood or other potentially infectious materials, the garment(s) shall be removed immediately or as soon as feasible.

(vii) All personal protective equipment shall be removed prior to leaving the work area.

(viii) When personal protective equipment is removed it shall be placed in an appropriately designated area or container for storage, washing, decontamination or disposal.

(ix) Gloves. Gloves shall be worn when it can be reasonably anticipated that the employee may have hand contact with blood, other potentially infectious materials, mucous membranes, and non-intact skin; when performing vascular access procedures except as specified in paragraph (d)(3)(ix)(D); and when handling or touching contaminated items or surfaces.

(A) Disposable (single use) gloves such as surgical or examination gloves, shall be replaced as soon as practical when contaminated or as soon as feasible if they are torn, punctured, or when their ability to function as a barrier is compromised.

(B) Disposable (single use) gloves shall not be washed or decontaminated for re-use.

(C) Utility gloves may be decontaminated for re-use if the integrity of the glove is not compromised. However, they must be discarded if they are cracked, peeling, torn, punctured, or exhibit other signs of deterioration or when their ability to function as a barrier is compromised.

(D) If an employer in a volunteer blood donation center judges that routine gloving for all phlebotomies is not necessary, then the employer shall: {1} Periodically reevaluate this policy; {2} Make gloves available to all employees who wish to use them for phlebotomy; {3} Not discourage the use of gloves for phlebotomy; and {4} Require that gloves be used for phlebotomy in the following circumstances:

{i} When the employee has cuts, scratches, or other breaks in his or her skin;

{ii} When the employee judges that hand contamination with blood may occur, for example, when performing phlebotomy on an uncooperative source individual; and

{iii} When the employee is receiving training in phlebotomy.

(x) Masks, Eye Protection, and Face Shields. Masks in combination with eye protection devices, such as goggles or glasses with solid side shields, or chin-length face shields, shall be worn whenever splashes, spray, spatter, or droplets of blood or other potentially infectious materials may be generated and eye, nose, or mouth contamination can be reasonably anticipated.

(xi) Gowns, Aprons, and Other Protective Body Clothing. Appropriate protective clothing such as, but not limited to, gowns, aprons, lab coats, clinic jackets, or similar outer garments shall be worn in occupational exposure situations. The type and characteristics will depend upon the task and degree of exposure anticipated.

(xii) Surgical caps or hoods and/or shoe covers or boots shall be worn in instances when gross contamination can reasonably be anticipated (e.g., autopsies, orthopaedic surgery).

(4) Housekeeping.

(i) General. Employers shall ensure that the worksite is maintained in a clean and sanitary condition. The employer shall determine and implement an appropriate written schedule for cleaning and method of decontamination based upon the location within the facility, type of surface to be cleaned, type of soil present, and tasks or procedures being performed in the area.

(ii) All equipment and environmental and working surfaces shall be cleaned and decontaminated after contact with blood or other potentially infectious materials.

(A) Contaminated work surfaces shall be decontaminated with an appropriate disinfectant after completion of procedures; immediately or as soon as feasible when surfaces are overtly contaminated or after any spill of blood or other potentially infectious materials; and at the end of the work shift if the surface may have become contaminated since the last cleaning.

(B) Protective coverings, such as plastic wrap, aluminum foil, or imperviously-backed absorbent paper used to cover equipment and environmental surfaces, shall be removed and replaced as soon as feasible when they become overtly contaminated or at the end of the workshift if they may have become contaminated during the shift.

(C) All bins, pails, cans, and similar receptacles intended for reuse which have a reasonable likelihood for becoming contaminated with blood or other potentially infectious materials shall be inspected and decontaminated on a regularly scheduled basis and cleaned and decontaminated immediately or as soon as feasible upon visible contamination.

(D) Broken glassware which may be contaminated shall not be picked up directly with the hands. It shall be cleaned up using mechanical means, such as a brush and dust pan, tongs, or forceps.

(E) Reusable sharps that are contaminated with blood or other potentially infectious materials shall not be stored or processed in a manner that requires employees to reach by hand into the containers where these sharps have been placed.

(iii) Regulated Waste.

(A) Contaminated Sharps Discarding and Containment.

{1} Contaminated sharps shall be discarded immediately or as soon as feasible in containers that are:

[a] Closable;

[b] Puncture resistant;

[c] Leakproof on sides and bottom; and

[d] Labeled or color-coded in accordance with paragraph (g)(1)(i) of this standard.

{2} During use, containers for contaminated sharps shall be:

[a] Easily accessible to personnel and located as close as is feasible to the immediate area where sharps are used or can be reasonably anticipated to be found (e.g., laundries);

[b] Maintained upright throughout use; and

[c] Replaced routinely and not be allowed to overfill.

{3} When moving containers of contaminated sharps from the area of use, the containers shall be:

[a] Closed immediately prior to removal or replacement to prevent spillage or protrusion of contents during handling, storage, transport, or shipping;

[b] Placed in a secondary container if leakage is possible. The second container shall be:

[i] Closable;

[ii] Constructed to contain all contents and prevent leakage during handling, storage, transport, or shipping; and

[iii] Labeled or color-coded according to paragraph (g)(1)(i) of this standard.

{4} Reusable containers shall not be opened, emptied, or cleaned manually or in any other manner which would expose employees to the risk of percutaneous injury.

(B) Other Regulated Waste Containment.

{1} Regulated waste shall be placed in containers which are:

[a] Closable;

[b] Constructed to contain all contents and prevent leakage of fluids during handling, storage, transport or shipping; and

[c] Labeled or color-coded in accordance with paragraph (g)(1)(i) of this standard; and

[d] Closed prior to removal to prevent spillage or protrusion of contents during handling, storage, transport, or shipping.

{2} If outside contamination of the regulated waste container occurs, it shall be placed in a second container. The second container shall be:

[a] Closable;

[b] Constructed to contain all contents and prevent leakage of fluids during handling, storage, transport or shipping;

[c] Labeled or color-coded in accordance with paragraph (g)(1)(i) of this standard; and

[d] Closed prior to removal to prevent spillage or protrusion of contents during handling, storage, transport, or shipping.

(C) Disposal of all regulated waste shall be in accordance with applicable regulations of the United States, States and Territories, and political subdivisions of States and Territories.

(iv) Laundry.

(A) Contaminated laundry shall be handled as little as possible with a minimum of agitation.

{1} Contaminated laundry shall be bagged or containerized at the location where it was used and shall not be sorted or rinsed in the location of use.

{2} Contaminated laundry shall be placed and transported in bags or containers labeled or color-coded in accordance with paragraph (g)(1)(i) of this standard. When a facility utilizes universal precautions in the handling of all soiled laundry, alternative labeling or color-coding is sufficient if it permits all employees to recognize the containers as requiring compliance with universal precautions.

{3} Whenever contaminated laundry is wet and presents a reasonable likelihood of soak-through of or leakage from the bag or container, the laundry shall be placed and transported in bags or containers which prevent soak-through and/or leakage of fluids to the exterior.

(B) The employer shall ensure that employees who have contact with contaminated laundry wear protective gloves and other appropriate personal protective equipment.

(C) When a facility ships contaminated laundry off-site to a second facility which does not utilize universal precautions in the handling of all laundry, the facility generating the contaminated laundry must place such laundry in bags or containers which are labeled or color-coded in accordance with paragraph (g)(1)(i).

(e) HIV and HBV Research Laboratories and Production Facilities.

(1) This paragraph applies to research laboratories and production facilities engaged in the culture, production, concentration, experimentation, and manipulation of HIV and HBV. It does not apply to clinical or diagnostic laboratories engaged solely in the analysis of blood, tissues, or organs. These requirements apply in addition to the other requirements of the standard.

(2) Research laboratories and production facilities shall meet the following criteria:

(i) Standard Microbiological Practices. All regulated waste shall either be incinerated or decontaminated by a method such as autoclaving known to effectively destroy bloodborne pathogens.

(ii) Special Practices.

(A) Laboratory doors shall be kept closed when work involving HIV or HBV is in progress.

(B) Contaminated materials that are to be decontaminated at a site away from the work area shall be placed in a durable, leakproof, labeled or color-coded container that is closed before being removed from the work area.

(C) Access to the work area shall be limited to authorized persons. Written policies and procedures shall be established whereby only persons who have been advised of the potential biohazard, who meet any specific entry requirements, and who comply with all entry and exit procedures shall be allowed to enter the work areas and animal rooms.

(D) When other potentially infectious materials or infected animals are present in the work area or containment module, a hazard warning sign incorporating the universal biohazard symbol shall be posted on all access doors. The hazard warning sign shall comply with paragraph (g)(1)(ii) of this standard.

(E) All activities involving other potentially infectious materials shall be conducted in biological safety cabinets or other physical-containment devices within the containment module. No work with these other potentially infectious materials shall be conducted on the open bench.

(F) Laboratory coats, gowns, smocks, uniforms, or other appropriate protective clothing shall be used in the work area and animal rooms. Protective clothing shall not be worn outside of the work area and shall be decontaminated before being laundered.

(G) Special care shall be taken to avoid skin contact with other potentially infectious materials. Gloves shall be worn when handling infected animals and when making hand contact with other potentially infectious materials is unavoidable.

(H) Before disposal all waste from work areas and from animal rooms shall either be incinerated or decontaminated by a method such as autoclaving known to effectively destroy bloodborne pathogens.

(I) Vacuum lines shall be protected with liquid disinfectant traps and high-efficiency particulate air (HEPA) filters or filters of equivalent or superior efficiency and which are checked routinely and maintained or replaced as necessary.

(J) Hypodermic needles and syringes shall be used only for parenteral injection and aspiration of fluids from laboratory animals and diaphragm bottles. Only needle-locking syringes or disposable syringe-needle units (i.e., the needle is integral to the syringe) shall be used for the injection or aspiration of other potentially infectious materials. Extreme caution shall be used when handling needles and syringes. A needle shall not be bent, sheared, replaced in the sheath or guard, or removed from the syringe following use. The needle and syringe shall be promptly placed in a puncture-resistant container and autoclaved or decontaminated before reuse or disposal.

(K) All spills shall be immediately contained and cleaned up by appropriate professional staff or others properly trained and equipped to work with potentially concentrated infectious materials.

(L) A spill or accident that results in an exposure incident shall be immediately reported to the laboratory director or other responsible person.

(M) A biosafety manual shall be prepared or adopted and periodically reviewed and updated at least annually or more often if necessary. Personnel shall be advised of potential hazards, shall be required to read instructions on practices and procedures, and shall be required to follow them.

(iii) Containment Equipment.

(A) Certified biological safety cabinets (Class I, II, or III) or other appropriate combinations of personal protection or physical containment devices, such as special protective clothing, respirators, centrifuge safety cups, sealed centrifuge rotors, and containment caging for animals, shall be used for all activities with other potentially infectious materials that pose a threat of exposure to droplets, splashes, spills, or aerosols.

(B) Biological safety cabinets shall be certified when installed, whenever they are moved and at least annually.

(3) HIV and HBV research laboratories shall meet the following criteria:

(i) Each laboratory shall contain a facility for hand washing and an eye wash facility which is readily available within the work area.

(ii) An autoclave for decontamination of regulated waste shall be available.

(4) HIV and HBV production facilities shall meet the following criteria:

(i) The work areas shall be separated from areas that are open to unrestricted traffic flow within the building.

Passage through two sets of doors shall be the basic requirement for entry into the work area from access corridors or other contiguous areas. Physical separation of the high-containment work area from access corridors or other areas or activities may also be provided by a double-doored clothes-change room (showers may be included), airlock, or other access facility that requires passing through two sets of doors before entering the work area.

(ii) The surfaces of doors, walls, floors, and ceilings in the work area shall be water resistant so that they can be easily cleaned. Penetrations in these surfaces shall be sealed or capable of being sealed to facilitate decontamination.

(iii) Each work area shall contain a sink for washing hands and a readily available eye wash facility. The sink shall be foot, elbow, or automatically operated and shall be located near the exit door of the work area.

(iv) Access doors to the work area or containment module shall be self-closing.

(v) An autoclave for decontamination of regulated waste shall be available within or as near as possible to the work area.

(vi) A ducted exhaust-air ventilation system shall be provided. This system shall create directional airflow that draws air into the work area through the entry area. The exhaust air shall not be recirculated to any other area of the building, shall be discharged to the outside, and shall be dispersed away from occupied areas and air intakes. The proper direction of the airflow shall be verified (i.e., into the work area).

(5) Training Requirements. Additional training requirements for employees in HIV and HBV research laboratories and HIV and HBV production facilities are specified in paragraph (g)(2)(ix).

(f) Hepatitis B Vaccination and Post-exposure Evaluation and Follow-up.

(1) General.

(i) The employer shall make available the hepatitis B vaccine and vaccination series to all employees who have occupational exposure, and post-exposure evaluation and follow-up to all employees who have had an exposure incident.

(ii) The employer shall ensure that all medical evaluations and procedures including the hepatitis B vaccine and vaccination series and post-exposure evaluation and follow-up, including prophylaxis, are:

(A) Made available at no cost to the employee;

(B) Made available to the employee at a reasonable time and place;

(C) Performed by or under the supervision of a licensed physician or by or under the supervision of another licensed healthcare professional; and

(D) Provided according to recommendations of the U.S. Public Health Service current at the time these evaluations and procedures take place, except as specified by this paragraph (f).

(iii) The employer shall ensure that all laboratory tests are conducted by an accredited laboratory at no cost to the employee.

(2) Hepatitis B Vaccination.

(i) Hepatitis B vaccination shall be made available after the employee has received the training required in paragraph (g)(2)(vii)(I) and within 10 working days of initial assignment to all employees who have occupational exposure unless the employee has previously received the complete hepatitis B vaccination series, antibody testing has revealed that the employee is immune, or the vaccine is contraindicated for medical reasons.

(ii) The employer shall not make participation in a prescreening program a prerequisite for receiving hepatitis B vaccination.

(iii) If the employee initially declines hepatitis B vaccination but at a later date while still covered under the standard decides to accept the vaccination, the employer shall make available hepatitis B vaccination at that time.

(iv) The employer shall assure that employees who decline to accept hepatitis B vaccination offered by the employer sign the statement in Exhibit 1.

(v) If a routine booster dose(s) of hepatitis B vaccine is recommended by the U.S. Public Health Service at a future date, such booster dose(s) shall be made available in accordance with section (f)(1)(ii).

(3) Post-exposure Evaluation and Follow-up. Following a report of an exposure incident, the employer shall make immediately available to the exposed employee a confidential medical evaluation and follow-up, including at least the following elements:

(i) Documentation of the route(s) of exposure, and the circumstances under which the exposure incident occurred;

(ii) Identification and documentation of the source individual, unless the employer can establish that identification is infeasible or prohibited by state or local law;

(A) The source individual's blood shall be tested as soon as feasible and after consent is obtained in order to determine HBV and HIV infectivity. If consent is not obtained, the employer shall establish that legally required consent cannot be obtained. When the source individual's consent is not required by law, the source individual's blood, if available, shall be tested and the results documented.

(B) When the source individual is already known to be infected with HBV or HIV, testing for the source individual's known HBV or HIV status need not be repeated.

(C) Results of the source individual's testing shall be made available to the exposed employee, and the employee shall be informed of applicable laws and regulations concerning disclosure of the identity and infectious status of the source individual.

(iii) Collection and testing of blood for HBV and HIV serological status;

(A) The exposed employee's blood shall be collected as soon as feasible and tested after consent is obtained.

(B) If the employee consents to baseline blood collection, but does not give consent at that time for HIV serologic testing, the sample shall be preserved for at least 90 days. If, within 90 days of the exposure incident, the employee elects to have the baseline sample tested, such testing shall be done as soon as feasible.

(iv) Post-exposure prophylaxis, when medically indicated, as recommended by the U.S. Public Health Service;

(v) Counseling; and

(vi) Evaluation of reported illnesses.

(4) Information Provided to the Healthcare Professional.

(i) The employer shall ensure that the healthcare professional responsible for the employee's hepatitis B vaccination is provided a copy of this regulation.

(ii) The employer shall ensure that the healthcare professional evaluating an employee after an exposure incident is provided the following information:

(A) A copy of this regulation;

(B) A description of the exposed employee's duties as they relate to the exposure incident;

(C) Documentation of the route(s) of exposure and circumstances under which exposure occurred;

(D) Results of the source individual's blood testing, if available; and

(E) All medical records relevant to the appropriate treatment of the employee including vaccination status which are the employer's responsibility to maintain.

(5) Healthcare Professional's Written Opinion. The employer shall obtain and provide the employee with a copy of the evaluating healthcare professional's written opinion within 15 days of the completion of the evaluation.

(i) The healthcare professional's written opinion for hepatitis B vaccination shall be limited to whether hepatitis B vaccination is indicated for an employee, and if the employee has received such vaccination.

(ii) The healthcare professional's written opinion for post-exposure evaluation and follow-up shall be limited to the following information:

(A) That the employee has been informed of the results of the evaluation; and

(B) That the employee has been told about any medical conditions resulting from exposure to blood or other potentially infectious materials which require further evaluation or treatment.

(iii) All other findings or diagnoses shall remain confidential and shall not be included in the written report.

(6) Medical Recordkeeping. Medical records required by this standard shall be maintained in accordance with paragraph (h)(1) of this section.

(g) Communication of Hazards to Employees.

(1) Labels and Signs.

(i) Labels.

(A) Warning labels shall be affixed to containers of regulated waste, refrigerators and freezers containing blood or other potentially infectious material; and other containers used to store, transport or ship blood or other potentially infectious materials, except as provided in paragraph (g)(1)(i)(E), (F) and (G).

(B) Labels required by this section shall include the following legend:

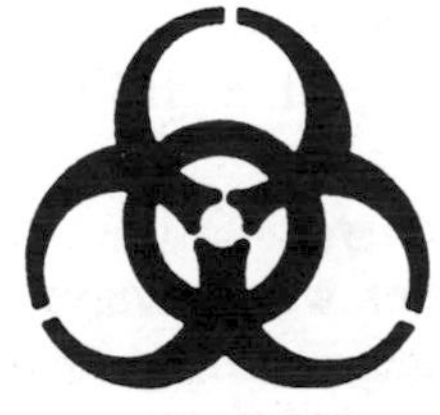

BIOHAZARD

(C) These labels shall be fluorescent orange or orange-red or predominantly so, with lettering and symbols in a contrasting color.

(D) Labels shall be affixed as close as feasible to the container by string, wire, adhesive, or other method that prevents their loss or unintentional removal.

(E) Red bags or red containers may be substituted for labels.

(F) Containers of blood, blood components, or blood products that are labeled as to their contents and have been released for transfusion or other clinical use are exempted from the labeling requirements of paragraph (g).

(G) Individual containers of blood or other potentially infectious materials that are placed in a labeled container during storage, transport, shipment, or disposal are exempted from the labeling requirement.

(H) Labels required for contaminated equipment shall be in accordance with this paragraph and shall also state which portions of the equipment remain contaminated.

(I) Regulated waste that has been decontaminated need not be labeled or color-coded.

(ii) Signs.

(A) The employer shall post signs at the entrance to work areas specified in paragraph (e), HIV and HBV Research Laboratory and Production Facilities, which shall bear the following legend: (BIOHAZARD SYMBOL as above, with wording: Name of infectious agent; special requirements for entering area; name and telephone number of laboratory director or other responsible person).

(B) These signs shall be fluorescent orange-red or predominantly so, with lettering and symbols in a contrasting color.

(2) Information and Training.

(i) Employers shall ensure that all employees with occupational exposure participate in a training program which must be provided at no cost to the employee and during working hours.

(ii) Training shall be provided as follows:

(A) At the time of initial assignment to tasks where occupational exposure may take place;

(B) Within 90 days after the effective date of the standard; and

(C) At least annually thereafter.

(iii) For employees who have received training on bloodborne pathogens in the year preceding the effective date of the standard, only training with respect to the provisions of the standard which were not included need be provided.

(iv) Annual training for all employees shall be provided within one year of their previous training.

(v) Employers shall provide additional training when changes such as modification of tasks or procedures or institution of new tasks or procedures affect the employee's occupational exposure. The additional training may be limited to addressing the new exposures created.

(vi) Material appropriate in content and vocabulary to educational level, literacy, and language of employees shall be used.

(vii) The training program shall contain at a minimum the following elements:

(A) An accessible copy of the regulatory text of this standard and an explanation of its contents;

(B) A general explanation of the epidemiology and symptoms of bloodborne diseases;

(C) An explanation of the modes of transmission of bloodborne pathogens;

(D) An explanation of the employer's exposure control plan and the means by which the employee can obtain a copy of the written plan;

(E) An explanation of the appropriate methods for recognizing tasks and other activities that may involve exposure to blood and other potentially infectious materials;

(F) An explanation of the use and limitations of methods that will prevent or reduce exposure including appropriate engineering controls, work practices, and personal protective equipment;

(G) Information on the types, proper use, location, removal, handling, decontamination, and disposal of personal protective equipment;

(H) An explanation of the basis for selection of personal protective equipment;

(I) Information on the hepatitis B vaccine, including information on its efficacy, safety, method of administration, the benefits of being vaccinated, and that the vaccine and vaccination will be offered free of charge;

(J) Information on the appropriate actions to take and persons to contact in an emergency involving blood or other potentially infectious materials;

(K) An explanation of the procedure to follow if an exposure incident occurs, including the method of reporting the incident and the medical follow-up that will be made available;

(L) Information on the post-exposure evaluation and follow-up that the employer is required to provide for the employee following an exposure incident;

(M) An explanation of the signs and labels and/or color coding required by paragraph (g)(1); and

(N) An opportunity for interactive questions and answers with the person conducting the training session.

(viii) The person conducting the training shall be knowledgeable in the subject matter covered by the elements contained in the training program as it relates to the workplace that the training will address.

(ix) Additional Initial Training for Employees in HIV and HBV Laboratories and Production Facilities. Employees in HIV or HBV research laboratories and HIV or HBV production facilities shall receive the following initial training in addition to the above training requirements.

(A) The employer shall ensure that employees demonstrate proficiency in standard microbiological practices and techniques and in the practices and operations specific to the facility before being allowed to work with HIV or HBV.

(B) The employer shall ensure that employees have prior experience in the handling of human pathogens or tissue cultures before working with HIV or HBV.

(C) The employer shall provide a training program to employees who have no prior experience in handling human pathogens. Initial work activities shall not include the handling of infectious agents. A progression of work activities shall be assigned as techniques are learned and proficiency is developed. The employer shall ensure that employees participate in work activities involving infectious agents only after proficiency has been demonstrated.

(h) Recordkeeping.

(1) Medical Records.

(i) The employer shall establish and maintain an accurate record for each employee with occupational exposure, in accordance with 29 CFR 1910.20.

(ii) This record shall include:

(A) The name and social security number of the employee;

(B) A copy of the employee's hepatitis B vaccination status including the dates of all the hepatitis B vaccinations and any medical records relative to the employee's ability to receive vaccination as required by paragraph (f)(2);

(C) A copy of all results of examinations, medical testing, and follow-up procedures as required by paragraph (f)(3);

(D) The employer's copy of the healthcare professional's written opinion as required by paragraph (f)(5); and

(E) A copy of the information provided to the healthcare professional as required by paragraphs (f)(4)(ii)(B), (C), and (D).

(iii) Confidentiality. The employer shall ensure that employee medical records required by paragraph (h)(1) are:

(A) Kept confidential; and

(B) Not disclosed or reported without the employee's express written consent to any person within or outside the workplace except as required by this section or as may be required by law.

(iv) The employer shall maintain the records required by paragraph (h) for at least the duration of employment plus 30 years in accordance with 29 CFR 1910.20.

(2) Training Records.

(i) Training records shall include the following information:

(A) The dates of the training sessions;

(B) The contents or a summary of the training sessions;

(C) The names and qualifications of persons conducting the training; and

(D) The names and job titles of all persons attending the training sessions.

(ii) Training records shall be maintained for 3 years from the date on which the training occurred.

(3) Availability.

(i) The employer shall ensure that all records required to be maintained by this section shall be made available upon request to the Assistant Secretary and the Director for examination and copying.

(ii) Employee training records required by this paragraph shall be provided upon request for examination and copying to employees, to employee representatives, to the Director, and to the Assistant Secretary.

(iii) Employee medical records required by this paragraph shall be provided upon request for examination and copying to the subject employee, to anyone having written consent of the subject employee, to the Director, and to the Assistant Secretary in accordance with 29 CFR 1910.20.

(4) Transfer of Records.

(i) The employer shall comply with the requirements involving transfer of records set forth in 29 CFR 1910.20(h).

(ii) If the employer ceases to do business and there is no successor employer to receive and retain the records for the prescribed period, the employer shall notify the Director, at least three months prior to their disposal, and transmit them to the Director, if required by the Director to do so, within that three-month period.

(i) Dates.

(The entire standard has been in effect since July 6, 1992.)

Exhibit 1: Hepatitis B Vaccine Declination (Mandatory)

I understand that due to my occupational exposure to blood or other potentially infectious materials I may be at risk of acquiring hepatitis B virus (HBV) infection. I have been given the opportunity to be vaccinated with hepatitis B vaccine, at no charge to myself. However, I decline hepatitis B vaccination at this time. I understand that by declining this vaccine, I continue to be at risk of acquiring hepatitis B, a serious disease. If in the future I continue to have occupational exposure to blood or other potentially infectious materials and I want to be vaccinated with hepatitis B vaccine, I can receive the vaccination series at no charge to me.

APPENDIX A–3

Directories

REGIONAL OFFICE ADDRESSES AND TELEPHONE NUMBERS

REGION I (Connecticut, Maine, Massachusetts, New Hampshire, Rhode Island, and Vermont)

Cindy A. Coe, Acting Regional Administrator
U.S. Department of Labor - OSHA
133 Portland St., 1st Floor
Boston, MA 02114
Telephone: (617) 565-7164 Fax: (617) 565-7157

REGION II (New Jersey, New York, and Puerto Rico, and the Virgin Islands)

Patricia K. Clark, Regional Administrator
U.S. Department of Labor - OSHA
201 Varick St., Room 670
New York, NY 10014
Telephone: (212) 337-2325 Fax: (212) 337-2378

REGION III (Delaware, District of Columbia, Maryland, Pennsylvania, Virginia, and West Virginia)

Linda R. Anku, Regional Administrator
U.S. Department of Labor - OSHA
3535 Market St., Room 2100
Philadelphia, PA 19104
Telephone: (215) 596-1201 Fax: (215) 596-4872

REGION IV (Alabama, Florida, Georgia, Kentucky, Mississippi, North Carolina, South Carolina, and Tennessee)

R. Davis Layne, Regional Administrator
U.S. Department of Labor - OSHA
1375 Peachtree St., NE, Room 587
Atlanta, GA 30367
Telephone: (404) 347-3573 Fax: (404) 347-0181

REGION V (Illinois, Indiana, Michigan, Minnesota, Ohio, and Wisconsin)

Michael G. Connors, Regional Administrator
U.S. Department of Labor - OSHA
230 S. Dearborn St., Room 3244
Chicago, IL 60604
Telephone: (312) 353-2220 Fax: (312) 353-7774

REGION VI (Arkansas, Louisiana, New Mexico, Oklahoma, and Texas)

Gilbert J. Saulter, Regional Administrator
U.S. Department of Labor - OSHA
525 Griffin St., Room 602
Dallas, TX 75202
Telephone: (214) 767-4731 Fax: (214) 767-4693

REGION VII (Iowa, Kansas, Missouri, and Nebraska)

John T. Phillips, Regional Administrator
U.S. Department of Labor - OSHA
911 Walnut St., Room 406
Kansas City, MO 64106
Telephone: (816) 426-5861 Fax: (816) 426-2750

REGION VIII (Colorado, Montana, North Dakota, South Dakota, Utah, and Wyoming)

Byron R. Chadwick, Regional Administrator
U.S. Department of Labor - OSHA
1961 Stout St., Room 1576
Denver, CO 80294
Telephone: (303) 844-3061 Fax: (303) 844-5310

REGION IX (America Samoa, Arizona, California, Guam, Hawaii, Nevada, and the Pacific Islands)

Frank Strasheim, Regional Administrator
U.S. Department of Labor - OSHA
71 Stevenson St., Suite 415
San Francisco, CA 94105
Telephone: (415) 744-6670 Fax: (415) 774-7114

REGION X (Alaska, Idaho, Oregon, and Washington)

James Lake, Regional Administrator
U.S. Department of Labor - OSHA
1111 Third Ave., Suite 715
Seattle, WA 98101-3212
Telephone: (206) 553-5930 Fax: (206) 553-6499

The location and telephone number of your local area office can be obtained from your regional office.

STATE CONSULTATION PROJECT DIRECTORY

State	Telephone	State	Telephone
Alabama	205-348-3033	Nebraska	402-471-4717
Alaska	907-264-2599	Nevada	702-688-1474
Arizona	602-255-5795	New Hampshire	603-271-3170
Arkansas	501-682-4522	New Jersey	609-292-0404
California	415-737-2843	New Mexico	505-827-2885
Colorado	303-491-6151	New York	518-457-5468
Connecticut	203-566-4550	North Carolina	919-733-3949
Delaware	302-571-3908	North Dakota	701-221-5188
Dist. of Columbia	202-576-6339	Ohio	614-644-2631
Florida	904-488-3044	Oklahoma	405-528-1500
Georgia	404-894-8274	Oregon	503-378-3272
Guam	671-646-9246	Pennsylvania	800-382-1241
Hawaii	808-548-4155		(Toll-free in state)
Idaho	208-385-3283		412-357-2561
Illinois	312-814-2339	Puerto Rico	809-754-2171
Indiana	317-232-2688	Rhode Island	401-277-2438
Iowa	515-281-5352	South Carolina	803-734-9599
Kansas	913-296-4386	South Dakota	605-688-4101
Kentucky	502-564-6895	Tennessee	615-741-7036
Louisiana	504-342-9601	Texas	512-440-3809
Maine	207-289-6460	Utah	801-530-6868
Maryland	410-333-4218	Vermont	802-828-2765
Massachusetts	617-727-3463	Virginia	804-786-6613
Michigan	517-335-8250(H)	Virgin Islands	809-772-1315
	517-322-1809(S)	Washington	206-586-0961
Minnesota	612-297-2393	West Virginia	304-348-7890
Mississippi	601-987-3981	Wisconsin	608-266-8579(H)
Missouri	314-751-3403		414-521-5063(S)
Montana	406-444-6401	Wyoming	307-777-7786

APPENDIX A–4

Resource List

Video

"As It Should Be Done" Item #: A19111-VNBI
National Audio Visual Center
8700 Edgeworth Drive
Capitol Heights, MD 20743
(301) 763-1896
Cost $45.00

Booklets

(Request by Title and Publication Number)
Occupational Exposure to Bloodborne Pathogens OSHA # 3127
Spanish Version: Exposicion a Patogenos OSHA # 3134
Transmitidos por la Sangre en el Trabajo

Fact Sheets

(One page each, request by title)
Bloodborne Facts: Reporting Exposure Incidents
Bloodborne Facts: Hepatitis B Virus Vaccine–Protection for You
Bloodborne Facts: Protect Yourself When Handling Sharps
Bloodborne Facts: Personal Protective Equipment Cuts Risk
Bloodborne Facts: Holding the Line on Contamination

Booklet and Fact Sheet Ordering Information

OSHA - Publications Office
U.S. Department of Labor, Rm. N3101
200 Constitution Ave., NW
Washington, DC 20210
Phone: (202) 219-4667 Fax: (202) 275-0019

Single copies of booklets and fact sheets are free.
Please send a self-addressed mailing label.

Index

Page numbers in *italics* denote figures and exhibits; those followed by "t" denote tables.

F

G

I

N